Recent Titles in Race, Ethnicity, Culture, and Health Series

Mexican American Psychology: Social, Cultural, and Clinical Perspectives
Mario A. Tovar

Better Health through Spiritual Practices

A Guide to Religious Behaviors and Perspectives That Benefit Mind and Body

Dean D. VonDras, PhD, Editor

Race, Ethnicity, Culture, and Health
Regan A.R. Gurung, Series Editor

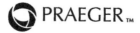 PRAEGER™

An Imprint of ABC-CLIO, LLC
Santa Barbara, California • Denver, Colorado

Library of Congress Cataloging-in-Publication Data

Names: VonDras, Dean D., editor.
Title: Better health through spiritual practices : a guide to religious behaviors and
    perspectives that benefit mind and body / Dean D. VonDras, PhD, editor.
Description: 1 [edition]. | Santa Barbara : Praeger, An Imprint of ABC-CLIO, LLC, 2017. |
    Series: Race, ethnicity, culture, and health | Includes index.
Identifiers: LCCN 2017018518 (print) | LCCN 2017024526 (ebook) |
    ISBN 9781440853685 (ebook) | ISBN 9781440853678 (hard copy : alk. paper)
Subjects: LCSH: Health—Religious aspects.
Classification: LCC BL65.M4 (ebook) | LCC BL65.M4 B435 2017 (print) |
    DDC 201/.6613—dc23
LC record available at https://lccn.loc.gov/2017018518

ISBN: 978-1-4408-5367-8
EISBN: 978-1-4408-5368-5

21 20 19 18 17   1 2 3 4 5

This book is also available as an eBook.

Praeger
An Imprint of ABC-CLIO, LLC

ABC-CLIO, LLC
130 Cremona Drive, P.O. Box 1911
Santa Barbara, California 93116-1911
www.abc-clio.com

This book is printed on acid-free paper ∞

Manufactured in the United States of America

Contents

Series Foreword

There are clearly many different cultural approaches to health, and it is of great importance for healthcare workers, psychologists, and the administrations that support them to be culturally aware. Knowing about the different approaches to health can also help the lay consumer be better appraised of cultural variations; this awareness can in turn lead to a reduction in stereotyping or prejudicial attitudes toward behaviors that may be seen as different from the norm.

Each book in this series—Race, Ethnicity, Culture, and Health—provides a comprehensive introduction to a particular group of people, or varied peoples with a shared overall approach, such as those in the current volume featuring spiritual and religious approaches to health. It is important to acknowledge that many cultural variations exist within ethnic communities. Knowing how different cultural groups approach health, and having a better understanding of how factors such as acculturation are important, can help clinicians, healthcare workers, and others with an interest in the ways lifestyle decisions are made to become more culturally competent. The efforts to increase cultural competence in the treatment of mental and physical health are promising, but the wider healthcare arena and the general public also need to pay attention to the causes of health disparities and the role played by multicultural approaches to health. We need a better connection between health care and the community, so individuals can seek out treatments that best fit their cultural needs and the manifold health disparities that currently exist in our society can be reduced.

Regan A.R. Gurung
Ben J. and Joyce Rosenberg Professor of Human
Development and Psychology
University of Wisconsin, Green Bay

Preface: The Prospect of Our Journey

Dean D. VonDras

As we take up the prospect of better health through spiritual practices, it is important to identify key points of destination for the reader. The primary aim of this book is to illuminate the orienting worldviews of religio-spiritual systems, and how these systems may compel healthy ways of living. Another goal is to become aware of various lifestyle practices and health behaviors found within different religio-spiritual orientations, and consider how they may be effectively coordinated beyond their native contexts to improve health and prevent disease. The hope is that the reader will travel to new places of understanding, and discover a variety of methods for maintaining health and preventing disease.

To provide a roadmap for the reader, we begin with a brief historical outline that introduces the model of religio-spiritual contextualism (Chapter 1). This theoretical viewpoint provides a lens of analysis for the exploration of Eastern and Western religio-spiritual traditions, as well as those of primal faiths, atheistic, agnostic, and nonreligious orientations, and their influences on lifestyle practices and health behaviors. We then launch into a deeper exploration of religio-spiritual contextualism in the discussion by Vibha Agnihotri and Vinamrata Agnihotri (Chapter 2), who describe the great faiths of India: Hinduism, Jainism, and Sikhism. These authors note the rich history of these worldviews, and various ways in which each tradition is incorporated into daily life routines and health behaviors. A subsequent discussion by Dana Dharmakaya Colgan, Nina J. Hidalgo, and

Paul E. Priester (Chapter 3) broadens our scope of investigation, and provides a very rich discussion of Buddhist values and practices. A key feature here is the various applications and therapeutic potential of mindfulness training, and how essential Buddhist precepts are linked to healthy living.

An intertwining of health with spirituality is also a central focus within Confucianism and Daoism, as noted by Robert Santee (Chapter 4). His discussion immerses us in Eastern thought, describing the dynamism and symbiosis of the Yin and Yang principle, and challenging the reader to contemplate the aphorisms for healthy living found within the classic texts of China. An allied discussion by Carl Olson (Chapter 5) deepens our excursion into Eastern thought, examining the symbolic meaning of narrative myth found within the naturalistic traditions of Shintoism and Shamanism in Japan. Cross-cultural interchanges with Buddhism and Hinduism are recognized here, and a broader sociological perspective becomes illuminated which emphasizes community practices that support healthfulness and well-being.

Shifting our focus to Western perspectives, we take up consideration of the Abrahamic religions in the discussions of Judaism by Miriam Korbman, Moses Appel, and David H. Rosmarin (Chapter 6), Catholic and Seventh-day Adventist Christian traditions by Arndt Büssing and Désirée Poier (Chapter 7), and Islamic traditions by Mona M. Amer (Chapter 8). These monotheistic faiths share a common history that traces back to Adam and the patriarchs Abraham, Isaac, and Jacob. In these chapters we find deep and profound expression of faith beliefs that powerfully orient ways of living, and that guide and direct health behaviors. Further exploration of traditions that emanate from the Abrahamic root are found in discussions of Islamic Sufism by Saloumeh Bozorgzadeh, Nasim Bahadorani, and Mohammad Sadoghi (Chapter 9), and in the Bahá'í, Rastafari, and Zoroastrian faiths by Holly Nelson-Becker, Leanne Atwell, and Shannan Russo (Chapter 10). These relatively younger traditions are noted to have developed through the actions of heroic figures and teaching of spiritual guides, and describe practices for healthy living that reflect an individual and collective search for wellness, balance, and spiritual unity.

There is a return to the exploration of naturalistic traditions in Chapters 11 (by Jeff King) and 12 (by Kevin A. Harris), as these authors consider the spiritualities of the indigenous peoples of North America. It should be recognized that the spiritualities of these First Nation peoples reflect humankind's earliest transcendent yearnings, sense of connection to the earth and all its inhabitants, and expression of basic values and morals for living. Here there is illumination of a shared historical narrative—one involving hardship, oppression, and expression of a mystical cosmology—that defines an awe-inspiring spirituality and coordinates a holistic approach to healthy living. These chapters focus on psychological well-being and the importance of cultural respect and use of religio-spiritual sensitive therapies to attain personal healing and communal restoration.

Next we consider the secular and humanistic styles of spirituality expressed in atheistic, agnostic, and nonreligious orientations in the discussion of Karen Hwang and Ryan T. Cragun (Chapter 13). Despite the eschewing of theistic beliefs within these orientations, we again find deep expression of virtues and values, and guiding ethical principles that direct lifestyle choices and shape health behaviors. This discussion underscores the importance of including all types of spirituality—even those that have nothing to do with theological beliefs—in appreciating how religio-spiritual influences may moderate lifestyle choices and healthy ways of living. A concluding final discussion by Scott F. Madey (Chapter 14) explores the relationship between science and religion. In a poignant reflection on the limitations of both scientific and religious understandings, the reader is asked to consider if a balance or integration might be sought between the two, and how we might then go about constructing a personal health-illness orientation.

A key feature throughout all the chapters is the religio-spiritual context in which we find the person, and the implicit expression of mind-body-spirit relationships that orient everyday living and guide and direct health behaviors. Further, although it is anticipated that the reader will discern that not all spiritual practices may be beneficial to health (indeed, certain practices such as fasting may exacerbate illness risk for some individuals), each chapter elucidates the potential for better health through spiritual practices.

Acknowledgments

I wish to thank ABC-CLIO acquisitions editor Debbie Carvalko and series editor Regan A.R. Gurung for their foresight and assistance in bringing together the possibility of this project. I also want to thank ABC-CLIO project managers Michelle Scott and Robin Tutt, and, at Antares Publishing Services, project manager Uma Maheswari and copyeditor Brooke D. Graves for their superb guidance and very skillful assistance in final editing and production of the book.

I also want to thank the contributing authors, who provide us opportunity to look across a diverse landscape of religio-spiritual perspectives, and describe for us how spirituality and health are intertwined. Lastly, I want to thank parents and families, teachers and guides, and all who have continued to offer assistance and support in our trek to find deeper insight and understanding in our living. I especially want to thank my family, Mary Elizabeth and Jack, for their ongoing support and assistance throughout this project, and in our life journey together.

Dean D. VonDras

Chapter 1

The Religio-Spiritual Context of Lifestyle Practices and Health Behaviors

Dean D. VonDras

A person's religious or spiritual orientation is one of the most basic and universal aspects of his or her psychological life (Emmons and Paloutzian 2003; Norenzayan and Heine 2005; Paloutzian 2016; Piedmont 1999), and perhaps the most central attribute of one's culture (Mead 1955). Even in our present age, when secular and materialistic orientations are increasingly seen as replacements for traditional nonsecular worldviews, religious perspectives and spiritual beliefs are still recognized as providing a basic framework that guides and directs the way people live (Smith 2001; Taylor 2011). Accordingly, religion and spirituality are noted to provide and import multiple levels of meaning for the person that broadly influence lifestyle practices and health behaviors (Park 2007). Moreover, it is well established that religious and spiritual beliefs are an important influence on a person's healthy living, and a key component in the effective programming and provision of health care (Aldwin, Park, Jeong, and Nath 2014; Brémault-Phillips, Olson, et al. 2015; Koenig 2012). Despite this recognition, however, many healthcare professionals and laypersons often lack an understanding of religious and spiritual traditions beyond their own native context, and thus are not able to adequately comprehend health behaviors associated with other belief systems, or employ both subtle and obvious health-maintenance and illness interventions that utilize or are based on principles found within various religions or spiritualities (Koenig, King, and Carson 2012; Nelson 2010). The intent of this book is to provide a description of the ways of living within religious and spiritual contexts found across the globe, and to elucidate health-associated practices that occur within each perspective, as well as potential health interventions that may be coordinated and used beyond a particular religious or spiritual context.

What we hope to show is that each religious and spiritual orientation instructively promotes key health-associated values and best practices for successful and healthy living (Koenig 2013; Puchalski 2013; Smith, Bartz, and Scott Richards 2007). For example, the Buddhist concerns for simple living, kindness toward and care for other beings, and the seeking of personal insight and growth illuminate a path of positive lifestyle practices and health behaviors (Murti 1955; H. Smith 1991). Descriptively, Buddhism offers a stress-reducing method noted in its espousal of pacifism as a way to approach interpersonal and social relations, a lowering of a variety of disease risks through the nutritional practice of vegetarianism, and the embrace and development of mindfulness as a means to improve both physical and emotional well-being of the individual (e.g., Baer 2003; Ludwig and Kabat-Zinn 2008). Similarly, many primal religions recognize that nature provides a necessary element of connection and pastoral relief for the individual (H. Smith 1991); hence, as epitomized in the beliefs of oneness of being and oneness with nature expressed in indigenous spiritualities, a holistic and healthy style of living is cultivated that benefits the individual as well as the broader community (e.g., Coyhis and Simonelli 2008; Gone 2013). What these examples begin to tell us is that faith beliefs and practices constitute foundational elements of a contextualism that directs thought; compels action; and links mind, body, and spirit (e.g., Mark and Lyons 2010; Nesdole, Voigts, Lepnurm, and Roberts 2014; Shea, Poudrier, Chad, Jeffery, Thomas, and Burnouf 2013).

As we begin, it is important to mention the orienting tack of this discussion and text. It is inspired by the work of Huston Smith (1991; 2001), who long championed and taught about the values and ethics found within the world's religions. Moreover, it embraces Smith's (2001) postulate that along with scientific explanations of life processes and events, there is enlightenment and further wisdom to be found within the traditional narratives of the world's religions. Therefore, without attempting to resolve controversies or to quell debate involving the existential problems the individual may incur and the interpretive limitations of religion (e.g., Freud 1918, 1928; Kirkpatrick 1999; McCullough and Willoughby 2009; McKinnon 2002; Paloutzian and Park 2005), or the East-versus-West concerns for how spirituality may be conceptualized (e.g., Forsyth, O'Boyle, Jr., and McDaniel 2008; Jung 1969a; Hill, Pargament, Hood, et al. 2000), or the historical influence of deism and science after Darwin (e.g., Byrne 2013; Thomson 2007), or other controversies (e.g., epistemological conflict; Evans and Evans 2008), this text seeks to illuminate the contextual features (e.g., ideologies, social norms, attributional frames, etc.) of various religious and spiritual worldviews, and the healthy ways of living that are embodied within these worldviews. Thus, across the various religious and spiritual worldviews described in the chapters that follow, a characterization of the tenets of faith, communal values, and social forces that are contextually present and expressed will be provided. This is accompanied by a delineation of living habits that suggest positive health interventions that individuals and healthcare workers may utilize (e.g., the embrace of religious creeds, suggestive religious exhortations to avoid or limit alcohol or drug use so as to prevent addiction; Blakeney, Blakeney, and Reich 2005; Hazel and Mohatt 2001), as well as potentially negative outcomes that may occur (e.g., fasting rituals that may produce negative health effects; Cherif, Roelands, Meeusen, and Chamari 2016; Farooq, Herrera, Almudahka, and Mansour 2015). Further, as Smith (1991) points out, while there are certainly differences to be found between various religious and spiritual orientations, there are also many commonalities to be recognized. For example, all religions and spiritualities provide a powerful form of connection to an Ultimate Truth, and espouse values and ethics that influence health behaviors and lifestyle practices of individuals and their communities (e.g., Kumar et al. 2015; Modell, Citrin, King, and Kardia 2014; Whitbeck 2006; Yalom 2002). Without emphasizing a better-or-worse comparison between different religious and spiritual orientations, a further goal of this text is to promote an awareness of these commonalities, and of the shared communal health values that may inspire individuals to live healthfully, offer potential to prevent illness and find healing, and enhance positive management of disorders and diseases.

CONCEPTUAL RELATIONSHIPS AND DISTINCTIONS BETWEEN RELIGION, SPIRITUALITY, AND ASSOCIATED CONSTRUCTS

There is a growing awareness within the social sciences of the importance of religion and spirituality, and their influence on the individual and society (e.g., Dillon 2003; Furness 2016; Gorsuch 1988; Idler 2014; Saroglou 2013). Indeed, considered from a psychological perspective, a person's religio-spiritual orientation is suggested to reveal a repository of unconscious motives (Jung 1933, 1938) that arouse an awareness of personal responsibility (Frankl 1963), and that offer a means for attaining wholeness, healing, and adaptation (Koenig 2005). Further, religio-spiritual beliefs and practices have been suggested to induce positive emotions such as joy, wonder, awe, and gratitude (Campbell 1968; Emmons and Paloutzian 2003), as well as negative emotions of anxiety and depression (Chatters 2000; Exline, Yali, and Lobel 1999; Pargament, Smith, Koenig, and Perez 1998). These beliefs and practices also make available rituals that assist the individual in major life transitions (e.g., the celebration of transitioning from childhood into adulthood, the exchange of vows as one enters into marriage, the process of bereavement when parents die, preparation for one's own death). Thus, beyond a healthy skepticism that questions nonscientific explanations of human experience and behavior (e.g., Feigl 1945; Skinner 1953; Spilka, Shaver, and Kirkpatrick 1985; Weber 1963), the person's religio-spiritual orientation has been suggested to function as a social control mechanism (Weber 1963), acting to compel and motivate health-promoting behaviors (Koenig 2001; Hill and Pargament 2008) and thus influence health practices and outcomes (e.g., Cotton, Zebracki, Rosenthal, Tsevat, and Drotar 2006; Park et al. 2016; Seeman, Dubin, and Seeman 2003; Seybold and Hill 2001). As we begin to explore the religio-spiritual and health relationship, however, it is important to clarify conceptual relationships between religion, spirituality, and their associated constructs of faith and belief.

The first distinction to note is that *religion* and *spirituality* are distinct concepts, although both have dimensions that are highly intertwined with one another (Griffiths 2015; Hill et al. 2000; Moberg 2001; Zinnbauer et al. 1997). For example, whereas religion is often thought to connote one's affiliation with a particular theology and community, and spirituality is suggested to reflect the individual's sense of and involvement with the sacred, both are reflected in one another and have as a central focus entities and processes that are revered and transcendent (Masters 2008). As described by Fowler (1981, 1996), and by Sulmasy (2002), religion is characterized as a cumulative tradition that includes the practice of spirituality and the embrace of specific beliefs, social customs, rituals, and language that affords the search for transcendent meaning. For example, religion may be defined by one's membership in a faith congregation, or regular attendance at religious services. Further, religion may be defined by adherence to a particular theological text (e.g., the Qur'an): its narrative stories, explanations and interpretations of life experiences, and guiding principles for living. In addition, the word *religion* refers to descriptive customs and rites (e.g., formulary for worship services, healing prayer, observance of holy days, fasting), texts (e.g., Vedas in Hinduism, Torah in Judaism, Daodejing in Daoism), forms of art (e.g., sacred architectural design, ceremonial dress, sculptures, paintings, music), and exclusive terminology to describe a variety of behaviors and rituals. Thus, it should be recognized that there is great diversity in the way religion is conceptualized, understood, and expressed (Griffiths 2015; McKinnon 2002).

The term *religion*, as Griffiths (2015) describes, also suggests a deeply bounded intimacy with an Ultimate Concern, and is dynamically characterized by its comprehensiveness, inability of abandonment, and centrality. All of these are also reflected in and associated with constructs such as spirituality, faith, and belief. As Griffiths (2015) explicates, religion holds a *comprehensiveness* for the individual; that is, a system of meaning that is foundational to the person's understanding in that it is relevant to everything and all aspects of life. Along with this comprehensiveness, the religious orientation lived by the person is incapable of abandonment; it so powerfully possesses the person, that if one were to leave this foundational point of life reference one would also take leave of a vital sense of one's own self. In addition to these features of comprehensiveness and incapability of abandonment, Griffiths (2015) also suggests that religion expresses and designates a centrality to one's living, in that it addresses the paramount concerns of existence and provides an essential structuring of one's life.

Similar to Griffiths's (2015) elucidation of the term *religion*, spirituality is also noted to be conceptually diverse, with many different descriptions, and representing a unique personal connection with something revered beyond one's self (*cf.* Armatowski 2001; Hill et al. 2000; Moberg 2001). Thus, *spirituality* can be defined as persons' expression of ultimate meaning and concerns of life, of their faith beliefs or affiliation with religious institution, their sense of the sacred and connection with nature, and/or their attitudes about their relation to others. For example, for some persons spirituality may be synonymous with a personal philosophy, a way-of-living, or the practice of a particular theological doctrine. For others, spirituality may reflect their affection for and connection with nature or other people, or of being in the here-and-now, or their practice of atheism. Thus, a key understanding here is that while *religion* refers to the past and ongoing traditions of particular belief systems and their practices, *spirituality* may also be conceptualized as a reflection of one's religious orientation, or devoid of any theological tradition or religious orientation, and thus shaped and defined in accordance with one's own system of ultimate meaning. Despite these distinctions, however, it should be understood that there is still substantial overlap between these constructs; thus, for the ongoing discussion, religion and spirituality will be considered as one and the same so as to respect the diversity of beliefs and behaviors found within and across different traditions and orientations (Hill et al. 2000; Moberg 2002).

Two constructs closely associated with religion and spirituality are faith and belief. Many people often understand *faith* and *belief* to be synonymous in meaning, and both subordinate referents of religion or spirituality. But again, conceptual clarification is needed. The distinction to make here is that faith and belief each reflect different and separate constructs with reference to their fusion with religion and spirituality. Key to our understanding, as Tillich (1957) notes, is the recognition that faith is not exclusively religious in its subject matter, teleological background, or phenomenological framework, but rather the most basic way that the individual perceives of self in relation to others against a background of shared meaning and purpose. Therefore, as Fowler (1981; 1996) describes, whether the person expresses acceptance of a specific theology; or is a practitioner of a particular spiritual behavior; or is agnostic, nonreligious, or atheist, the individual conceptualizes and constructs a personal meaning and holds to a basic set of principles and descriptions of purpose about life, and thus expresses some trust or faith in this constellation of metaphorical meaning, life principles, and reason. Moreover, a person's faith comprises and reflects an understanding of an ultimate reality that can be structured and organized in coordination with religious traditions, or with scientific principles and theories, or with distinctive philosophical systems of understanding and knowing.

In contrast, *belief* is defined as the holding of specific doctrinal and ideological claims about and with reference to a particular religious or nonreligious faith perspective. Beliefs are also recognized as being formed from and reflective of unconscious dynamics as well as the conscious awareness of religious and nonreligious traditions. Consequently, the expression of faith and its associated set of coordinated beliefs are found in many different forms of spirituality, and in the variety of religious and nonreligious systems of meaning making. For example, one person may describe his faith as Islam and ascribe an ultimate meaning about his life based on the teachings of the Prophet Muhammad. Another person may say her faith is in humanity, and profess a belief in humankind's altruistic potential and benevolent concern for others and the environment. Yet another person may describe her essential faith in terms of probability theorem and the truth of science, or of metaphysics. Therefore, it is important to understand that just as there are diverse ways of defining *religion* and *spirituality*, there are also a variety of ways of expressing one's faith, and a wide array of beliefs espoused and followed within these different orientations (*cf.* Hill et al. 2000; Moberg 2002). The great diversity in how faith and belief may be characterized and expressed is noted and discussed in the chapters that follow.

A BRIEF HISTORICAL OVERVIEW: THE FOUNDATIONAL IMPORTANCE OF RELIGIO-SPIRITUAL CONTEXTUALISM

Religious and spiritual concerns have long been at the epicenter of meaning making and self-understanding, signifying that these are foundational elements directing thought and action. Indeed, as early as 5000 to 3200 BCE, Egyptian hieroglyphs reveal that religio-spiritual beliefs and practices have been an important concern of humankind, providing a referent in depicting and understanding life processes, and in resolving our existential dilemma of finding meaning and wholeness (Nardo 2001). Thus, within all cultures and at all times in history, we find narratives constructed to explain the deepest meanings of our existence, of life events, and the occurrence of death (Campbell 1968, 1972; Heelas 1993; Malinowski 1954; McMullin 1989). Further, since the earliest of times, religio-spiritual beliefs have been used to explain the cause of illness, and in prescribing methods of illness prevention, healing, and adaptation (Benson 1996; Koenig 1999). Even in the rational approach of Hippocrates, the ancient Greek physician and father of modern medicine, religio-spiritual concerns were recognized, and divine solicitation embraced along with the prescription of drug and other therapies as viable treatments in a holistic style of health care (Kleisiaris, Sfakianakis, and Papathanasiou 2014; Orfanos 2007; Yapijakis 2009). Moreover, in establishing religion and spirituality as basic contextual elements, a very early description of their influence on thought and action is found in the philosophy of another ancient Greek, Aristotle. Alluding to the essential religio-spiritual context in which the interpretation of life processes and actions of the person occur, Aristotle suggests that our "first thought" involves a question about "what is good?" (Barnes 1984, vol. 2, pp. 1694–1695), and notes that "[o]ur forefathers, in the most remote ages, have handed down to us their posterity, a tradition in the form of a myth . . . with a view to the persuasion of the multitude, and to its legal and utilitarian expediency" (Barnes 1984, vol. 2, p. 1698). Further, postulating the interrelationship of mind, body, and spirit, Aristotle proposes that, "[s]oul and body . . . are affected sympathetically by one another" (Barnes 1984, vol. 1, p. 1242). Thus, Aristotle's characterization of a "first thought," recognition of the power of myth, and embrace of a divinely inspired existential expression provide a logical groundwork for considering religion and spirituality as foundational contextual elements that shape and influence health perceptions, lifestyle practices, and associated health behaviors of the individual. Later thinkers of the Middle and Enlightenment Ages also put forward the ideas of a "first thought" and religio-spiritual concerns as primary and essential aspects of our thinking and living. For example, St. Thomas Aquinas (Pegis 1945) provides another portrayal of this first principle in his description of "natural law," suggesting that the first precept of natural law is that "good is to be done and promoted and evil avoided . . . and that, all other psychological proclivities flow from this first inclination" (Pegis 1945, p. 637). Later, foreshadowing the emergence of the transcendental movement, Immanuel Kant (Ellington 1981) put forth the "moral imperative."

Again, like the notion of a "first thought," Kant's moral imperative suggests that reason alone may provide and reflect the voice of an *a priori*, transcendent, and ultimate authority that coordinates our thinking and guides our behavior.

Similar to the Western philosophical assumptions of Aristotle, Aquinas, and Kant that specify mind-body-spirit relationships, the ancient philosophies of Eastern societies and indigenous cultures also embraced a spirituality that was primary and central, residing within the person, and descriptive of relationship with a transcendent force beyond the self (*cf.* Davies 2000; Jung 1969a; Grieves 2009; H. Smith 1991; Yijie 1991). Moreover, these non-Western orientations, like the transcendental thinking of Aristotle and others in the West, also espoused a "first thought" that informs positive communal values and provides basic guiding principles for the individual and society (cf. Jung 1969a; Grieves 2009; H. Smith 1991, Yijie 1991). For example, Confucianism and Daoism (both originating around 400 to 300 BCE) similarly express a connection to a transcendent reality (heaven) that coordinates with and gives shape to social and moral philosophy (Smith 1991). As Yijie (1991, p. 26) describes, the early Confucian scholar, Dong Zhongshu, "preached the idea that heaven and man respond to each other and his argument was that the two were integrated." Further, recognizing the Confucian objective of societal and moral reform, Yijie (1991, p. 26) notes that early in the Common Era (220–420), "the metaphysics of the Wei and Jin dynasties focused its discussion on the relationship between nature and the Confucian ethical code." This moral concern is advanced somewhat differently in Daoism, which emphasizes a supernatural cosmology that directs refinement of personal habit, instructing that, "If you can keep the dao (tao) in your body, if you do not waste your vital energy, do not torture your spirit, then, you can attain immortality" (Yijie 1991, p. 184). In a similar way, as described by Grieves (2009, p. 7), the philosophies of indigenous peoples established the holistic idea of "the interconnectedness of the elements of the earth and the universe, animate and inanimate, whereby people, the plants and animals, landforms and celestial bodies are interrelated." This interconnectedness is symbolically encoded in the sacred stories created and passed down by ancestors who not only provided a description for the foundation of all life, but also of the Law (Grieves 2009). Thus, much like the social norms and moral principles found in Confucianism and Daoism that sustain the social order, as Grieves (2009, p. 7) notes, within indigenous societies the Law is given to ensure "that each person knows his or her connectedness and responsibilities for other people (their kin), for country (including watercourses, landforms, the species and the universe), and for their ongoing relationship with the ancestor spirits themselves."

In our present time, and especially in the West, further theorizing about the person's connection with the religio-spiritual, and the triumvirate of mind-body-spirit, has been strongly influenced by the psychoanalytic movement. Major influences here include the theories of Carl Jung (1933; 1938), who posited the "the religious unconscious"; as well as Viktor Frankl's (1963) suggestion of an unconscious motivation to "responsibility," and the work of other leading thinkers who noted religio-spiritual experiences to be a vital aspect and concern of the psyche (*see, e.g.,* Allport 1950; Fromm 1950; James 1985; Maslow 1964; Rank 1996). Taken as a whole, these theories suggest that religion and spirituality arise from deep, unconscious psychological processes. Thus, apart from philosophical or metaphysical considerations, modern psychology provides a phenomenological account that recognizes religion as "one of the most essential manifestations of the human mind" (Jung 1969b, p. 289). Indeed, from the theoretical viewpoint of Jungian psychology, religion and spirituality are posited as being reflections of the individual's "relationship to the highest or most powerful value, be it positive or negative . . . that is both accepted voluntarily, as well as involuntarily, that is to say you can accept consciously, the value by which you are possessed unconsciously" (Jung 1969a, p. 81). In so doing, again a dialecticism involving the interaction of religio-spiritual concerns and behavior is suggested. Describing this dynamic interaction, Jung (1969a) notes that religion and spirituality describe and inform a transcendental awareness and altering of consciousness, and thus the enactment of faith practices, religious rituals, and the following of theologic creeds "are codified and dogmatized forms of original religious experience" (pp. 8–9). Further, considering both Western and Eastern traditions, Jung (1969a) posits that religious and spiritual experiences (e.g., thoughts, emotions, actions) "come upon man from inside as well as outside" (p. 366), suggesting a symbiotic intertwining of the religio-spiritual with the psyche, and expressing an all-encompassing dialecticism as a basis for understanding human existence. Moreover, using Buddhist metaphor in describing this religio-spiritual and psychological symbiosis, Jung (1969a) suggests, "The psyche is therefore all-important; it is the all-pervading Breath, the Buddha-essence; it is the Buddha-Mind, the One, the Damakaya. All existence emanates from it, and all separate forms dissolve back into it" (p. 482).

As we consider religion and spirituality to be deeply and interdependently connected to our perceiving, reasoning, and acting, the viewpoint of Campbell (1968, 1972; *see also* Griffiths 2015; McKinnon 2002) is also illuminating, in that it further describes and gives a modern interpretation as to how religious and spiritual beliefs are intimately represented in our culture and reflected in our behavior. As Campbell (1968, 1972) describes, religions and spirituality provide a basic structure to life: a structure for living that is animated in the shared communal beliefs, ritual behaviors, and collective values that script out and announce our most revered life goals and dreams. Indeed, religion and spirituality are "embedded in broader cultural and intellectual traditions, narratives, and worldviews" (Nord 2010, pp. 203–204), so that, as Hofstede (2010, 2011) describes, religion and spirituality are inherent in the mental programming or *software of the mind* that directs our thinking, feeling, and acting. Therefore, it should be understood that in all cultures people speak about faith of some type, and articulate various styles of spirituality, demonstrating this culturally generic phenomenon of meaning making and construction of ultimate concern (e.g., God, natural or supernatural forces), and in doing so again underscore religion and spirituality as significant aspects of our psychology, intimately linked with and underpinning our perceiving, thinking, and acting so as to represent a very powerful and foundational contextualism.

This notion of religion and spiritual phenomena as key elements of the mind's programming language (Hofstede 2010, 2011), and their extensive influence on the individual, is further advanced by empirical investigations suggesting that religion and spirituality may organize (e.g., Bulbulia and Schjoedt 2013; Seitz and Angel 2011) and activate neural circuits (e.g., Barnby, Bailey, Chambers, and Fitzgerald 2015; Inzlicht, McGregor, Hirsh, and Nash 2009; Kapogiannis et al. 2009); mediate social cognition processes (e.g., Goplen and Plant 2015; Holbrook, Fessler, and Pollack 2016; Norenzayan, Atran, Faulkner, and Schaller 2006; Shariff and Norenzayan 2007); constitute a source of identity, life purpose, and guide for character development (e.g., Fowler 1981, 1996; King 2008; Mariano and Damon 2008; Roeser, Issac, Abo-Zeno, Brittian, and Peck 2008); and affect health behaviors and health outcomes (e.g., Galen and Rogers 2004; Hayward, Krause, Ironson, and Pargament 2016; Koenig 2012, Koenig, King, and Carson 2012; Van Cappellen, Toth-Gauthier, Saroglou, and Fredrickson 2016). Thus, similar to the philosophical and psychological theories discussed earlier, empirical investigations further suggest that one's religio-spiritual orientation, regardless of how it may be individually defined and expressed, is a most basic and powerful influence on one's living.

TOWARD A PARADIGM OF DEEP AND PENETRATING SYMBIOSIS: DIALECTICAL CONTEXTUALISM

The concern for understanding contextual influences on behavior was recognized early on in experimental psychology by Bruner (1957; *see also* Lewin 1951). In accord with the ancient wisdom that "we do not see things the way they are, rather, we see things the way *we are*" expressed in the Talmud,[1] Bruner (1957) proposed the construct of perceptual readiness, positing that the person perceives and behaves in coordination with earlier experiences, characteristics, habits, and current needs and states. Within the zeitgeist of social psychology, however, explanations of behavior have historically reflected assumptions of economic, information processing, and statistical sciences, advancing theories based on actor-observer differences, social inferencing, and whether or not the behavior is caused by external/internal or global/specific factors, or under personal control (Malle 2011). Further, this long-established tradition has often omitted explanation of how a person's religious or spiritual orientation may influence thinking and action (Hill et al. 2000). Nevertheless, Bruner (1990) and others (e.g., Biglan and Hayes 1997; Herbert and Padovani 2015; Lerner 1978; Staw 2016) have continued to suggest that to fully comprehend a person's behavior, there must also be a deep understanding of the cultural and environmental setting in which that behavior occurs. As a result, recent theories have begun to recognize the deep and penetrating symbiosis of one's sociocultural and religio-spiritual background with thinking and acting. This view recognizes a broader and more extensive historical influence, and posits that a person's deeper unconscious concerns; personal characteristics, culture, and acculturation processes; along with immediate context, should all be considered key factors that direct thought and action (e.g., Kraus, Piff, Mendoza-Denton, Rheinschmidt, and Keltner 2012; Malle 1999; Malle, Knobe, O'Laughlin, Pearce, and Nelson 2000; Owe et al. 2013).

In a similar manner, although previous investigations have reported the importance of social norms and expectations as critical influences on health behaviors and practices (e.g., D'Blasi, Harkness, Ernst, Georgiou, and Kleijnen 2010; Reid, Cialdini, and Aiken 2010), there has also been recent acknowledgment of the need for a new paradigm that emphasizes the multiple influences on and dimensions of behavior, and the usefulness of an interdisciplinary approach to aid explication and understanding of these relationships (*cf.* Emmons and Paloutzian 2003; Masters 2008; Hexham 2011). In sympathetic response, a conceptual model of dialectical contextualism is put forth here, seeking to broaden the path toward a shift in paradigm that emphasizes a multilevel and interdisciplinary approach (e.g., Emmons and Paloutzian 2003; Masters 2008). The central assumption of this model is that the person's religio-spiritual orientation represents a foundational and basic point of reference that directs lifestyle practices and health-related behaviors. Thus, as described by Ratner (2007), religio-spiritual concerns in conjunction with lifestyle and associated health practices are recognized as interdependent, interpenetrating, and internally related, taking on qualities of each other as they exert and allow reciprocal influence and change. Dynamically, then, this dialectical contextualism promotes a shift in paradigm beyond psychological positivism—where there is an assumption of an independence and isolation of factors, and where religio-spiritual phenomena are implicitly understood to be separate, self-contained, simple, and homogenous—toward a description of contextual-behavioral relationships that reflects the emic approach of Echensberger (2015), embracing an understanding of a phenomenon framed from within its religio-spiritual context, as opposed to a method of description and understanding framed from an outside and external scheme. To expand understanding of religio-spiritual orientations and their involvement with lifestyle practices and health behaviors, a hypothetical model portraying this dialectical contextualism is shown in Figure 1.1. As informed by a similar model of cultural influences (VonDras, Pouliot, Malcore, and Iwahashi 2008), and incorporating health-behavior relationships noted by Aldwin et al. (2013), Masters (2008), and Bonelli and Koenig (2013), along with orienting contextual elements and dimensions suggested by Spilka (1993), Hofstede (2010, 2011), and Ratner (2007), this model seeks to portray the all-encompassing, interdependent, and penetrating influence of religio-spiritual orientation on social, cognitive, and behavioral elements, and resultant health outcomes.

Further, this model of dialectical contextualism, analogous to the manifold levels of meaning that Grice (1989) posits to be found within language, should be understood as multifaceted, made up of a personally significant and communally complex system of meaning and understanding. In addition, emphasizing dialectical relations, this religio-spiritual contextualism should be understood as both verbal (e.g., containing scriptural exhortations, theological tenets, dynamic pastoral directives and guidance, etc.), as well as nonverbal (e.g., involving ritualistic behavior, creative expressions, social contagion, etc.), and—again in analogy with Grice's logic of communication (1989)—reflecting a type of *implicature*. That is, the religio-spiritual orientation of the person provides an interpretive meaning beyond the literal that reflects an interdependent communal point of reference, and which instills beliefs and encourages specific actions by the individual and the community. Thus, as similarly suggested by Jung (1969a) and Griffiths (2015), the implicature of the person's religio-spiritual orientation embodies a comprehensiveness, with every aspect of life tacitly understood and comprised within it. Accordingly, this dialectical contextual model affords the construction and embrace of a paradigm in which a person's religio-spiritual orientation is recognized as archetypal and foundational, and understood as a most important point of reference that universally

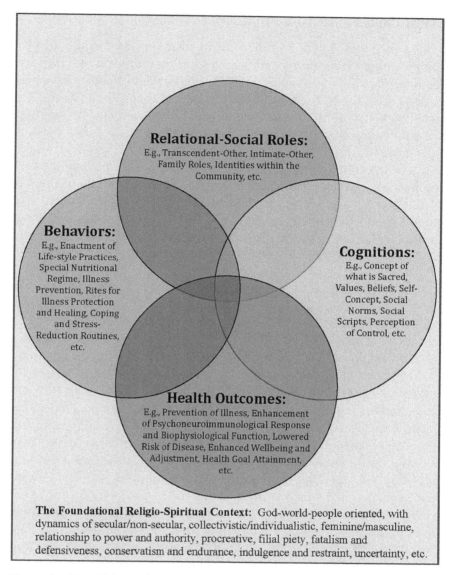

Figure 1.1 The Dialectical Contextual Model of Religio-Spirituality, Behavior, and Health

shapes ways of living and guides health-related behaviors. As we consider religious and spiritual influences on lifestyle practices and health behaviors in the following chapters, this model will help us to draw into focus and distinguish unique practices and relationships within religio-spiritual orientations, as well as to find commonalities across them.

SEVEN CHALLENGES TO OUR UNDERSTANDING

Given the theory of dialectical contextualism proposed in this chapter, there is a need to recognize potential challenges to the model, and the varying interpretation of ontological relationships and epistemological explanations that may be suggested here. The first challenge to be realized, as noted by Watts (1951), is that "science and religion are talking about the same universe, but using different kinds of language" (pp. 135–136). Both offer profound insights, but of particular concern will be how these insights might be integrated by the person and society so as to deepen understanding and provide intellectual enlightenment. Thus the reader should beware of the interpretive problems inherent in understanding the nature of subjective experience versus objective reality that exists within the topography of dialectic contextualism (Kincaid 2004; Little 1995; Malterud 2001; Morgan and Smircich 1980) and, indeed, found within the chapters of this book.

A second related challenge involves the feasibility of moving beyond the limit of understanding offered by Freedland (2004), who suggested that even if there were solid evidence suggesting relationship between religious and spiritual activities and health, "it would relegate religious beliefs to a distal node in the causal pathways . . . one far removed from the dominion of the physicians, surgeons and nurses in charge of preventing and managing illness" (p. 240). In contrast, the chapters of this text hope to echo and champion the response to Freedland offered by Contrada et al. (2004): that religious and spiritual beliefs and practices *are* immediate (i.e., proximal), important to the individual, and quite plausible influences on preventative behaviors and disease-reducing psychophysicological processes. Therefore, following Masters (2008) and Seeman, Dubin, and Seeman (2003), who have suggested that religious and spiritual beliefs and practices are linked with health-related biophysiological processes that include cardiovascular, immune, and neuroendocrine functions, the chapters of this text seek to illuminate the many ways religio-spiritual beliefs and practices may lead to positive as well as potentially negative health outcomes. In doing so, this book raises the question of how we might consider the positivism of science and the transcendentalism expressed in religio-spiritual philosophies as complements of one another. Thus, when using a dialectical contextual approach (e.g., Capstick, Norris, Sopoaga, and Tobata 2009; Wilson 2000), this second challenge is to take into account how the empirical and material may be connected to and in interaction with the intuitive and spiritual, so as to gain deeper insight into how religio-spiritual orientations may affect the person's pattern of living, and resultant physical health and mental well-being.

The third challenge is to recognize the type of relationship we construct between science and religion, and the valuing of both in this dynamic union. Thus, as we consider the influence of religio-spiritual orientation on health behavior, it should also be noted that in the moments of our deepest intimacies and greatest comfort, we understand our experience to be connected with a wholeness-making and euphoria-producing spirituality (e.g., Chirban 1992; Galanter 2008; Krägeloh, Billington, Henning, and Chai 2014; Tyler and Raynor, Jr. 2006). Indeed, evidence of this close association of spirituality with well-being and wholeness appears in the various prescriptive guides for living found throughout the world religions. For example, the halal and haram laws in Islam, emphasizing what foods may be consumed and how they must be prepared, underscores the closeness of religio-spiritual belief and lifestyle practice (Bonne and Verbeke 2008). Similarly, the abstinence from tobacco and alcohol as proscribed within various religious traditions (e.g., Merrill, Folsom, and Christopherson 2005; Michalak, Trocki, and Bond 2007), and the suggested reliance on or belief in a higher power to maintain sobriety and battle addictions (e.g., Dermatis and Galanter 2016; Li, Feifer, and Strohm 2000), also suggest a union of religio-spiritual faith and belief with health behaviors and practices. Further, with regard to preventative programs, it is suggested that the greatest likelihood of success for health behavior change is through the application of culturally specific approaches that recognize and include spirituality as part of the psychological orientation of the person (e.g., Nebelkopf and Wright 2011). As noted by H. Smith (1991, 2001), the values, ethics, and philosophies of religion, along with the scientific approach of medicine, offer a variety of resources and tools for promoting healthy living and in finding healing. However, while elevating the importance of religious and spiritual phenomena so as to enhance our understanding, it should be noted that the intention is not to diminish the utility or authority of science. Rather, we hope to promote a balance between scientific and religious understandings, embracing the insight to which Jung (1969a) alludes: "While science is seen as a replacement for religio-spirituality in the West, and with great conflict, in the East there is no conflict between religion and science, because no science is there based upon the passion for facts, and no religion upon mere faith; there is religious cognition and cognitive religion . . . in the East, man is God and he redeems himself" (p. 480). Thus, the third challenge includes re-thinking how we construct a relationship between science and religio-spiritual understandings, and how this constructed relationship may aid the individual and family in making healthy lifestyle choices, and help the clinician to provide a style of optimal care that is sensitive to the individual's religio-spiritual orientation (Koenig 2004).

Although previous works have illuminated relationships between religio-spiritual practices and health (e.g., Plante and Sherman 2001; Koenig, King, and Carson 2012), this text seeks to expand beyond those earlier works by looking more closely within the cultural contexts of the world's religions; this is our fourth challenge. In doing so, it is intended to serve as a counterpoint to perspectives that merely suggest religious and faith beliefs as independent factors, to be partitioned or controlled so as understand their relationship between more relevant behaviors and health outcomes (e.g., T. W. Smith 2001). Answering the call of Piedmont (2014) for a deeper and more coherent understanding of the numinous ground of religion and spirituality, and its penetrating and interdependent influence on all behavior, the chapters that follow seek to broaden comprehension of the contextual ground of religion and spirituality, and elucidate how these foundational elements may powerfully influence and direct lifestyle practices and health behaviors. Of central concern, however, is that for any given individual there may be a myriad of contextual influences, or, as Fowler (1981) has suggested, a polytheistic pattern of faith-identity relationships, that lacks one center of power and guiding influence that focuses the individual's living and directs their life. Hence, the question arises as to how we may understand the weight of religio-spiritual influences, whether faintly or strongly, within and across the diverse dialectical contexts in which people are oriented. This challenge involves how we advance our thinking and research so as to recognize and understand both the micro and macro processes of congruence and discord, tranquility and tension, constructive and destructive compromise (Adams, Day, Dyk, Frede, and Rogers 1992) that are communally present, and that powerfully impact the lifestyle practices and health outcomes of the individual, the family, the community, and broader society (Adams and Marshall 1996; Lerner 1992).

A fifth challenge involves a concern for whether any prospective implementation of religio-spiritual-associated interventions (e.g., mindfulness training, yoga) may also tacitly reflect, or explicitly suggest, a religious indoctrination, and the associated ethical concerns that are inherent in this issue (e.g., Brown 2015; Kabat-Zinn 2003; Van Gordon, Shonin, and Griffiths 2016). A related sixth challenge concerns the potential for adverse effects of religio-spiritual-associated interventions (e.g., Koenig 2012; Reeves, Beazley, and Adams 2011). For both of these issues, as noted in the guidance offered by Van Gordon et al. (2016), Koenig (2008), and Reeves et al. (2011), it should be understood that religious or spiritual interventions may reflect or intentionally support nonsecular beliefs, or be procedures claiming a strict secularism and intention, and in both instances result in positive or negative effects for the individual. Thus, the careful ethical consideration of potential effects of any religio-spiritual-associated intervention, along with close adherence to professional ethical codes and standards in implementing any intervention, is warranted. Further, just as it is expected that there may be variation in the efficacy of any intervention (e.g., Yeaton and Sechrest 1981), there is also a need to weigh the probable risk of any religio-spiritual associated intervention, and to understand its potential costs versus benefits (Garfield, Isacco, and Sahker 2013). Combined, these challenges ask us to consider what is possible and what is practical with regard to religio-spiritual-associated interventions.

A seventh and final challenge aligns with the recognition of religious expression as a basic need and universal human right (Davis 2002; United Nations General Assembly 1948). The full address of this challenge in some ways involves the degree to which it is possible to embrace a religio-spiritual pluralism, to see beyond our own boundaries of spirituality, and to view other religious and nonreligious orientations in a respectful, and equally valid and valuing, way. Certainly, there may be long distances to span here, as most religio-spiritual orientations embrace the notion that they are the one true path to enlightenment or salvation (Smith 1991). Yet, in cultures where religious faith is common and national support high, greater subjective well-being is reported (Lun and Bond 2013), highlighting the centrality and importance of religio-spiritual expression in people's living. Thus, this challenge involves deep personal introspection into one's inner dialogue, and the confrontation of cognitive frameworks that sustain religio-spiritual centrism, support ideological chauvinism, or, in the extreme, perpetuate prejudices and biases toward different or unfamiliar religio-spiritual orientations. The upholding of freedom of religious expression as a basic need and universal human right, and the respecting and equal valuing of the religio-spiritual orientation of the person, are all needed to foster an accommodation of religio-spiritual practices in health care, and in tailoring illness prevention programs, health interventions, and other healthcare services so that they are culturally appropriate and accessible (Francis, Griffith, and Leser 2014; Kim et al. 2008; Koenig 2008).

CONCLUSION

Religion and spirituality are central aspects of one's culture and psychological life (Mead 1955; Griffiths 2015; Norenzayan and Heine 2005), and are found at the core of healthy lifestyle practices and behaviors (e.g., Koenig 2005; Koenig, King, and Carson 2012, Koenig, McCullough, and Larson 2001; Miller and Thoresen 2003). However, healthcare professionals as well as laypersons often lack knowledge of religious and spiritual traditions beyond their own (Koenig 2004; Nelson 2010). Thus, a primary focus of this book is the illumination of the orienting worldviews of religious and nonreligious systems, and the associated psychological and social forces that support programs of wellness maintenance and illness prevention. Moreover, the text is intended to foster the reader's consideration of how different worldviews compel positive health behaviors that may be effectively coordinated beyond their native context to improve health and prevent disease. The chapters that follow are intended to provide a mosaic of understanding, showing how the world's religious, spiritual, and nonreligious traditions guide and direct lifestyle practices and health behaviors. A further hope is that there will be an advancement of the notion that there are many avenues of understanding, all illuminating a constellation of core truths made clear through a deeper understanding of the person, and the religio-spiritual context in which they live.

NOTE

1. See also Aristotle's *Metaphysics* (Barnes, 1984, vol. 2, pp. 1552–1728) for an early discussion of how one's perceptions are of the individual.

REFERENCES

Adams, G. R., T. Day, P. H. Dyk, E. Frede, and D. R. B. Rogers. 1992. "On the Dialectics of Pubescence and Psychosocial Development." *Journal of Early Adolescence* 12: 348–365.

Adams, G. R., and S. K. Marshall. 1996. "A Developmental Social Psychology of Identity: Understanding the Person-in-Context." *Journal of Adolescence* 19: 429–442.

Aldwin, C. M., C. L. Park, Y.J. Jeong, and R. Nath. 2014. "Differing Pathways Between Religiousness, Spirituality, and Health: A Self-Regulation Perspective." *Psychology of Religion and Spirituality* 6: 9–21.

Allport, G.W. 1950. *The Individual and His Religion: A Psychological Interpretation.* Oxford, UK: MacMillan.

Armatowski, J. 2001. "Attitudes toward Death and Dying Among Persons in the Fourth Quarter of Life." In D. O. Moberg, ed., *Aging and Spirituality: Spiritual Dimensions of Aging Theory, Research, Practice, and Policy*, pp. 71–83. New York: Haworth Pastoral Press.

Baer, R. A. 2003. "Mindfulness Training as a Clinical Intervention: A Conceptual and Empirical Review." *Clinical Psychology: Science and Practice* 10: 125–143.

Barnby, J. M., N. W. Bailey, R. Chambers, and P. B. Fitzgerald. 2015. "How Similar Are the Changes in Neural Activity Resulting from Mindfulness Practice in Contrast to Spiritual Practice?" *Consciousness and Cognition* 36: 219–232.

Barnes, J., ed. 1984. *Complete Works of Aristotle, Volumes 1 and 2: The Revised Oxford Translation.* Princeton, NJ: Princeton University Press.

Benson, H. 1996. *Timeless Healing: The Power and Belief of Biology.* New York: Simon and Schuster.

Biglan, A., and S. C. Hayes. 1997. "Should the Behavioral Sciences Become More Pragmatic? The Case for Functional Contextualism in Research on Human Behavior." *Applied and Preventive Psychology* 5: 47–57.

Blakeney, C. D., R. F. Blakeney, and H. Reich. 2005. "Leaps of Faith: The Role of Religious Development in Recovering Integrity among Jewish Alcoholics and Drug Addicts." *Mental Health, Religion, and Culture* 8: 63–77.

Bonelli, R. M., and H. G. Koenig. 2013. "Mental Disorders, Religion and Spirituality 1990 to 2010: A Systematic Evidence-Based Review." *Journal of Religion and Health* 52: 657–673.

Bonne, K., and W. Verbeke. 2008. "Religious Values Informing Halal Meat Production and the Control and Delivery of Halal Credence Quality." *Agriculture and Human Values* 25: 35–47.

Brémault-Phillips, S., J. Olson, P. Brett-MacLean, D. Oneschuk, S. Sinclair, R. Magnus, . . . C. M. Puchalski. 2015. "Integrating Spirituality as a Key Component of Patient Care." *Religions* 6: 476–498.

Brown, C. G. 2015. "Textual Erasures of Religion: The Power of Books to Redefine Yoga and Mindfulness Meditation as Secular Wellness Practices in North American Public Schools." *Mémoires du Livre/Studies in Book Culture* 6(2). doi:0.7202/1032713ar

Bruner, J. S. 1957. "On Perceptual Readiness." *Psychological Review* 64: 123–152.

Bruner, J. S. 1990. *Acts of Meaning.* Cambridge, MA: Harvard University Press.

Bulbulia, J., and U. Schjoedt. 2013. "The Neural Basis of Religion." In F. Krueger and J. Grafman, eds., *The Neural Basis of Human Belief Systems*, pp. 169–190. New York: Psychology Press.

Byrne, P. 2013. *Natural Religion and the Nature of Religion: The Legacy of Deism.* New York: Routledge.

Campbell, J. 1968. *The Hero with a Thousand Faces* (2nd ed.). New York: Princeton University Press.

Campbell, J. 1972. *Myths to Live By.* New York: Viking.

Capstick, S., P. F. Norris, F. Sopoaga, and W. Tobata. 2009. "Relationships Between Health and Culture in Polynesia: A Review." *Social Science & Medicine* 7: 1341–1348.

Chatters, L. M. 2000. "Religion and Health: Public Health Research and Practice." *Annual Review of Public Health* 21: 335–367.

Cherif, A., B. Roelands, R. Meeusen, and K. Chamari. 2016. "Effects of Intermittent Fasting, Caloric Restriction, and Ramadan Intermittent Fasting on Cognitive Performance at Rest and During Exercise in Adults." *Sports Medicine* 46: 35–47.

Chirban, J. T. 1992. "Healing and Spirituality." *Pastoral Psychology* 40(4): 235–244.

Contrada, R. J., E. L. Idler, C. Cather, T. M. Goyal, L. Rafalson, and T. J. Krause. 2004. "Why Not Find Out Whether Religious Beliefs Predict Surgical Outcomes?

If They Do, Why Not Find Out Why? Reply to Freedland (2004)." *Health Psychology* 23: 243–246.

Cotton, S., K. Zebracki, S. L. Rosenthal, J. Tsevat, and D. Drotar. 2006. "Religion/Spirituality and Adolescent Health Outcomes: A Review." *Journal of Adolescent Health* 38: 472–480.

Coyhis, D., and R. Simonelli. 2008. "The Native American Healing Experience." *Substance Use & Misuse* 43: 1927–1949.

Davies, M. B. 2000. *Following the Great Spirit: Exploring Aboriginal Belief Systems.* Hamilton, Ontario, Canada: Manor House.

Davis, D. H. 2002. "The Evolution of Religious Freedom as a Universal Human Right: Examining the Role of the 1981 United Nations Declaration on the Elimination of All Forms of Intolerance and of Discrimination Based on Religion or Belief." *Brigham Young University Law Review* 2002(2): 217–236.

D'Blasi, Z., E. Harkness, E. Ernst, A. Georgiou, and J. Kleijnen. 2010. "Influence of Context Effects on Health Outcomes: A Systematic Review." *The Lancet* 357: 757–762.

Dermatis, H., and M. Galanter. 2016. "The Role of Twelve-Step-Related Spirituality in Addiction Recovery." *Journal of Religion and Health* 55(2): 510–521.

Dillon, M. 2003. *Handbook of the Sociology of Religion.* Cambridge, UK: Cambridge University Press.

Echensberger, L. H. 2015. "Integrating the Emic (Indigenous) with the Etic (Universal): A Case of Squaring the Circle or for Adopting a Culture Inclusive Action Theory Perspective." *Journal for the Theory of Social Behaviour* 45: 108–140.

Ellington, J. W., ed. 1981. *Grounding for the Metaphysics of Morals* (2nd ed.). Indianapolis: Hackett.

Emmons, R. A., and R. F. Paloutzian. 2003. "The Psychology of Religion." *Annual Review of Psychology* 54: 377–402.

Evans, J. H., and M. S. Evans. 2008. "Religion and Science: Beyond the Epistemological Conflict Narrative." *Sociology* 34: 87–105.

Exline, J. J., A. M. Yali, and M. Lobel. 1999. "When God Disappoints: Difficulty Forgiving God and Its Role in Negative Emotion." *Journal of Health Psychology* 4: 365–379.

Farooq, A., C. P. Herrera, F. Almudahka, and R. Mansour. 2015. "A Prospective Study of the Physiological and Neurobehavioral Effects of Ramadan Fasting in Preteen and Teenage Boys." *Journal of the Academy of Nutrition and Dietetics* 115: 889–897.

Feigl, H. 1945. "Operationism and Scientific Method." *Psychological Review* 52: 250–259.

Forsyth, D. R., E. H. O'Boyle Jr., and M. A. McDaniel. 2008. "East Meets West: A Meta-Analytic Investigation of Cultural Variations in Idealism and Relativism." *Journal of Business Ethics* 83: 813–833.

Fowler, J. W. 1981. *Stages of Faith: The Psychology of Human Development and the Quest for Meaning.* San Francisco: Harper & Row.

Fowler, J. W. 1996. *Faithful Change: The Personal and Public Challenges of Postmodern Life*. Nashville: Abingdon Press.

Francis, S. A., F. M. Griffith, and K. A. Leser. 2014. "An Investigation of Somali Women's Beliefs, Practices, and Attitudes about Health, Health Promoting Behaviours and Cancer Prevention." *Health, Culture and Society* 6(1). doi:10.5195/hcs.2014.119.

Frankl, V. E. 1963. *Man's Search for Meaning: An Introduction to Logotherapy: Or From Death-camp to Existentialism*. Translated by Ilse Lasch. Pref. by Gordon W. Allport. Boston: Beacon Press.

Freedland, K. E. 2004. "Religious Beliefs Shorten Hospital Stay? Psychology Works in Mysterious Ways. Comments on Contrada, et al. (2004)." *Health Psychology* 23(3): 239–242.

Freud, S. 1918. *Totem and Taboo*. New York: Moffat, Yard.

Freud, S. 1928. *The Future of an Illusion*. London: Hogarth Press.

Fromm, E. 1950. *Psychoanalysis and Religion*. New Haven, CT: Yale University.

Furness, S. 2016. "Religion, Spirituality and Social Work." In M. de Souza, J. Bone, and J. Watson, eds., *Spirituality across Disciplines: Research and Practice*, pp. 179–190. Berlin, Germany: Springer International Publishing.

Galanter, M. 2008. "The Concept of Spirituality in Relation to Addiction Recovery and General Psychiatry." In L. E. Kastkutis and M. Galanter, eds., *Recent Developments in Alcoholism*, pp. 125–140. New York: Springer.

Galen, L. W., and W. M. Rogers. 2004. "Religiosity, Alcohol Expectancies, Drinking Motives and Their Interaction in the Prediction of Drinking Among College Students." *Journal of Alcohol Studies* 66: 469–476.

Garfield, C. F., A. Isacco, and E. Sahker. 2013. "Religion and Spirituality as Important Components of Men's Health and Wellness: An Analytic Review." *American Journal of Lifestyle Medicine* 7: 27–37.

Gone, J. P. 2013. "A Community-Based Treatment for Native American Historical Trauma: Prospects for Evidence-Based Practice." *Journal of Consulting and Clinical Psychology* 77: 751–762.

Goplen, J., and E. A. Plant. 2015. "A Religious Worldview Protecting One's Meaning System Through Religious Prejudice." *Personality and Social Psychology Bulletin* 41: 1474–1487.

Gorsuch, R. L. 1988. "Psychology of Religion." *Annual Review of Psychology* 39: 201–221.

Grice, P. 1989. *Studies in the Way of Words*. Cambridge, MA: Harvard University Press.

Grieves, V. 2009. *Aboriginal Spirituality: Aboriginal Philosophy as the Basis of Aboriginal Social and Emotional Well-Being*. Casuarina, Australia: Cooperative Research Centre for Aboriginal Health.

Griffiths, P. J. 2015. *Problems of Religious Diversity*. Oxford, UK: John Wiley & Sons.

Hayward, R. D., N. Krause, G. Ironson, and K. I. Pargament. 2016. "Externalizing Religious Health Beliefs and Health and Well-Being Outcomes." *Journal of Behavioral Medicine* 39: 887–895.

Hazel, K. W., and G. V. Mohatt. 2001. "Cultural and Spiritual Coping in Sobriety: Informing Substance Abuse Prevention for Alaska Native Communities." *Journal of Community Psychology* 29: 541–562.

Heelas, P. 1993. "The New Age in Cultural Context: The Premodern, the Modern and the Postmodern." *Religion* 23: 103–116.

Herbert, J. D., and F. Padovani. 2015. "Contextualism, Psychological Science, and the Question of Ontology." *Journal of Contextual Behavioral Science* 4: 225–230.

Hexham, I. 2011. *Understanding World Religions: An Interdisciplinary Approach.* Grand Rapids, MI: Zondervan.

Hill, P. C., and K. I. Pargament. 2008. "Advances in the Conceptualization and Measurement of Religion and Spirituality: Implications for Physical and Mental Health Research." *American Psychologist* 58: 64–74.

Hill, P. C., K. I. Pargament, R. W. Hood, Jr., M. E. McCullough, J. P. Swyers, D. B. Larson, and B. J. Zinnbauer. 2000. "Conceptualizing Religion and Spirituality: Points of Commonality, Points of Departure." *Journal of the Theory of Social Behavior* 30: 51–77.

Hofstede, G. 2010. *Cultures and Organizations: Software of the* Mind (3rd ed.). New York: McGraw-Hill.

Hofstede, G. 2011. "Dimensionalizing Cultures: The Hofstede Model in Context." *Online Readings in Psychology and Culture* 2(1). http://dx.doi.org/10.9707 /2307-0919.1014

Holbrook, C., D. M. Fessler, and J. Pollack. 2016. "With God on Our Side: Religious Primes Reduce the Envisioned Physical Formidability of a Menacing Adversary." *Cognition* 146: 387–392.

Idler, E. 2014. "Religion and Spirituality as Social Determinants of Health over the Life Course." In *142nd APHA Annual Meeting and Exposition* (November 15-November 19, 2014). APHA, 2014.

Inzlicht, M., I. McGregor, J. B. Hirsh, and K. Nash. 2009. "Neural Markers of Religious Conviction." *Psychological Science* 20: 385–392.

James, W. 1985. *The Varieties of Religious Experience.* Cambridge, MA: Harvard University Press.

Jung, C. G. 1933. *Modern Man in Search of a Soul.* New York: Harvest.

Jung, C. G. 1938. *Psychology and Religion.* New Haven, CT: Yale University Press.

Jung, C. G. 1964. *Man and His Symbols.* New York: Dell.

Jung, C. G. 1969a. *Collected Works of C.G. Jung, Volume 11: Psychology and Religion: West and East.* Princeton, NJ: Princeton University Press.

Jung, C. G. 1969b. *Collected Works of C.G. Jung, Volume 18: The Symbolic Life: Miscellaneous Writings.* Princeton, NJ: Princeton University Press.

Kabat-Zinn, J. 2003. "Mindfulness-Based Interventions in Context: Past, Present, and Future." *Clinical Psychology: Science and Practice* 10: 144–156.

Kapogiannis, D., A. K. Barney, M. Su, G. Zamboni, F. Krueger, and J. Grafman. 2009. "Cognitive and Neural Foundations of Religious Belief." *Proceedings of the National Academy of Science USA* 106: 4876–4881.

Kim, K. H., L. Linnan, M. K. Campbell, C. Brooks, H. G. Koenig, and C. Wiesen. 2008. "The WORD (wholeness, oneness, righteousness, deliverance): a Faith-Based Weight-Loss Program Utilizing a Community-Based Participatory Research Approach." *Health Education & Behavior* 35: 634–650.

Kincaid, H. 2004. "Contextualism, Explanation and the Social Sciences." *Philosophical Explorations* 7: 201–218.

King, P. E. 2008. "Spirituality as a Fertile Ground for Positive Youth Development." In R. M. Lerner, R. W. Roeser, and E. Phelps, eds. *Positive Youth Development & Spirituality*, pp. 55–73. Philadelphia: Templeton Foundation Press.

Kirkpatrick, L. A. 1999. "Toward an Evolutionary Psychology of Religion." *Journal of Personality* 67: 921–952.

Kleisiaris, C. F., C. Sfakianakis, and I. V. Papathanasiou. 2014. "Health Care Practices in Ancient Greece: The Hippocratic Ideal." *Journal of Medical Ethics and History of Medicine* 7(6). PMCID: PMC4263393.

Koenig, H. G. 1999. *The Healing Power of Faith: Science Explores Medicine's Last Great Frontier.* New York: Simon & Schuster.

Koenig, H. G. 2001. "Religion and Medicine II: Religion, Mental Health, and Related Behaviors." *International Journal of Psychiatry in Medicine* 31: 97–109.

Koenig, H. G. 2004. "Religion, Spirituality, and Medicine: Research Findings and Implications for Clinical Practice." *Southern Medical Journal* 97: 1194–1200.

Koenig, H. G. 2005. *Faith & Mental Health: Religious Resources for Healing.* Philadelphia: Templeton Foundation Press.

Koenig, H. G. 2008. "Religion and Mental Health: What Should Psychiatrists Do?" *Psychological Bulletin* 132: 201–203.

Koenig, H. G. 2012. "Religion, Spirituality, and Health: The Research and Clinical Implications." *ISRN Psychiatry*, 2012: 1–33. doi:10.5402/2012/278730

Koenig, H. G. 2013. *Spirituality in Patient Care: Why, How, When, and What.* Philadelphia: Templeton Foundation Press.

Koenig, H. G., D. King, and V. B. Carson. 2012. *Handbook of Religion and Health* (2nd ed.). New York: Oxford University Press.

Koenig, H. G., M. E. McCullough, and D. B. Larson. 2001. *The Handbook of Religion and Health.* New York: Oxford University Press.

Krägeloh, C. U., D. R. Billington, M. A. Henning, and P. P. Chai. 2014. "Spiritual Quality of Life and Spiritual Coping: Evidence for a Two-Factor Structure of the WHOQOL Spirituality, Religiousness, and Personal Beliefs Module." *Health and Quality of Life Outcomes* 13: 26–26.

Kraus, M. W., P. K. Piff, R. Mendoza-Denton, M. L. Rheinschmidt, and D. Keltner. 2012. "Social Class, Solipsism, and Contextualism: How the Rich Are Different from the Poor." *Psychological Review* 119: 546–572.

Kumar, V., A. Kumar, A. K. Ghosh, R. Samphel, R. Yadav, D. Yeung, D., and G. L. Darmstadt. 2015. "Enculturating Science: Community-Centric Design of Behavior Change Interactions for Accelerating Health Impact." *Seminars in Perinatology* 39: 393–415.

Lerner, R. M. 1978. "Nature, Nurture, and Dynamic Interactionism." *Human Development* 21: 1–20.

Lerner, R. M. 1992. "Dialectics, Developmental Contextualism, and the Further Enhancement of Theory about Puberty and Psychosocial Development." *Journal of Early Adolescence* 12: 366–388.

Lewin, K. 1951. *Field Theory in Social Science.* New York: Harper.

Li, E. C., C. Feifer, and M. Strohm. 2000. "A Pilot Study: Locus of Control and Spiritual Beliefs in Alcoholics Anonymous and SMART Recovery Members." *Addictive Behaviors* 25: 633–640.

Little, D. 1995. "Objectivity, Truth and Method: A Philosopher's Perspective on the Social Sciences." *Anthropology Newsletter* 36(8): 42–43.

Ludwig, D. S., and J. Kabat-Zinn. 2008. "Mindfulness in Medicine." *Journal of the American Medical Association* 300: 1350–1352.

Lun, V. M., and M. H. Bond. 2013. "Examining the Relation of Religion and Spirituality to Subjective Well-Being Across National Cultures." *Psychology of Religion and Spirituality* 5: 304.

Malinowski, B. 1954. *Magic, Science, and Religion.* New York: Doubleday.

Malle, B. F. 1999. "How People Explain Behavior: A New Theoretical Framework." *Personality and Social Psychology Review* 3: 23–48.

Malle, B. F. 2011. "Attribution Theories: How People Make Sense of Behavior." In D. Chadee, ed., *Theories in Social Psychology,* pp. 72–95. Hoboken, NJ: Wiley-Blackwell.

Malle, B. F., J. Knobe, M. O'Laughlin, G. E. Pearce, and S. E. Nelson. 2000. "Conceptual Structure and Social Functions of Behavior Explanations: Beyond Person–Situation Attributions." *Journal of Personality and Social Psychology* 79: 309–326.

Malterud, K. 2001. "Qualitative Research: Standards, Challenges, and Guidelines." *The Lancet* 358: 483–488.

Mariano, J. M., and W. Damon. 2008. "The Role of Spirituality and Religious Faith in Supporting Purpose in Adolescence." In R. M. Lerner, R. W. Roeser, and E. Phelps, eds., *Positive Youth Development & Spirituality,* pp. 210–230. Philadelphia: Templeton Foundation Press.

Mark, G. T., and A. C. Lyons. 2010. "Maori Healers' Views on Wellbeing: The Importance of Mind, Body, Spirit, Family and Land." *Social Science & Medicine* 70: 1756–1764.

Maslow, A. H. 1964. *Religions, Values, and Peak-Experiences* (vol. 35). Columbus, OH: Ohio State University Press.

Masters, K. S. 2008. "Mechanisms in the Relation Between Religion and Health with Emphasis on Cardiovascular Reactivity Stress." *Research in the Social Scientific Study of Religion* 19: 91–116.

McCullough, M. E., and B. L. B. Willoughby. 2009. "Religion, Self-Regulation, and Self-Control: Associations, Explanations, and Implications." *Psychological Bulletin* 135: 69–93.

McKinnon, A. M. 2002. "Sociological Definitions, Language Games, and the 'Essence' of Religion." *Method & Theory in the Study of Religion* 14: 61–83.

McMullin, N. 1989. "Buddhism and the State in Sixteenth-Century Japan." *Japanese Journal of Religious Studies* 16: 3–40.

Mead, M., ed. 1955. *Cultural Patterns and Technical Change.* New York: United Nations Educational, Scientific and Cultural Organization.

Merrill, R. M., J. A. Folsom, and S. S. Christopherson. 2005. "The Influence of Family Religiosity on Adolescent Substance Use According to Religious Preference." *Social Behavior and Personality: An International Journal* 33: 821–836.

Michalak, L., K. Trocki, and J. Bond. 2007. "Religion and Alcohol in the US National Alcohol Survey: How Important Is Religion for Abstention and Drinking?" *Drug and Alcohol Dependence* 87(2–3): 268–280.

Miller, W. R., and C. E. Thoresen. 2003. "Spirituality, Religion and Health. An Emerging Research Field." *American Psychologist* 58(1): 24–35.

Moberg, D. O. 2001. "The Reality and Centrality of Spirituality." In D. O. Moberg, ed., *Aging and Spirituality: Spiritual Dimensions of Aging Theory, Research, Practice, and Policy,* pp. 3–20. New York: Haworth Pastoral Press.

Moberg, D. O. 2002. "Assessing and Measuring Spirituality: Confronting Dilemmas of Universal and Particular Evaluative Criteria." *Journal of Adult Development* 9: 47–60.

Modell, S. M., T. Citrin, S. B. King, and S. L. Kardia. 2014. "The Role of Religious Values in Decisions about Genetics and the Public's Health." *Journal of Religion and Health* 53: 702–714.

Morgan, G., and L. Smircich. 1980. "The Case for Qualitative Research." *Academy of Management Review* 5: 491–500.

Murti, T. R. V. 1955. *The Central Philosophy of Buddhism: A Study of the Madhyamika System.* London: Routledge.

Nardo, D. 2001. *Egyptian Mythology.* Berkeley Heights, CA: Enslow.

Nebelkopf, E., and S. Wright. 2011. "Holistic System of Care: A Ten-Year Perspective." *Journal of Psychoactive Drugs* 43: 302–308.

Nelson, J. M. 2010. *Psychology, Religion, and Spirituality.* New York: Springer.

Nesdole, R., D. Voigts, R. Lepnurm, and R. Roberts. 2014. "Reconceptualizing Determinants of Health: Barriers to Improving the Health Status of First Nations Peoples." *Canadian Journal of Public Health* 105: 209–213.

Nord, W. A. 2010. *Does God Make a Difference? Taking Religion Seriously in Our Schools and Universities.* New York: Oxford University Press.

Norenzayan, A., S. Atran, J. Faulkner, and M. Schaller. 2006. "Memory and Mystery: The Cultural Selection of Minimally Counterintuitive Narratives." *Cognitive Science* 30: 531–553.

Norenzayan, A., and S. J. Heine. 2005. "Psychological Universals: What Are They and How Can We Know." *Psychological Bulletin* 131: 763–784.

Orfanos, C. 2007. "From Hippocrates to Modern Medicine." *Journal of the European Academy of Dermatology and Venereology* 21: 852–858.

Owe, E., V. L. Vignoles, M. Becker, R. Brown, P. B. Smith, S. W. Lee, . . . and P. Baguma. 2013. "Contextualism as an Important Facet of Individualism-Collectivism Personhood Beliefs Across 37 National Groups." *Journal of Cross-Cultural Psychology* 45: 24–45.

Paloutzian, R. F. 2016. *Invitation to the Psychology of Religion.* New York: Guilford Press.

Paloutzian, R. F., and C. L. Park. 2005. "Integrative Themes in the Current Science of the Psychology of Religion." In R. F. Paloutzian and C. L. Park, eds., *Handbook of the Psychology of Religion and Spirituality,* pp. 3–20. New York: Guilford Press.

Pargament, K. I., B. W. Smith, H. G. Koenig, and L. Perez. 1998. "Patterns of Positive and Negative Religious Coping with Major Life Stressors." *Journal for the Scientific Study of Religion* 37: 710–724.

Park, C. L. 2007. "Religiousness/Spirituality and Health: A Meaning Systems Perspective." *Journal of Behavioral Medicine* 30: 319–328.

Park, C. L., K. S. Masters, J. M. Salsman, A. Wachholtz, A. D. Clements, E. Salmoirago-Blotcher, K. Trevino, and D. M. Wischenka. 2016. "Advancing Our Understanding of Religion and Spirituality in the Context of Behavioral Medicine." *Journal of Behavioral Medicine* (2017): 1–13. doi:10.1007/s10865-016-9755-5

Pegis, A. C., ed. 1945. *Introduction to St. Thomas Aquinas: The Summa Theologica, The Summa Contra Gentiles.* New York: Modern Library.

Piedmont, R. L. 1999. "Does Spirituality Represent the Sixth Factor of Personality? Spiritual Transcendence and the Five-Factor Model." *Journal of Personality* 67: 985–1013.

Piedmont, R. L. 2014. "Looking Back and Finding Our Way Forward: An Editorial Call to Action." *Psychology of Religion and Spirituality* 6: 265–267.

Plante, T. G., and Sherman, A. C. (eds.). 2001. *Faith and Health: Psychological Perspectives.* New York: Guilford Press.

Puchalski, C. M. 2013. "Integrating Spirituality into Patient Care: An Essential Element of Person-Centered Care." *Polish Archives of Internal Medicine* 123: 491–497.

Rank, O. 1996. "Psychology and the Soul." *Journal of Religion and Health* 35: 193–201.

Ratner, C. 2007. "Contextualism versus Positivism in Cross-Cultural Psychology." In G. Zheng, K. Leung, and J. G. Ardair, eds., *Perspectives and Progress in Contemporary Cross-cultural Psychology,* pp. 35–48. Beijing: China Light Industry Press.

Reeves, R. R., A. R. Beazley, and C. E. Adams. 2011. "Religion and Spirituality: Can It Adversely Affect Mental Health Treatment?" *Journal of Psychosocial Nursing and Mental Health Services* 49(6): 6–7.

Reid, A. E., R. B. Cialdini, and L. S. Aiken. 2010. "Social Norms and Health Behavior." In K. E. Freedland, J. R. Jennings, M. M. Llabre, S. B. Manuck, and

E. J. Susman, eds., *Handbook of Behavioral Medicine: Methods and Applications*, pp. 263–274. New York: Springer.

Roeser, R. W., S. S. Issac, M. Abo-Zeno, A. Brittian, and S. C. Peck. 2008. "Self and Identity Processes and Positive Youth Development." In R. M. Lerner, R. W. Roeser, & E. Phelps, eds., *Positive Youth Development & Spirituality*, pp. 74–105. Philadelphia: Templeton Foundation Press.

Saroglou, V. 2013. "Religion, Spirituality, and Altruism." In K. I. Pargament, ed., *APA Handbook of Psychology, Religion and Spirituality*, pp. 439–457. Washington, DC: American Psychological Association.

Seeman, T. E., L. F. Dubin, and M. Seeman. 2003. "Religiosity/Spirituality and Health: A Critical Review of the Evidence for Biological Pathways." *American Psychologist* 58: 53–63.

Seitz, R. J., and H. F. Angel. 2011. "Processes of Believing—A Review and Conceptual Account." *Reviews in Neuroscience* 23(3): 303–309.

Seybold, K. S., and P. C. Hill. 2001. "The Role of Religion and Spirituality in Mental and Physical Health." *Current Directions in Psychological Science* 10: 21–24.

Shariff, A, F., and A. Norenzayan. 2007. "God Is Watching You: Priming God Concepts Increases Prosocial Behavior in an Anonymous Economic Game." *Psychological Science* 18: 803–809.

Shea, J. M., J. Poudrier, K. Chad, B. Jeffery, R. Thomas, and K. Burnouf. 2013. "In Their Own Words: First Nations Girls' Resilience as Reflected Through Their Understandings of Health." *Pimatisiwin* 11: 1–15.

Skinner, B. F. 1953. *Science and Human Behavior*. New York: Free Press.

Smith, H. 1991. *The World's Religions*. New York: HarperCollins.

Smith, H. 2001. *Why Religion Matters*. New York: Harper-Collins.

Smith, T. B., J. Bartz, and P. Scott Richards. 2007. "Outcomes of Religious and Spiritual Adaptations to Psychotherapy: A Meta-Analytic Review." *Psychotherapy Research* 17: 643–655.

Smith, T. W. 2001. "Religion and Spirituality in the Science and Practice of Health Psychology: Openness, Skepticism, and the Agnosticism of Methodology." In T. G. Plante and A. C. Sherman, eds., *Faith and Health: Psychological Perspectives*, pp. 355–380. New York: Guilford Press.

Spilka, B. 1993. "Spirituality: Problems and Direction in Operationalizing a Fuzzy Concept." Paper presented at the annual meeting of the American Psychology Association, Toronto, Ontario, August, 1993.

Spilka, B., P. Shaver, and L. A. Kirkpatrick. 1985. "A General Attribution Theory for the Psychology of Religion." *Journal for the Scientific Study of Religion* 24:1–20.

Staw, B. M. 2016. "Stumbling Toward a Social Psychology of Organizations: An Autobiographical Look at the Direction of Organizational Research." *Annual Review of Organizational Psychology and Organizational Behavior* 3: 1–19.

Sulmasy, D. P. 2002. "A Biopsychosocial-Spiritual Model of the Care of Patients at the End of Life." *The Gerontologist* 42, Special Issue III: 24–33.

Taylor, C. 2011. *Dilemmas and Connections.* Cambridge, MA: Harvard University Press.

Thomson, K. S. 2007. *Before Darwin: Reconciling God and Nature.* New Haven, CT: Yale University Press.

Tillich, P. 1957. *The Dynamics of Faith.* New York: Harper & Row.

Tyler, I. D., and J. E. Raynor, Jr. 2006. "Spirituality in the Natural Sciences and Nursing: An Interdisciplinary Perspective." *ABNF Journal* 17: 63–66.

United Nations General Assembly. 1948. Universal Declaration of Human Rights. Retrieved from http://www.un.org/en/universal-declaration-human-rights/

Van Cappellen, P., M. Toth-Gauthier, V. Saroglou, and B. L. Fredrickson. 2016. "Religion and Well-Being: The Mediating Role of Positive Emotions." *Journal of Happiness Studies* 17: 485–505.

Van Gordon, W., E. Shonin, and M. D. Griffiths. 2016. "Are Contemporary Mindfulness-Based Interventions Unethical?" *British Journal of General Practice* 66: 94–95.

VonDras, D. D., G. S. Pouliot, S. A. Malcore, and S. Iwahashi. 2008. "Effects of Culture and Age on the Perceived Exchange of Social Support Resources." *International Journal of Aging and Human Development* 67: 63–100.

Watts, A. W. 1951. *The Wisdom of Insecurity.* New York: Pantheon.

Weber, M. 1963. *The Sociology of Religion* (4th ed.). Boston: Beacon Press.

Whitbeck, L. B. 2006. "Some Guiding Assumptions and a Theoretical Model for Developing Culturally Specific Preventions with Native American People." *Journal of Community Psychology* 34: 183–192.

Wilson, H. J. 2000. "The Myth of Objectivity: Is Medicine Moving Towards a Social Constructivist Medical Paradigm?" *Family Practice* 17: 203–209.

Yalom, I. 2002. "Religion and Psychiatry." *American Journal of Psychotherapy* 56: 301–316.

Yapijakis, C. 2009. "Hippocrates of Kos, the Father of Clinical Medicine, and Asclepiades of Bithynia, the Father of Molecular Medicine." *In Vivo* 23: 507–514.

Yeaton, W. H., and L. Sechrest. 1981. "Critical Dimensions in the Choice and Maintenance of Successful Treatments: Strength, Integrity, and Effectiveness." *Journal of Consulting and Clinical Psychology* 49: 156–167.

Yijie, T. 1991. *Confucism, Buddhism, Daoism, Christianity, and Chinese Culture.* Washington, DC: Council for Research on Values and Philosophy.

Zinnbauer, B. J., K. I. Pargament, B. Cole, M. S. Rye, E. M. Butter, T. G. Belavich, . . . and J. L. Kadar. 1997. "Religion and Spirituality: Unfuzzying the Fuzzy." *Journal for the Scientific Study of Religion* 36: 549–564.

Chapter 2

Hinduism, Jainism, and Sikhism

Vibha Agnihotri and Vinamrata Agnihotri

Durkheim (1986) maintained that religion served not just the social order, but health functions as well. In this chapter we discuss key aspects of Hinduism, Jainism, and Sikhism, and their influences on physical health and psychological well-being. As we begin, it is noted that religion/spirituality is an important part of one's cultural milieu, and imparts a sense of meaning, significance, and control over life. A number of findings point toward a constructive relationship of religio-spiritual orientation and superior health. For example, research has indicated that people who have conventional spiritual traditions tend to live longer (e.g., Strawbridge, Cohen, Shema, and Kaplan 1997); this suggests that they may apply or rely on their beliefs when dealing with sickness, suffering, and tensions in life. Other research has indicated that those who are spiritual tend to develop a more encouraging attitude and an enhanced quality of life. For instance, patients with terminal cancer who find contentment in their devout spiritual beliefs report having less pain and being pleased and happier with their lives (Yates et al. 1981). In a related manner, it is noted that pain may be perceived differently within various religious orientations (Lee and Newberg 2005), and that spiritual activities such as prayer offer a way of coping with and finding relief from pain (Wachholtz, Pearce, and Koenig 2007). One study indicated that the holding of Hindu beliefs moderated the experience of pain, so that it is more accepted, tolerated, and viewed as part of life experience (Whitman 2007). Another investigation, involving individuals dying from HIV/AIDS, reported a positive correlation between patients' spiritual welfare and their appreciation of life and ability to cope with the suffering brought on by this disease (Mehr et al. 2014). Importantly, this research shows spirituality to be of great significance for the individual, and eminently worthy of clinical focus. Noting the important connection between spirituality and health, the 37th World Health Assembly, in 1998, adopted a historic resolution that recognized health as comprising four domains: physical, mental, social, and spiritual (Chirico 2016). This resolution established that health is not merely the absence of illness, but rather a state of full physical, mental, social, and spiritual well-being. In response, several religious and spiritually affiliated organizations established hospitals and health care services as a part of their activities. In India, the Satya Sai Institute of Higher Medical Sciences (Whitefield and Puttaparthy), the Amrita Institute of Medical Sciences (Cochin), and the Aravind Eye Care System (Madurai) are a few examples of hospitals where care provision is deeply rooted in spirituality.

OVERVIEW

In previous centuries, technological expansion has led to overall improvement in a variety of health practices. However, as we consider spirituality and health, we note that *healing* embraces not only traditional medical treatments, but alternative therapies as well. Ancient theory held that a sickness begins in the mind, and from places deeper in the soul, and is cured through the process of spiritual healing. In seeking spiritual healing, the person yields to the divine with the assistance of a healer who is the sole agent assisting the person seeking healing. The healer absorbs the flow of spiritual energy through a channel. This disturbs all aspects of life: mental, physical, emotional, and spiritual. Thus, in past as well as in current times, there has been great public curiosity about and desire to understand the relationships among spirituality, health, and illness, and the power of spiritual belief in healing. This concern, reflecting development of both personal and societal attendant beliefs, is reflected in investigations reporting that individuals who attended church expect to have less severe stages of illness (Derrickson 1996). Similarly, concern for how spirituality may influence health is discernible in research suggesting that faith convictions act to diminish the magnitude of stress reported, as well as the conviction that spiritual beliefs offer the individual the supremacy of control (Park 2005). Spiritual beliefs are also seen to aid in recovery from illness (as well as preventive practice). For example, research on Brahmins of North India indicated that spiritual persons heal relatively faster in contrast to nonspiritual people (Agnihotri

2014). Given this history and many studies, spirituality and health have become linked in a very profound way. Indeed, basic philosophies found within all the world's religions suggest a positive connection between spirituality and the physical and psychological welfare of the individual person.

It should also be noted that religion and spirituality play an important role in the lives of healthcare professionals as well. As medical students advance through their medical training, many tend to develop decreasing virtue, increasing sarcasm, and growing apathy toward the medical profession (Smith and Weaver 2006). Practicing medicine takes a toll on life. Thus, during their professional journey, some physicians may feel burnt out and disheartened, lack motivation, encounter mental disorder and physical illness, harbor suicidal thoughts, and turn to alcohol and drug abuse (Center et al. 2003). It has been recognized that physicians may use religion and spirituality as a health-promotion practice for their own well-being (Weiner, Swain, Wolf, and Gottlieb 2001). Indeed, research suggests that regular spiritual exercises may diminish physical, cognitive, and emotional burnout in medical and mental health practitioners (Holland and Neimeyer 2005). Consequently, healthcare professionals have come to recognize religion and spirituality not only as a central concern of their patients, but also as a key feature in their own renewal and healing processes (Pattison 2006).

India is one of the most religiously diverse countries of the world. Historically, between the seventh and fifth centuries BCE, the intellectual life of India was in commotion. It has been pointed out that this age was a turning point in the intellectual and spiritual advancement of the entire world. In India, this time period in the world's history is described by the Vedas. It was also a time when many other religions, such as Sikhism and Jainism, emerged from the Hindu religion. Although Sikh and Jain ideologies are very similar to those of Hinduism, each religion has its unique features. One distinction to promote cultural understanding is that all the major Indian languages use the word *dharma* in place of *religion*. However, dharma and religion are etymologically distinct. Dharma is closer to spirituality than to religion as an organized institution. Dharma derives from the Sanskrit root "*dhri*," meaning to uphold, support, or sustain. So, the primary connotation of the word dharma is what maintains existence: life, and growth, being and becoming. Brief descriptions of Hinduism, Jainism, and Sikhism, and their relations to various dimensions of health and well-being, are presented in this chapter.

HINDUISM

As described by King and Brockington (2005) and others (Lipner 2012; Partridge 2003), Hinduism is one of the oldest religions in the world. To gain perspective at the outset, Hinduism should be understood as something much more than just a religion: it is a way of life. As one of the earliest religions, the dates and authors of most of the Hindu sacred texts and scriptures are unknown. However, several historians and scholars describe Hinduism as the consequence of the religious development that occurred in India between 4000 and 2500 BCE and can be traced back to the Indus Valley civilization. Hinduism should be viewed as a fusion of various traditions. Traditionally, all Hindus respected the authority of the Vedas (the oldest sacred Hindu text) and the Brahmins (the priestly class). However, with changing times and traditions, some Hindus nowadays reject one or both of these authorities. Thus, Hinduism cannot be characterized as a homogeneous, organized system. A large population of Hindus are ardent devotees of the *Trimurti* (the three gods Brahma, Vishnu, and Shiva/Mahesh), whom they consider as their only true god. Brahma is the god of creation; Vishnu is considered the god of preservation; and Shiva, the third of the Trimurti, is the god of destruction. Because millions of gods and goddesses are believed to exist, many Hindus worship deities that have been passed down to them by their ancestry and tradition, whereas other Hindus look inward to the divine Self (Soul). Nonetheless, most Hindus recognize the existence of Brahman, the Unifying Principle and the Supreme Reality behind all that exists.

The Hindu system of medicine had its origin in the ancient religious texts of *Atharvaveda*. The Vedic system of healing has a rich methodology that can be utilized to interpret the occurrence of events, diseases, and psychological well-being in the present context, as well as their timing, quite accurately. Centuries before the World Health Organization acknowledged that health is not merely physical well-being or the absence of disease, Ayurveda had been dealing with the many aspects of subjective and spiritual well-being of the individual. The word *ayur* means life, and *veda* means science. Therefore, *Ayurveda* literally means the "science of life," and as a method involves the use of homeopathic remedies such as herbs, oils, massage, exercise, and purging (*see* Bhishagratna 1907, 1911, 1916; Dash and Junius 1997). Further, while giving Ayurvedic treatment to cure any particular disease, the practitioner also takes the person's well-being into consideration, and thus spiritual concerns and practices are interwoven into the various alternative-medicine treatments that may be used. It should also be noted that Ayurvedic treatments may be applied in the form of *Karmakand*, or spiritual rituals performed by the Brahmin. With further consideration of medicine and medical practice, the Ayurveda points out that the knowledge of life is closely linked to the science of astrology. In olden times every Ayurveda practitioner was supposed to be an astrologer as well. Indeed, the famous surgeon of ancient India, Sushruta, was said to consult the patient's horoscope before subjecting the individual to any major operation.

Ayurveda has eight main branches (*see* Bhishagratna 1907, 1911, 1916; Dash and Junius 1997):

- *Shalyachikitsh*, which includes instruction for surgical training, surgical procedures, and protocols for medical hygiene
- *Salakyam*, the study and treatment of diseases of the head, nose, and throat, and treatments such as massage, herbs, and oils
- *Kaaya-chikitsa*, the branch concerned with internal medicine and diseases of the body, and treatments such as herbal remedies, sweating, medicated enemas, nasal administration of oils, and others
- *Bhuta vidya*, the classification and treatment of spiritual and psychiatric disorders, and therapeutic interventions which include use of herbal remedies, ritual ceremonies, fumigations, and other means
- *Kaumarabhrtyam*, the study and treatment of the mother's health during neonatal and immediate post-birth stages of the child's development, and also the study of normative pediatric growth and pediatric illnesses and diseases and their treatments
- *Agadatantram*, the branch concerned with the toxicologic effects of plants and poisons that may be ingested, and various homeopathic remedies
- *Rasayanam*, the branch concerned with illness prevention and building of immunity through herbal medications, meditation, religious ceremonies, exercise, and use of oils and massage
- *Vajikaranam*, which involves the study of fertility/infertility and sexual dysfunction, educational literature such as the *Kama sutra*, herbal potions, aphrodisiacs, hypnotherapy, and other alternative-medicine interventions

Ayurveda techniques are holistic in orientation, and focused on promoting wellness and illness prevention. Research on the use of plant-based medications suggests that micronutrients contained in some herbal remedies may enhance anti-stress metabolic regulation and produce regeneration of neural tissues in the aging brain (Rhoda 2014; R. H. Singh, Narsimhamurthy, and Singh 2008). However, other research has indicated that ingestion of some herbal remedies may increase bodily levels of heavy metals and other neurotoxins (Saper et al. 2004; Suchday et al. 2014). Further, Ayurveda techniques such as massage and meditation may also be used as therapy for mental illness (Dube 1978; Juthani 2001; Mamtani and Cimino 2001; Nichter 1981); however, these have yet to undergo much double-blind experimental investigation, and a cautious approach is recommended in using meditation for patients with schizophrenic or bipolar disorder (Arias, Steinberg, Banga, and Trestman 2006).

The Hindu belief system also incorporates energy centers known as *chakras*. This is a system that explains interaction and relationships among mind, matter, and spirit (R. P. B. Singh 1993). As described by Singh (1993), the chakras serve to amass, absorb, and transfer physical, psychic, and spiritual energies within the individual, and beyond to the individual's surroundings. The chakras can be conceptualized as lotus blossoms or spinning wheels. They are believed to align and travel through the center of the body, connected by two crisscrossing *nadis* (channels) called the *Sushumna*. One nadi is called the *ingla* (left nadi represented by the moon), and the other nadi, *pingala* (right nadi represented by the sun). These nadis carry life force, or *prana*, throughout the body. Neither the chakras nor the nadis are visible; however, they are believed to transmit energy that envelops and interpenetrates the body and mind.

As Singh (1993) describes, the chakras orient from the base of the spine to the top of the head. The first chakra is *muladhara,* located in the genital area and represented by *kundalini,* or snake energy. This chakra is associated with the male reproductive system and male sexuality, and represents a grounding of the human body. The second chakra is *svadhisthana,* located in the stomach area. This chakra is believed to be associated with gut feelings and emotions such as anger, anxiety, animosity, and fear. It is believed that when psychic problems arise, these difficulties are manifested by this chakra in the form of ulcers, indigestion, and nausea. The third chakra is *manipuraka,* located in the area of the navel. It is associated with women's reproductive organs, and relationship activities (e.g., service to others); trauma in this chakra is suggested to manifest in low-self esteem and co-dependency. The fourth chakra is *anahata,* located near the heart. This chakra is identified as the seat of our love: giving and receiving love, loving and respecting self, and feelings of loss when we lose loved ones (animal or human). It is believed that repressing one's feelings for any reason may disrupt the energy of this chakra, and lead to hypertension and risk for heart attack. The fifth chakra is *vishuddha,* located in the neck area. This chakra is believed to be involved with self-assertion, and the quivering of the voice during stress or trauma. The sixth chakra is *agya,* located in the middle of the forehead. This chakra is believed to be one's "third eye," capable of extrasensory perceptions. The seventh chakra is *sahasrara,* located on the top of the head. This chakra is believed to gather higher consciousness energy from God/cosmos. If this chakra is disrupted, mental and emotional trauma may occur. The alternative medicine approaches of chakra-focused meditation, breath control, and yoga postures have been generally suggested to enhance and maintain health and wellness (Becker 2000; Edwards 2006; Raub 2002); however, there is report of increased risk for physical injury from prolonged participation in extreme yoga postures or exercise (Arias et al. 2006).

Along with the richness of the Ayurveda and chakra systems, the ceremonial rites and rituals of Hindus are infinite. Indeed, there are traditions and rituals for every action and event in one's life. From the time a person wakes up, right up to when he goes to sleep, he has certain rituals that he needs to perform. The rituals performed in a Hindu Brahmin house symbolize and celebrate the various stages of life. For example, a ceremony is performed, even before the birth of a child, for the expectant mother. The prayers recited and holy ceremonies performed by the officiating priest are offered for the good health of the mother and the unborn child. There are also other ceremonies that are seen as health promoting. For example, from birth onward Hindus are trained that it is good for their health to wake up before sunrise, as the sun is the source of energy. Thus, *Surya Darshan,* the ceremony of seeing and welcoming the morning sun, is believed to be good for health, and indeed sunlight is associated with the synthesis of vitamin D (Engelsen 2010). In general, and according to Brahmin teaching, it is believed that if a person is religious and follows the Hindu practices, it will lead to better mental health and greater adaptability to stress. Indeed, Hindu religious beliefs and practices have been found to be associated with lower levels of anxiety and depression, and higher levels of psychological well-being (e.g., Joshi, Kumari, and Jain 2008; Paikkatt, Singh, Singh, Jahan, and Ranjan 2015; Varambally and Gangadhar 2012).

It is thought that the religious life of Hindu persons decides their life satisfaction and happiness in many ways. Children learn from their parents that they should wash their feet when they come into the house after they have been playing outside, and before they say a prayer. Daily living entails regular bathing, cleaning of teeth, skin care, and eye washing. Many of these rituals, which are linked to religion, foster cleanliness and personal hygiene. Thus, there is strong belief among Hindus that hygiene is an important component of religious virtue. Many folk beliefs are also incorporated into family living. For example, as Dwivedi (2004) describes, children may be told right from childhood that while sleeping they should keep their feet toward the north, as that direction is considered to be the seat of *Kuber* (the Indian wealth god), and that they may attain blessing for more wealth by doing so. In the opposite orientation (feet to the south), a person is thought to march toward death and loss of wealth. It is also believed that the individual will also feel discomfort by sleeping in the opposite way (feet toward the south), because the earth's magnet will pull their energy away. Children are also instructed to pray in front of the deities before they study or take an examination. Thus, young people become indoctrinated in a way that links religious beliefs and practices with the scientific principle of causation. Other daily life practices include regularly sweeping and mopping the floor of the house, along with the daily bath and washing of one's feet (especially after entering the house from outside). These practices ensure that dust and germs are reduced within the house.

Fasting is also a prescribed spiritual and health-related activity. It is believed that during fasting, the toxins from the body are released, and that this allows the negativity of the mind to be released from the body and soul as well. Fasting is also believed to help the mind and willpower become strong. Karmic (deed) debts can be purified by fasting as well. In addition, it is believed that the *prana*—the vital force—usually engaged in digesting food can be employed in healing the body and flowing to the higher chakras of the body during fasting. Another type of fasting occurs when there is an eclipse of the sun. Hindus are prohibited from consuming any food at this time. The reason for this fast is that the sun is believed to be the source of energy and responsible for the metabolic activities of all living beings, including plants. Thus, when an eclipse occurs, one is cut off from its life-giving rays, and consequently metabolic activity declines. The sun is also believed to regulate the activities of gastric glands that secrete digestive juices; in the absence of sunlight, these juices become scarce and digestion suffers. This is the reason why one's digestion becomes upset in the rainy season and whenever the sky is cloudy and blocking the rays of the sun. Clearly, Hindu fasting is undertaken for many reasons, and although fasting is believed to offer spiritual as well as physical benefits (Rajendran 2010), it may also exacerbate risk for individuals with diabetes (Kalra et al. 2015).

JAINISM

As described by Jaini (1916) and others (Dundas 2002; King and Brockington 2005; Partridge 2003), Jainism is one of the oldest extant religions, thought to have originated perhaps as early as 3000 to 3500 BCE. The main purpose of the Jain way of life is to attain salvation. Jains believe that all actions we perform throughout our lives ultimately affect the purification of the soul. The three main pillars of Jainism are *ahimsa* (nonviolence), *auekautauada* (nonabsolutism), and *aparigraha* (nonpossessiveness). Jains adhere to fruitarianism, the practice of eating only that which will not kill the plant or animal from which it is taken.

The Jain belief system associates many religious activities with health. For example, Jains perform meditations known as *samayika* and *pratikrman*. These types of meditation involve remaining calm and gradually detaching oneself from all external objects, which alleviate stress and promotes the release of catecholamine and adrenal hormones. Jains' dietary practice embraces vegetarianism to the extent that devout followers may avoid ingesting animal-derived food products even when they are unwell. Their pattern of eating is based on the key principle of *ahimsa* (nonviolence). The strictest forms of the Jain diet also excludes underground plants/vegetables such as potato, onion, and garlic, as well as mandating avoidance of honey and multiseeded fruit like guava. Such foods are believed to have a quality of darkness or lethargy, and a putrid smell. Jains who are strict in their practices do not consume milk or milk products. According to the days specified in a lunar calendar, Jains fast twice or thrice and only consume grains. During these fasts, no fruits or green vegetables are allowed. Many Jains take meals only after sunrise and before sunset. The use of contraception is not favored in Jainism, and abortion is forbidden. Even when the mother's life is in danger, abortion should be avoided, and if one undergoes it in even an emergency situation, one must repent. Jainism does not, under any conditions, permit assisted suicide or euthanasia. A decision to withdraw or withhold life support may be permissible, but such action is usually taken only after seeking counsel from a spiritual leader.

SIKHISM

As described by Kalsi (2014), Cole and Sambhi (1995), and others (Harr, Kalsi, and Barr 2005; King and Brockington 2005; S. H. Singh 2009; S. J. Singh 2011; Teece 2004), the word *Sikh* means a disciple or a learner. Historically, Sikhism was a reform movement, aimed at abolishing Hinduism as a structure for living. Essential beliefs are described in the *Guru Granth Sahib*. This text expresses a rather logical and humanistically oriented faith tradition. From this faith perspective, God is known as *Ik Onkar*, or One Supreme Reality. Sikhism emphasizes the power of prayer and meditation. It also proposes three main principles for living: *Naam Japna* (remember and meditate on God); *Dharm Di Kirt Karna* (give to the needy); and *Wand Chhakna* (earn by honest means). Further, followers of Sikhism are expected to adhere to the four cardinal commandments of their holy book: no consumption of alcohol, tobacco, or any such intoxicating substance; no cutting of hair on the body, face, or scalp; no eating of sacrificial meat; no performance of any act of adultery.

Sikh patients consider illness and disease to be the will of God, and also that God is merciful and benign. However, one has to make an effort to get better, which permits and includes medical treatment. Sikhs mostly refrain from consuming tobacco, alcohol, intoxicants, and other illicit drugs. The taboos of the cardinal commandments are a powerful illness-prevention mechanism that serves to reduce risk of lung disease and addiction to drugs or alcohol (Bhopal 1986). Sikhs also engage in meditation as an integral part of their religious practice, and believe that their prayers and hymns are meant for providing healing and peace. This gives them the strength to accept God's will and the patience to endure all suffering with courage and faith (K. Singh 2008). Death is considered to be an opportunity for the reunion of soul with the Almighty. Sikhs also believe in reincarnation or the theory of *Karma* (good deeds). During times of sickness and disease, Sikhs pray to seek God's help; remember *Wahe Guru* (God's name) to obtain peace; plead for forgiveness; and recite or listen to *Gurbani*, the sacred hymns, which are God's words, voiced through the Sikh gurus and enshrined in the *Guru Granth Sahib* (the Holy Scripture). It is believed that prayer and the recitation of sacred scriptures provide physical and spiritual vigor and nourishment. Thus, use of prayer by the Sikhs, as a way of coping with the uncertainty of illness, is similar to that found in other religious groups (Koenig 2013). Blood transfusions are allowed, but in accord with faith beliefs, assisted suicide and euthanasia are not encouraged. Birth control is acceptable, but some individuals may choose not to use it, as it may be regarded as disrupting the natural cycle of life as mentioned in the *Guru Granth Sahib*. Again in accord with faith beliefs, abortion is not sanctioned except in cases of medical necessity. Organ transplantation, both donation and receipt, is allowed. Because death with dignity is respected, maintaining a terminally ill patient on artificial life supports is discouraged.

COMPARISONS

Whereas most Hindus believe in a god (or goddess), and believe that entity to be the creator, preserver, and destroyer of the universe, Jainism rejects any such god (or goddess). Jains consider the universe to be an everlasting phenomenon, one that can be neither created nor destroyed. It is a self-sustained, automated phenomenon that runs on the principle of cause and effect (karma and reincarnation). The Sikh belief system of service to humanity has transformed the manner in which religions are advocated and followed. Further, while Hindus and Sikhs accept Karma philosophy, Jains describe karma as debris that adulterates the soul. For each soul to attain liberation, it must rely on its own efforts (*Purusharth*) to cleanse off these karma particles. An example of this liberation is found in the life of Mahavira, who was born as a prince but renounced his royal life at the age of 30 and became an ascetic. For the next 12 years, he practiced meditation to such an extent that he got accustomed to all the hardships, and torment ceased to trouble him; people tortured him to the level of piercing his ears with nails and casting stones at him, but they could not disturb his meditation. In due course, Mahavira attained sapience at the age of 42. However, he was not able to obtain *moksha* (enlightenment), as he retained some karma remaining from his prior existence. Finally, at the age of 72, he vacated his body and all the remaining karma, thus achieving moksha and freedom from the cycle of life and death. The stage of enlightenment in Jainism is the final borderline of the cosmos, and here the soul remains perpetually idyllic and disconnected eternally. For the followers of Jainism, Mahavira and the other Tirthankars are simply role models, and not deities or providers of worldly or spiritual rewards. Jains must depend only on their own individual efforts to achieve moksha. Sikhs incorporate sayings by prophets from other religions whose preaching corresponds with their own faith beliefs.

CONCLUSION

Certainly all three belief systems—Hinduism, Jainism, and Sikhism—can be appreciated, respected, and loved for their three unique influences and contributions to the world. Hinduism presents the view of Brahman that bonds the whole universe in a single transcendental reality that is hidden behind the worldly phenomena we perceive. Jainism demonstrates the ideology of nonviolence. Sikhism stresses the recognition of equality among all people, and the value of service to all humanity.

It is important to recognize the similarities and differences between these religions. All three religions originated in the Indian subcontinent, though at different periods, with Sikhism being one of the youngest religions. To a large extent, they all give equal status to women. Sikhism and Jainism are largely liberal religions, acknowledging and giving respect to other religions as well; even atheists are allowed to take part in their religious activities. Hinduism represents polytheism (belief in several gods/deities), whereas Sikhism and Jainism preach monotheism. Sikhism and Jainism both prohibit any practice of idol worship, nor do they believe in superstitions, unlike Hinduism.

The Hindu concept of the oneness of the universe and the Jain concept of nonviolence are most coveted in present times to save the planet from ultimate ecological destruction. The two leading causes of ecological destruction are overexhaustion and contamination of natural resources in the form of burning fossil fuels (including by automobiles) and consuming meat. Both are thought to cause, or at the least contribute to, climate change that will endanger our planet's survival. Only the devotion to and respect for other species and the various elements of Mother Earth, such as air and water, that Indian tradition teaches can salvage the planet. Similarly, only the teaching of the different religions' mindfulness and meditation practices can lead us to the ultimate bliss.

REFERENCES

Agnihotri, V. 2014. "Spirituality, Religious Belief and Practices Associated with the Health and Medicine among North Indian Brahmins." *Voice of Intellectual Man* 4: 97–108.

Arias, A. J., K. Steinberg, A. Banga, and R. L. Trestman. 2006. "Systematic Review of the Efficacy of Meditation Techniques as Treatments for Medical Illness." *Journal of Alternative & Complementary Medicine* 12: 817–832.

Becker, I. 2000. "Uses of Yoga in Psychiatry and Medicine." *Complementary and Alternative Medicine and Psychiatry* 19: 107–145.

Bhishagratna, K. K. L. 1907. *An English Translation of the Sushruta Smahita in Three Volumes* (Vol. 1). Archived by the University of Toronto.

Bhishagratna, K. K. L. 1911. *An English Translation of the Sushruta Smahita in Three Volumes* (Vol. 2). Archived by the University of Toronto.

Bhishagratna, K. K. L. 1916. *An English Translation of the Sushruta Smahita in Three Volumes* (Vol. 3). Archived by the University of Toronto.

Bhopal, R. S. 1986. "Asians' Knowledge and Behaviour on Preventive Health Issues: Smoking, Alcohol, Heart Disease, Pregnancy, Rickets, Malaria Prophylaxis and Surma." *Journal of Public Health* 8: 315–321.

Center, C., M. Davis, T. Detre, D. E. Ford, W. Hansbrough, H. Hendin, . . . J. Lazlo. 2003. "Confronting Depression and Suicide in Physicians: A Consensus Statement." *Journal of the American Medical Association* 289: 3161–3166.

Chirico, F. 2016. "Spiritual Well-Being in the 21st Century: It's Time to Review the Current WHO's Health Definition?" *Journal of Health and Social Sciences* 1(1): 11–16.

Cole, W. H., and P. S. Sambhi. 1995. *The Sikhs: Their Religious Beliefs and Practices.* Sussex, UK: Sussex Academic Press.

Dash, B., and A. M. M. Junius. 1997. *Handbook of Ayurveda.* Delhi, India: Concept Publishing.

Derrickson, B. S. 1996. "The Spiritual Work of the Dying: A Framework and Case Studies". *Hospice Journal* 11(2): 11–30.

Dube, K. C. 1978. "Nosology and Therapy of Mental Illness of Ayurveda." *American Journal of Chinese Medicine* 6(3): 209–228.

Dundas, P. 2002. *The Jains* (2d ed.). New York: Routledge Press.

Durkheim, E. 1986. *An Introduction to Four Major Works.* Beverly Hills, CA: Sage.

Dwivedi, B. 2004. *Vaastu Inquisitiveness & Solutions.* New Delhi, India: Diamond Books.

Edwards, S. 2006. "Experiencing the Meaning of Breathing." *Indo-Pacific Journal of Phenomenology* 6: 1–13.

Engelsen, O. 2010. "The Relationship Between Ultraviolet Radiation Exposure and Vitamin D Status." *Nutrients* 2: 482–495.

Haar, K., S. S. Kalsi and A. M. Barr. 2005. *Sikhism.* Philadelphia, PA: Chelsea House.

Holland, J. M., and R. A. Neimeyer. 2005. "Reducing the Risk of Burnout in End of Life Care Setting: The Role of Daily Spiritual Experiences and Training." *Palliative & Support Care* 3: 173–181.

Jaini, J. L. 1916. *Outlines of Jainism.* Cambridge, England: Cambridge University Press.

Joshi, S., S. Kumari, and M. Jain. 2008. "Religious Belief and Its Relation to Psychological Well-Being." *Journal of the Indian Academy of Applied Psychology* 34: 345–354.

Juthani, N. V. 2001. "Psychiatric Treatment of Hindus." *International Review of Psychiatry* 13(2): 125–130.

Kalra, S., S. Bajaj, Y. Gupta, P. Agarwal, S. K. Singh, S. Julka, . . . and N. Agrawal. 2015. "Fasts, Feasts and Festivals in Diabetes-1: Glycemic Management During Hindu Fasts." *Indian Journal of Endocrinology and Metabolism* 19: 198–203.

Kalsi, A. S. 2014. *Sikhism Yesterday Today & Tomorrow.* Lucknow, India: Abhyudaya Prakashan.

King, A. S., and J. L. Brockington, 2005. *The Intimate Other: Love Divine in Indic Religions.* Delhi, India: Orient Blackswan.

Koenig, H. G. 2013. *Spirituality in Patient Care: Why, How, When, and What.* Philadelphia, PA: Templeton Foundation Press.

Lee, B. Y., and A. B. Newberg. 2005. "Religion and Health: A Review and Critical Analysis." *Zygon®* 40: 443–468.

Lipner, J. 2012. *Hindus: Their Religious Beliefs and Practices.* New York: Routledge Press.

Mamtani, R., and A. Cimino. 2001. "A Primer of Complementary and Alternative Medicine and Its Relevance in the Treatment of Mental Health Problems." *Psychiatric Quarterly* 73: 367–381.

Mehr, S. E., A. Pirastehmotlagh, T. A. Aliabad, Y. Ansari, A. Rozeyan, A. Derakhsh, and F. Mohamadi. 2014. "The Relationship between Variables of Spirituality, Attitude Toward the Disease and Suffering in AIDS Cases." *Advances in Environmental Biology*: 655–661.

Nichter, M. 1981. "Negotiation of the Illness Experience: Ayurvedic Therapy and the Psychosocial Dimension of Illness." *Culture, Medicine and Psychiatry* 5: 5–24.

Paikkatt, B., A. R. Singh, P. K. Singh, M. Jahan, and J. K. Ranjan. 2015. "Efficacy of Yoga Therapy for the Management of Psychopathology of Patients Having Chronic Schizophrenia." *Indian Journal of Psychiatry* 57: 355–360.

Park, C. L. 2005. "Religion and Meaning." In R. F. Paloutzian and C. L. Park, eds., *Handbook of the Psychology of Religion and Spirituality,* pp. 295–314. New York: Guilford Press.

Partridge C., ed. 2003. *Introduction to World Religions.* Minneapolis, MN: Fortress Press.

Pattison, M. 2006. "Finding Peace and Joy in the Practice of Medicine." *Health Progress* 87(3): 22–24.

Rajendran, N. S. 2010. "Science of Fasting: Aspects from Hinduism Perspective." In R. Singh and A. M. C. Muhamed, eds., *Fasting and Sustainable Health Conference 2010,* pp. 29–35. Healthy Life Cluster, University of Malaysia.

Raub, J. A. 2002. "Psychophysiologic Effects of Hatha Yoga on Musculoskeletal and Cardiopulmonary Function: A Literature Review." *Journal of Alternative & Complementary Medicine* 8: 797–812.

Rhoda, D. 2014. "Ayurvedic Psychology: Ancient Wisdom Meets Modern Science." *International Journal of Transpersonal Studies* 33: 158–171.

Saper, R. B., S. N. Kales, J. Paquin, M. J. Burns, D. M. Eisenberg, R. B. Davis, and R. S. Phillips. 2004. "Heavy Metal Content of Ayurvedic Herbal Medicine Products." *Journal of the American Medical Association* 292: 2868–2873.

Singh, K. 2008. "The Sikh Spiritual Model of Counseling." *Spirituality and Health* 9: 32–43.

Singh, R. H., K. Narsimhamurthy, and G. Singh. 2008. "Neuronutrient Impact of Ayurvedic Rasayana Therapy in Brain Aging." *Biogerontology* 9(6): 369–374.

Singh, R. P. B. 1993. "Cosmos, Theos, Anthropos: An Inner Vision of Sacred Ecology in Hinduism." *National Geographic Journal* 39: 113–130.

Singh, S. H. 2009. *Faith & Philosophy of Sikhism.* Delhi, India: Kalpaz Publications.

Singh, S. J. 2011. *Study of the Sikhism Part-I.* Amritsar, India: Dharam Parchar Committee, Shiromani Gurdwara Parbandhak.

Smith, J. K., and D. B. Weaver. 2006. "Capturing Medical Student Idealism." *Annals of Family Medicine* 4 (Suppl. 1): 32–37.

Strawbridge, W. J., R. D. Cohen, S. J. Shema, and G. A. Kaplan. 1997 "Frequent Attendance at Religious Services and Mortality Over 28 years." *American Journal of Public Health* 87: 957–961.

Suchday, S., N. P. Ramanayake, A. Benkhoukha, A. F. Santoro, C. Marquez, and G. Nakao. 2014. "Ayurveda: An Alternative in the United States." In R. A.R. Gurung, ed., *Multicultural Approaches to Health and Wellness in America, Volume 1*, pp. 151–170. Santa Barbara, CA: Praeger.

Teece, G. 2004. *Sikhism: Religion in Focus.* Mankato, MN: Black Rabbit Books.

Varambally, S., and B. N. Gangadhar. 2012. "Yoga: A Spiritual Practice with Therapeutic Value in Psychiatry." *Asian Journal of Psychiatry* 5: 186–189.

Wachholtz, A. B., M. J. Pearce, and H. Koenig. 2007. "Exploring the Relationship Between Spirituality, Coping, and Pain." *Journal of Behavioral Medicine* 30: 311–318.

Weiner, E. L., G. R. Swain, B. Wolf, and M. Gottlieb. 2001. "A Qualitative Study of Physicians' Own Wellness Promotion Practices." *Western Journal of Medicine* 174: 19–23.

Whitman, S. M. 2007. "Pain and Suffering as Viewed by the Hindu Religion." *Journal of Pain* 8: 607–613.

Yates, J. W., B. J. Chalmer, P. St. James, M. Folansbee, and F. P. McKegney. 1981. "Religion in Patients with Advanced Cancer." *Medical and Pediatric Oncology* 9: 121–128.

Chapter 3

The Middle Path to Health: The Relationship between Buddhist Practices and Beliefs, and Health Outcomes

Dana Dharmakaya Colgan, Nina J. Hidalgo, and Paul E. Priester

Writing a book chapter on the topic of the relationship between Buddhist practices and beliefs and health outcomes is a daunting and humbling task, for several reasons. First, the Buddhist religion has a divergent range of expression in the world. Summarizing one of the world's great religions that is practiced in such divergent ways in a short book chapter risks the possibility of displaying a shallow image of a complex phenomenon. The second challenge in writing this chapter is related to the essence of Buddhism. Buddhism is unique in that it does not offer an authoritarian perspective on faith practices. Buddhism in general is not dogmatic in the demands placed on practitioners. In fact, dogmatic adherence to a doctrine would be rather un-Buddhist. Throughout this chapter, you will read a discussion of the middle path. When faced with the choice of two extremes, the path of the Buddha is the middle path. Hence, being overly dogmatic in belief or practices related to Buddhism would not be following such a middle path.

A third challenge in creating this chapter is laying out truth claims of a religious tradition for empirical examination. This is a complicated matter. Many scientifically minded individuals are drawn to Buddhism, as they feel that it is a tradition that is most compatible with the Western, empirical tradition. This is especially the case for American practitioners of Buddhism. From a broader perspective, it can be highly problematic to empirically challenge the truth claims of a religious tradition using scientific methods. Perhaps we should follow the Buddha's example and take the middle path here as well. Thus, we will attempt to explore what the current scientific literature says about the relationship between Buddhist practices and beliefs and health outcomes. These findings should always be taken respectfully and simultaneously lightly. To be dogmatic and renounce research that contradicts Buddhist traditions is as extreme as stating that research showing a paradoxical result disconfirms the value of the Buddhist tradition. In this chapter, we hope to demonstrate a high level of intellectual honesty and allow the research to speak for itself, especially when the findings run counter to core Buddhist principles. One such example is the research suggesting that gossip can have a positive impact on psychological health. Notably, the fourth precept of Buddhism encourages individuals to avoid the practice of gossip. This body of research does not "disprove" the Buddha's teachings. Rather, it demonstrates what complicated and messy creatures we humans are. In reviewing the research, we will attempt to be comprehensive and explore the impact of Buddhist practices and beliefs in a wide array of contexts: psychological, vocational, physical, and social.

The chapter begins with a review of the relationship between Buddhism broadly conceived, with an emphasis on the practices of meditation and mindfulness, and health outcomes. The author of this section is Colgan. Hidalgo then explores possible negative health outcomes associated with meditation and mindfulness. We then explore the relationship between behavioral practices recommended by the five precepts of Buddhism and health outcomes. Specifically, Priester examines empirical work related to vegetarianism, sexual misconduct, dishonesty and gossip, and avoidance of intoxicants. Priester also explores the relationship of tea consumption to Buddhism and associated health outcomes. Finally, Hidalgo explores commonalities between the Buddhist tradition and other faith traditions.

An appropriate metaphor from Japanese Buddhism is the concept of a "hungry ghost." A *hungry ghost* refers to a situation in which you try to fulfill a deeply desired goal, but through a short-sighted, insufficient attempt. Thus, the outcome is not satisfying, but rather spurs and deepens the initial desire. The hope is that in the following chapter we will provide some level of satisfaction to your curiosity regarding the relationship between

Buddhist practices and beliefs and health outcomes, thereby in some way providing you with some level of meaningful satiation, rather than merely the temporary feeding of a hungry ghost.

HEALTH-ORIENTED WORLDVIEWS OF BUDDHISM, MEDITATION, AND MINDFULNESS

Buddhism originated in Northwest India some 2,500 years ago, with the enlightenment of Siddhartha Gautama, who became known as the Buddha. His teaching spread throughout Asia, and Buddhist civilizations were established in China, Tibet, Japan, and East Asia. Unlike most religions, Buddhism, in its most conservative form, is a tradition that denies the existence of a God or creators. Within this tradition, there is no primary cause that works as a determinant, or a single originating event that took place. All existence is believed to have originated from numerous causes: Each cause or determinant relates to others, while all are interdependent. This is known as Dependent Arising (*pratityasamutpada*; Bodhi 2005). Further, existence is understood in terms of integrated factors or a combination of various elements, known as the Five Aggregates: material form (*rupa*), feeling (*vedanā*), perception (*saññā*), volitional impulse (*saṅkhāra*), and consciousness (*viññāṇa*). A person's existence depends upon processes of interdependent and causal relationships among these five groups, and is void of a stable, separate "self" (*anatta*). The Buddhist perspective instead offers a vision of radical interidentification: a philosophy in which all living beings are identified with all other living begins (*anicca*; Paonil and Sringernyuang 2002).

The Buddhist concept of *kamma* (also *Karma* in Sanskrit) is the process of mental proliferation and its consequences. In essence, good deeds are thought to bring about good results, whereas bad deeds are thought to bring about bad results (Payutto 1993). In the Buddhist view of kamma, when there is kamma, there are immediate results. Even a brief thought of unmonumental importance is not void of consequence. The primary agent or prompting force in all human creations and destructions is intention; therefore, one's intention is the true essence of kamma (Paonil and Sringernyuang 2002).

Grounded within these foundational principles, the meanings of health and illness are quite disparate from the Western biomedical understanding of health. Under Buddhist principles, the health of body and mind are, in part, a result of previous good actions, starting from the previous moment, the previous year, or a previous life. The individual, therefore, is ultimately responsible for his or her health. However, although each individual has a duty to maintain health, the responsibility is understood within the contextual framework that neither the body nor the mind exists as a separate self. Health and wellness, as well as diseases and death, originate from multiple and related factors and are determined by the natural law and Dependent Arising (Paonil and Sringernyuang 2002).

According to Buddhist thought, the wisdom deficit or ignorance that arises from being attached to an inherently existing self is the underlying cause of all forms of suffering, including the entire spectrum of physical and psychological disorders. The ultimate goal, therefore, is an unwavering understanding of impermanence of self (Shonin, Van Gordon, and Griffiths 2014a).

As noted by Smith (1991), the conceptual framework the Buddha provided to lead individuals from suffering was the *Four Noble Truths*: (a) life is suffering (*dukkha*); (b) the origins of suffering are our selfish cravings and desires (*tanha*); (c) the cure for suffering is overcoming selfish craving; and (d) the path that leads to the end of suffering is the *Noble Eightfold Path*. The eight aspects of the path to liberation can be grouped into three essential elements of Buddhist practice: (1) the development of ethical discipline, integrity, and virtues (Right Speech, Right Action, Right Livelihood); (2) mental discipline (Right Effort, Right Mindfulness, Right Concentration); and (3) wisdom (Right View, Right Thought/Intention). The term "Right" can be interpreted as skillful, and signifies that each element of the path leads to reduced suffering for self or others. For example, Right Livelihood means earning one's living in a way that is benevolent and causes no harm to self or others. Right View, which includes Dependent Arising, acts as an ethical compass for the other seven interdependent factors (Bodhi 2011). While Right View provides the inspiration, behavioral ethical disciplines (*sīla*) lay the foundation.

The Buddhist practice of mindfulness is a central aid in the journey along the Noble Path, and has gained considerable attention in the scientific literature over the past two decades due to its positive effects on health and health behaviors. *Mindfulness* is often translated as "seeing with discernment," and is a form of mental training that enhances one's ability to nonjudgmentally attend to the present moment. The teachings of mindfulness offer a process-oriented view of experience as a series of interdependent, cognitive events arising and dissolving each moment as the sense organs encounter incoming environmental data, with which the mind then constructs a world of meaning to interpret and cognitively, emotionally, and behaviorally respond (Olendzki 2011). This in-depth mind development is purported to alleviate, and ultimately eliminate, suffering by fostering sustainable changes in one's cognitive and emotional states that, subsequently, lead to changes in more permanent and stable behavioral, psychological, and physical traits (Dhargyey 1974), such as freedom from misperceptions, rigid and problematic thinking patterns, and problematic behaviors that interfere with optimal mental and physical health.

Explicit instructions on how to develop mindfulness are found in the *Satipaṭṭhāna Sutta*, a highly revered discourse of the Buddha. Foremost of the processes to foster mindfulness is to develop a clear awareness of one's present internal or "personal" experiences, including thoughts, emotions, sensations, and behaviors, as well as attention to perception of elements in the surrounding environment. For this reason, some have defined mindfulness as "bare attention," or "pure" or "lucid" awareness (Dass and Goleman 1990). These terms suggest that mindfulness reveals what is occurring before or beyond ideas, judgments, or analyses. This can be contrasted with "automatic" cognitive and behavioral reactivity that occurs without conscious awareness. Present-moment awareness is often at the forefront of contemporary explanations of and training in mindfulness, and is indeed a necessary and foundational element of mindfulness; however, most (if not all) individuals' awareness is shaped by conditioning, and contains both valence (positive or negative) and evaluations. Therefore, awareness may be better understood as a precondition to, or elemental factor for, mindfulness, rather than its complete definition (Witkiewitz, Roos, Colgan, and Bowen 2017).

A second inherent process of mindfulness is attentional allocation, which involves sustained attention, monitoring, and attentional shifting (Garland, Froeliger, and Howard 2014). As an individual attempts to attend to a "personal" experiences (the breath, bodily sensations; *sustaining*), one is also acknowledging discursive thoughts and emotions that may arise (*monitoring*). The ability to notice getting "caught up" in thoughts or emotions, and subsequently returning to the object of attention, requires a purposeful and fluid shifting of attention (*attentional shifting*). As the mind wanders off into concerns about the future, ruminations about events that occurred in the past, or evaluations of the present moment, the mindfulness practitioner notices these processes and then kindly redirects attention back to the sensations and experiences occurring in the present moment.

A third, and perhaps most important, aspect of mindfulness is the cultivation of particular qualities of awareness. Attitudes that exemplify this quality include curiosity, kindness, nonreactivity, and equanimity. A kind, curious, and nonreactive awareness is cultivated so that one simply notices the object, or series of emerging objects, and the secondary evaluations and appraisals that occur. With continued practice, this nonreactive awareness eventually allows for the de-automatization of habitual reactions to the present-moment experience and the associated secondary appraisals, predictions, critiques, or judgments about what has taken or is taking place. This process can be understood as the further development and temporal extension of bare attention, thereby adding clarity and depth to the typically shorter periods, or momentary flashes, of time occupied by bare attention (Olendzki 2011).

Furthermore, the mindfulness practitioner meets all internal experiences that arise—positive, negative, or neutral—with equal interest and equanimity. This is in contrast to the typical human tendency to pursue and hold onto pleasure and to avoid and escape from discomfort. Instead, the mindful practitioner remains aware of what is happening internally, with an even and unbiased deportment, as if gazing upon the internal landscape without interference (Desbordes et al. 2014). It is purported that it is only when one can regard an experience, or object of attention, with a balanced objectivity that one is free from emotional agitation, and the understanding of the experience is potentially transformative (Olendzki 2011). This is reflective of the elements of awareness, allocation of attention, and a nonjudgmental or equanimous stance toward all experience. Grossman (2015) describes this coalescing of awareness and attention with a particular set of attitudes as an act of unbiased, open-hearted, and equanimous experience of perceptible events and processes as they unfold from moment to moment.

Right mindfulness is the seventh aspect of the Noble Path, situated adjacent to right effort and right concentration. Mindfulness or *sati* (*smṛti* in Sanskrit) is derived from the verb "to remember" or the act of "calling to mind" (Ṭhānissaro 2012). This early definition reflects the philosophy that mindfulness is not the equivalent of the function of memory, but instead an active, purposeful, and particular way of attending and remembering. Therefore, the historical understanding of mindfulness is not merely a passive and nonjudgmental attentiveness, or an awareness exclusive to the present moment, but an actively engaged and discerning awareness that is capable of remembering and knowing skillful, as well as unskillful, phenomena and behaviors of the past and the present, with the intended purpose of abandoning those that lead to suffering, distress, and ill health (Purser and Milillo 2015).

This watchful, nonreactive receptivity forms the foundation for *satipatthana*, an awareness that is usually translated as clear comprehension, a middle path that neither suppresses the content of the present moment nor habitually reacts. Through the development of clear comprehension, one first develops a rudimentary knowing of what is happening in the present moment. This awareness may subsequently lead to an ability to discern wholesome from unwholesome, skillful from unskillful, healthy from unhealthy, and thoughts and behaviors as being within the present moment. This formula suggests that mindfulness is informed and influenced by many factors, such as one's view of reality; the nature of one's thoughts, speech, and actions; the methods of earning one's living; and the effort put forth in avoiding unwholesome and unskillful states while developing those that are skillful and favorable to health (Witkiewitz et al. 2017).

Mindfulness meditation differs from concentration-based meditation practices, though historically the two practices are intimately interwoven (Analayo 2004). Concentration practices, also called focused practices, require restricting one's attention to a single object, such as the breath, a repeated word or phrase (mantra), a visualization, or a sensation. When the mind wanders during a concentration practice, attention is brought back to the object of attention with little or no investigation of the "distraction." A concentration practice calms and stabilizes the wandering and distracted mind, and historically has been considered a perquisite for advanced mindfulness practices.

Preliminary concentration practices have several advantages. First, while attempting to focus the restless and wandering mind, an individual may become more aware of the mind's tendency to judge simple sensation (Sayadaw 1994). In noticing the mind's frequent tendency to judge and evaluate, an individual can become progressively aware of the mind as an intermediary or secondary interpreter (Dreeben, Mamberg, and Salmon 2013). Second, the calm mental state that often results from these practices provides the foreground from which one is most easily able to recognize and perceptually discriminate thoughts and feelings about sensation from direct perception of sensation. The ability to distinguish between sensation and cognition opens the opportunity to remain longer with the pure sensory experience before attention is once again overtaken by language-based judging, evaluation, and comparing. Third, a concentration practice creates the mental state in which delight and rapture are most acutely experienced (Dhargyey 1974).

With a concentration practice that has stabilized and strengthened attentional processes, participants then proceed to the practice of mindfulness. This permits an expansion of awareness from a restricted, focused attention to an open, receptive, nonjudgmental awareness where there is observation of the constantly changing stream of internal and external stimuli as they arise and dissolve, moment by moment. With continued practice and development, this expanded, nonjudgmental, nonreactive awareness embraces all thoughts, emotions, physical sensations, memories, fantasies, perceptions, and urges with a sense of equanimity and balance. Therefore, mind wandering is simply another event to witness (Witkiewitz et al. 2017).

Mindfulness practice cultivates an awareness of one's personal experiences without attachment to or investment in what or how particular experiences occur. The advantage of this perspective is that the self is experienced as an arena in which the internal content of consciousness is not threatening (Hayes, Pistorello, and Levin 2012). With practice, individuals begin to experience thoughts and emotions as temporary states, rather than as identifying characteristics, providing a sense of steadiness. This sort of mindfulness has been referred to as the ground of mental function or choiceless awareness (Kabat-Zinn, Lipworth, and Burney 1985). Therefore, a concentration practice that develops the capacity to cultivate attention in a more direct and deliberate manner can help the mindfulness practitioner begin to discern and understand the nature of the mind. With time and practice, wisdom arises.

THE IMPACT OF MINDFULNESS ON HEALTH BEHAVIORS

Health behaviors play a significant role in the prevention, diagnosis, and treatment of the most frequent chronic health conditions: heart disease, stroke, respiratory disease, diabetes, and hypertension (Heron and Tejada-Vera 2009). Research suggests that more than 50% of mortality from the leading causes of death could be reduced if people ate a healthy diet, maintained a reasonable weight, exercised regularly, refrained from problematic drug and alcohol consumption, adhered to their medication plans, and performed therapeutic exercises for chronic pain (Van Dam, Li, Spiegelman, Franco, and Hu 2008). Therefore, doctors often prescribe behavioral changes for people who seek medical care. Behavioral change, however, even with the strongest of intentions, can be difficult. As noted earlier, developing a kind, nonreactive awareness of the present moment may lead to a discriminative ability to discern wholesome from unwholesome, skillful from unskillful, and healthy from unhealthy thoughts and behaviors. Therefore, mindful awareness may serve as a preventative cognitive mechanism that fosters a wellness orientation and directs positive health behaviors.

As we consider health behaviors, it is important to recognize that even when individuals realize that their current behaviors are not optimal for their health, and try to make concerted efforts to change their behavior, failure to maintain any lasting change in behavior is relatively common. One reason why failure to change behavior is so common is that experiential avoidance occurs, which impedes behavior change. Experiential avoidance (EA) is defined as the (a) the unwillingness to remain in contact with aversive private experience (including bodily sensations, emotions, thoughts, memories, and behavioral predispositions), and (b) action taken to alter the aversive experiences or the events that elicit them (Bond et al. 2011). The phenomenon of EA is often proposed to undergird, and thus be critical in the development and maintenance of, psychopathology and other problematic health behaviors (Hayes, Wilson, Gifford, Follette, and Strosahl 1996). For example, it has been suggested that substance abuse is a highly effective short-term strategy for manipulation of the present-moment experience, and that a subgroup of substance abusers are experiential avoiders (Hayes et al. 1996). Even if individuals did not start their patterns of abuse as a method of experiential avoidance, the continuation of the abuse behavior is intended to avoid the uncomfortable withdrawal states; thus, EA helps to maintain the pattern of abuse (Marlatt and Gordon 1985). Related research has demonstrated that the same neurobiological pathways implicated in drug abuse also regulate food consumption, suggesting that effective interventions targeting the neural areas involved in EA and sustaining substance-use disorders may also prove beneficial in treating obesity, weight-related diseases such as diabetes, and binge eating (Acosta, Manubay, and Levin 2008).

Therefore, cultivating a deliberate and focused awareness, coupled with acceptance and curiosity, offers a great resource to counteract the tendency toward experiential avoidance. Indeed, mindful awareness permits the alteration of one's relationship with thinking and style of interaction with internal content, creating a sense of expansion and space around what is being experienced or observed. In this way, an individual is able to become familiar with, and perhaps even friendly toward, the nature and habits of the mind, even when they are uncomfortable. The person is then empowered to respond to the present-moment experience, rather than to habitual, and often unconscious, response. In this way, mindful awareness can allow for and help develop a broader, more adaptive, and potentially more skillful behavioral repertoire, freeing the person from the habitual cognitive, emotional, and behavioral patterns that perpetuate suffering and disease, and providing a path toward greater health (Witkiewitz et al. 2017).

Evidence of positive effects of mindful awareness has been demonstrated in several areas related to health and wellness. For example, Mindfulness-Based Eating Awareness (MB-EAT) was developed as a treatment for binge eating disorder (Kristeller, Wolever, and Sheets 2014). A central focus of MB-EAT is to cultivate a kind and curious awareness of one's eating experience and one's behavior in relation to food. Specifically, individuals engage in a variety of mindful eating practices designed to enhance awareness of subtle internal hunger and satiety cues, to slow down and savor the food experience, and to recognize the tendency of mindless eating, in order to increase conscious food choices. Further, participants learn to become familiar with cognitive, emotional, and situational triggers and increase their willingness to experience all of their internal experiences as they are—pleasant and unpleasant—in order to change eating behaviors.

Mindfulness-Based Relapse Prevention (MBRP; Bowen et al. 2009) is an outpatient aftercare treatment approach for individuals with substance use disorders who have completed initial inpatient or intensive outpatient treatment. MBRP is designed to target three factors that play a key role in returning to problematic substance use following treatment: (1) lack of awareness of various internal (thoughts, physical sensations, emotions) and external (environmental factors) aspects of the present moment; (2) reactivity to aversive internal or external experiences, and perceived lack of ability to withstand aversion without reacting; and (3) lack of kindness and compassion toward oneself and one's experience, or a sense of shame and self-blame. To address these three factors, MBRP aims to promote mindfulness processes, self-compassion, and nonjudgment toward oneself and one's experience, thus helping the individual cultivate and bring awareness to his or her inner resources (e.g., stability, dignity, and equanimity in the face of potentially triggering phenomena).

The practice of mindfulness can take many forms, including formal and informal practices. Formal practices create opportunities to experience mindfulness at its deepest levels. Mindfulness meditations are considered "formal" when they are typically practiced by dedicating a period of time in one's day to engage in the practice. A related formal and relatively common practice is *mindful breathing*. During this practice, participants are guided to become aware of physical sensations—especially those associated with the process of breathing—and to observe them without the intention of altering them. Participants are asked to notice in an accepting, nonjudgmental manner when their minds wander to something other than the breath, and to gently return focus to the sensations of breathing. Simply by observing the breath, the breath rate tends to slow. Slow and steady breathing has been shown to strengthen the vagal tone, affording a balanced and healthy nervous system and greater resilience to stress (Porges 1992). Proper breathing also enhances the immune system, memory, and concentration and reduces cardiovascular risk (Friedman 2002; Park and Park 2012; Rama, Ballentine, and Hymes 1998; Van Diest et al. 2014).

Mindfulness of breathing in daily life also is encouraged, as it promotes the generalization of self-awareness of the constantly fluctuating internal states experienced in ordinary activities. This increased self-awareness develops insight into and familiarity with the nature of the mind, and subsequently has the potential to connect individuals with a wider and broader perspective. Further, enhanced awareness of the breath is associated with decreased physiological arousal, stress reactivity, and emotion and reduced habitual, automatic, and maladaptive behaviors (Gard, Noggle, Park, Vago, and Wilson 2014).

Walking meditation is another formal practice frequently taught and practiced. During a walking meditation, the gaze is generally soft and straight ahead. One option for the practice is to have approximately 80% of the attention directed inward, while the remaining 20% is directed outward toward the external environment. Attention is directed to the sensations of movements, shifting of weight and balance, and sensations in the feet and legs associated with walking. As in other meditation exercises, participants are encouraged to notice when their minds wander off and to gently bring their attention back to the rhythm and physical sensations of walking. Walking meditation can similarly be incorporated into daily life, such as while running errands or walking between the car and the workplace. Recent research has shown that a mindful Buddhist walking meditation was more effective in reducing depressive symptoms, improving functional fitness, vascular reactivity, and overall improvements than a traditional walking program without a mindfulness component (Prakhinkit, Suppapitiporn, Tanaka, and Suksom 2014).

Mindful movement or mindful stretching is another formal mindfulness practice. Mindful movement often involves engaging in gentle and slow stretches or postures while focusing one's awareness on the bodily sensations that arise from moment to moment. In addition, while stretching or holding postures, the participant practices noticing any thoughts and emotions that arise with an attitude of openness and curiosity. A growing body of evidence supports the hypothesis that mindful movement practice, when compared to traditional exercise routines, benefits physical and mental health via downregulation of the hypothalamic–pituitary–adrenal axis and the sympathetic nervous system. For example, in a recent literature review comparing the effects of yoga and traditional exercise activities in both healthy and diseased populations, yoga was suggested to be as effective or more effective than traditional exercise at improving a variety of health-related symptoms associated with diabetes, multiple sclerosis, menopause, kidney disease, schizophrenia, and depression (Ross, Friedmann, Bevans, and Thomas 2013).

The term *informal practices* refers to the engagement of mindful awareness during daily activities, and supplements the meditative awareness cultivated in formal practices. Participants are encouraged to apply mindful awareness to routine activities, such as cleaning the house, washing the dishes, eating, driving, and shopping. Increased awareness of daily experiences is believed to lead to increased self-awareness and enhanced ability to make real-time, skillful decisions during difficult and problematic situations as they arise. Furthermore, applying mindfulness to daily living can increase the frequency and enjoyment of pleasant moments (Witkiewitz et al. 2017).

While the practice of mindfulness allows for a broader, and potentially more skillful, behavioral repertoire, Buddhism also aims to develop specific psychological qualities. Of specific interest is the development of the four immeasurable qualities (*Brahmavihara*) of loving-kindness (*metta*), compassion (*karuna*), empathic joy (*mudita*), and equanimity (*upe-kkha*). Loving-kindness is defined as the wish for all sentient beings to have happiness and its causes. Compassion is defined as the wish for all sentient beings to be free from suffering and its causes. Empathic joy consists of celebrating and finding joy in the happiness and success of others. Equanimity has been defined as an even-minded mental state that cannot be swayed by biases or preferences (Desbordes et al. 2014). These four deeply interrelated immeasurable attitudes are often generated and then directed toward all other sentient beings. Development of the Four Immeasurables is thought to be necessary to foster the wisdom of interdependence; in turn, the wisdom of interdependence facilitates the development of compassion and loving-kindness for others (Davidson, Harrington, and Rosch 2003). Buddhist training facilitates the development of nonreferential, or unbiased, compassion, or what is termed a universal compassion for all sentient beings (Halifax 2012).

Alternatively, from the perspective of Western science, there has been a focus on compassion for self, often called *referential compassion*. Self-compassion involves being touched by one's own suffering, generating the desire to alleviate one's suffering, and treating oneself with understanding and concern. It is also considered a common outcome, as well as a mechanism, of mindfulness. Self-compassion may assist one to nonjudgmentally witness the unfolding of a distressing experience, in order to embrace the self and the associated distressing experiences, with balance, equanimity, and kindness (Neff 2003). Among clinical and nonclinical populations, greater self-compassion has consistently been found to predict lower levels of anxiety and depression, more so than mindfulness (Van Dam, Sheppard, Forsyth, and Earleywine 2011). Self-compassion has also been shown to decrease cortisol levels and increase heart-rate variability, both associated with the ability to self-soothe when stressed (Rockliff, Gilbert, McEwan, Lightman, and Glover 2008). Greater self-compassion is also linked with less rumination, perfectionism, and fear of failure (Neff, Hsieh, and Dejitterat 2005). Furthermore, self-compassion has been found to be correlated with positive psychological strengths such as happiness, optimism, wisdom, curiosity and exploration, personal initiative, and emotional intelligence (Hollis-Walker and Colosimo 2011; Neff, Kirkpatrick, and Rude 2007). Relatedly, self-compassion is inversely associated with burnout among healthcare providers, and positively associated with resilience among medical residents (Olson, Kemper, and Mahan 2015). Researchers have also found that priming self-compassion enhances interpersonal functioning. For example, self-compassionate individuals have been described as being more emotionally connected, accepting, and autonomy-supporting while being less detached, controlling, and verbally or physically aggressive than those lacking self-compassion (Neff and Pommier 2013). Similarly, individuals with greater self-compassion were found to provide more social support and encouraged interpersonal trust when compared to those lacking in self-compassion (Crocker and Canevello 2008).

As a result of increased interest in the effects of mindfulness training on health and well-being, there is now a growing body of robust evidence from randomized clinical trials (RCTs) that demonstrates the effectiveness of mindfulness-based interventions (MBIs) in improving a wide range of physical and psychological health outcomes in comparison to control conditions. Many current MBIs are based on Mindfulness-Based Stress Reduction (MBSR; Kabat-Zinn, Lipworth, and Burney 1985), a secularized intervention approach developed to treat patients with chronic pain. MBSR is theoretically grounded in secularized Buddhist meditation practices, mind-body medicine, and the transactional model of stress, which suggests that people can be taught to manage stress by adjusting their cognitive perspective and increasing their coping skills. The primary aims of MBSR are to enhance attentional control and receptive awareness by focusing on internal (bodily sensations, breath, thoughts, emotions) and external (sights, sounds) stimuli in the present moment. With this enhanced attentional allocation and awareness, it is postulated that one may skillfully, rather than habitually or reactively, respond to the present-moment experience. This process allows for a larger, and potentially more skillful, behavioral repertoire in the presence of stress and adversity. As one of the first Western, secularized MBIs to be developed, MBSR has provided a foundation for the development of numerous other MBIs.

As a result, there is strong scientific support for the beneficial effects of MBIs on numerous medical conditions, including Type 2 diabetes (Rosenzweig et al. 2007), fibromyalgia (Grossman, Teifenthaler-Gilmer, Raysz, and Kesper 2007), rheumatoid arthritis (Pradhan et al. 2007), and attention-deficit hyperactivity disorder (Mitchell, Zylowska, and Kollins 2015). Recent reviews have also summarized the efficacy of MBIs for persons with cancer (Shennan, Payne, and Fenlon 2011), chronic pain, and chronic medical conditions (Bohlmeijer, Prenger, Taal, and Cuijpers 2010). Mindfulness training has further been shown to enhance immune response (Davidson, Kabat-Zinn, et al. 2003), decrease inflammatory responses (Rosenkranz et al. 2013), and accelerate skin healing in psoriasis (Kabat-Zinn et al. 1998). Clinical efficacy and durability have been indicated for eating disorders (Wanden-Berghe, Sanz-Valero, and Wanden-Berghe 2010) and insomnia (Ong and Sholtes 2010), as well as substance use disorders (Bowen et al. 2009). Further, recent meta-analyses estimated small- to medium-sized treatment effects for the impact of mindfulness training on symptoms of stress, anxiety, depression (Hoffman, Sawyer, Witt, and Oh 2010), and psychosis (Khoury, Sharma, Rush, and Fournier 2015). Additionally, MBIs have been shown to inhibit unhealthy adaptations or coping responses to chronic stress, such as smoking, decreased exercise, and poor sleep (Gross et al. 2011). Trials of MBIs with health providers and community samples demonstrate significant improvements in stress management and enhanced well-being (Irving, Dobkin, and Park 2009). Finally, MBIs have recently been adapted for first responders, such as police officers and physicians, with open trials evincing promising results (Christopher et al. 2015; Schroeder, Stephens, Colgan, Hunsinger, Rubin, and Christopher 2016).

The foremost intention of Buddhism is to promote well-being and prevent and alleviate suffering for all beings. The Buddha's comprehensive and penetrating teachings, which propose that behavioral, cognitive, affective, and biological experiences can be influenced through the practice of mental training, has forever changed the landscape of Western medicine. The contribution of the Buddhist tradition has been an exceptional influence in Western science—and this cultural phenomenon is likely still in its infancy.

POTENTIAL NEGATIVE OUTCOMES RELATED TO MINDFULNESS AND MEDITATION PRACTICE

As a recent meta-analysis demonstrates, there is little doubt that mindfulness mediation programs can effectively reduce negative or unpleasant psychological experiences (e.g., anxiety, depression, chronic pain; Goyal et al. 2014). This literature review demonstrated there was no empirical evidence of adverse health effects from participating in mindfulness meditation programs, although the authors noted that surprisingly few studies have examined and reported on harms (Goyal et al. 2014). Still, there remains a possibility that problematic health outcomes can result from MBIs as well as informal mindfulness meditation practice. Among some mindfulness scholars and researchers, there is concern regarding the absence of explicitly taught ethics (i.e., the Five Precepts) in secular MBIs because that lack could lead to the development of "wrong mindfulness," that is, mindfulness used for harmful purposes or leading to adverse effects (Monteiro, Musten, and Compson 2015). Recent qualitative findings indicate that MBI participants respond more favorably to therapeutic mindfulness interventions when they feel the mindfulness instructor is able to impart an authentically embodied transmission of the mindfulness teachings (Shonin, Van Gordon, and Griffiths 2014a). This suggests that at the very least, the level of perceived instructor competency and experience can affect participant response. Thus, it should be recognized that some MBI instructors may lack the necessary contextual (i.e., ethical) grounding in mindfulness meditation, which may contribute to a transmission of "wrong mindfulness" to the participants.

Despite these concerns, however, there is a dearth of empirical studies explicitly investigating nonsalutory effects of MBI participation. While the current review of the research literature may not yet be fully attuned to potentially harmful effects of mindfulness meditation, detailed accounts exist in the classical Buddhist meditation literature of how mindfulness and mindfulness meditation practice may have detrimental impacts on psychosocial functioning (Shonin, Van Gordon, and Griffiths 2014b). For example, as noted by Shonin et al. (2014b), the Buddhist literature provides descriptions of how "wrong mindfulness" can lead to deleterious health outcomes. These include social disinterest, nihilistic or defeatist attitudes, overextending oneself to engage in compassionate activities, and dysphoric mood states induced by incorrect breathing techniques. Additionally, there are also accounts of developing spiritual addiction, characterized by a dependency on the experience of "meditative bliss." This addiction may also develop such that the meditation practice becomes addictive and serves to increase attachment to ego and narcissistic behavior (Cutler and Newland 2015).

The scant reports of meditation-related adverse health outcomes in the empirical literature are limited to Transcendental Meditation (TM), Qigong, and nonspecific relaxation-based meditation. The documented adverse effects found related to practicing TM and Qigong include panic attacks, antisocial behavior, impaired reality testing, dissociation, musculoskeletal pain, uncomfortable kinesthetic sensations, suicidal feelings, exhaustion, and psychosocial distress related to addiction to meditation (Perez-De-Albeniz and Holmes 2000). In regard to nonspecific meditation, several distinct case studies have described unrelated instances in which participants experienced psychotic episodes precipitated by meditation that incorporated mindfulness components (Sethi and Bhargava 2003). Although different meditative approaches may reflect fundamentally different theoretical orientations, there are some shared attributes, such as attention to introspection, breath awareness, and parasympathetic activation. In meditative interventions that are not explicitly mindfulness-based, it is typical for such interventions to integrate common techniques, such as breath awareness, that are also present in MBIs (Shonin et al. 2014b).

Mindfulness meditation programs and MBIs generally aim to improve health and well-being by reducing unpleasant or negative psychological experiences and increasing the positive dimensions of health. The existing literature provides support for the effectiveness of MBIs in reducing negative experiences; however, a large-scale meta-analysis did not show any effects on positive affect or well-being from any meditation program. The authors concluded that there were no indications of increases in positive mood as a result of participating in meditation programs (Goyal et al. 2014).

A critical component of mindfulness meditation involves engendering *detachment*, that is, a dispassionate and nonevaluative stance toward internal and external experiences. The outcome is a general reduction in the intensity of emotional arousal, regardless of its positive or negative valence. In a Western cultural context, however, a healthful response to unpleasant or negative internal or external stimuli is not necessarily always flat or minimal affect (David 2014). When individuals encounter negative stimuli, such as social rejection, work failure, or chronic pain, unpleasant emotional experiences (e.g., sadness, concern, remorse) can elicit the motivation needed to develop adaptive coping or problem-solving approaches. David (2014) posits that indiscriminate practice of mindfulness meditation may unintentionally create an unhealthy detachment from the very feelings that make us human.

Although traditional Buddhist texts delineate the potentially harmful effects of practicing "wrong mindfulness," it should be noted there is little empirical research to date exploring these harms. Most existing research literature has focused on other types of meditation practices, including TM and Qigong, as well as unspecified meditation. In general, these studies have yielded results indicating that harmful effects can arise from engaging in meditation practices. Thus, although more research is needed to better understand potentially harmful effects of participation in MBIs as well as informal mindfulness meditation practices, there is very good reason to believe that mindfulness meditation, if used wisely by a facilitator who has proper contextual grounding, and special regard for the individual and the specific problem being treated, may provide some level of beneficial health outcome.

HEALTH OUTCOMES RELATED TO BEHAVIORAL PRACTICES SUGGESTED OR PROSCRIBED BY THE FIVE PRECEPTS

The Five Precepts are the basic code of ethics for Buddhists. They include: (1) avoid harming living organisms; (2) do not take what is not given; (3) avoid sexual misconduct; (4) avoid false speech; and (5) avoid the use of intoxicants (Thich Nat Hanh 2007). The following section of this chapter explores the relationship between these behaviors and associated health outcomes. However, due to an insufficiently developed research literature, we do not explore the second precept.

The First Precept: Avoid the Harming of Living Things

Many Buddhists respect this precept through the practice of vegetarianism. It is ironic that the best current thinking on the evolution of humans was only possible when humans began eating flesh. Domínguez-Rodrigo et al. (2012), based on archaeological research, asserts that it was the protein-, nutrient-, and fat-rich diet of consuming animal flesh that led to the expansion of the brain and the rise of humans as we now know them.

There is an extensive body of research examining the impact of vegetarianism on health outcomes. Although there are some contradictory findings, in general the conclusion is that those with a diet that relies heavily on plant sources had better health outcomes than meat eaters. Specifically, vegetarians were 12% less likely to die from all causes when compared to meat eaters (Orlich, Singh, and Sabate 2013). This exhaustive study, which tracked the dietary patterns of 73,000 Seventh-day Adventists, also found that there were lower death rates associated with cardiovascular disease, diabetes, and renal disorders. There were no differential death rates associated with cancer when comparing vegetarians and meat eaters. Another study established that vegetarians had decreased mortality when compared to meat eaters, but only when examining cardiovascular disease (Key et al. 1999). This study suggested that for all other causes of mortality, there were no differences between vegetarians and meat eaters. Thus, it seems safe to conclude that there are potential positive health outcomes associated with the vegetarian diet.

Thich Nat Hanh (2007) makes an excellent point that it is impossible to absolutely follow this precept. He points out that in order to cook a carrot, I must pull the carrot out of the ground, thereby killing a living organism. Furthermore, I must boil water. In boiling the water, I am killing the bacteria that live in the water. Thus, it is impossible to fully commit to this precept. Once again, the Buddha calls his followers to the middle path in this precept.

The Third Precept: Avoid Sexual Misconduct

There is considerable controversy within the different Buddhist traditions as how to interpret this precept. Some traditions view adherence to this precept as requiring Buddhist clergy to abstain from all sexual activities. Other traditions expand it beyond the sexual realm to include overly developed attachments to objects such as chocolate. In Western Buddhism, the focus is on a moral expression of sexual activity for lay Buddhists. Expressing one's sexuality within a moral framework may include behaviors such as monogamy, and the avoidance of the use of force or pain in sexual expression (as this would run counter to the first precept).

It is self-evident that limiting an individual's sexual activity to the boundaries of a monogamous relationship will result in lower rates of sexually transmitted infections. Even within a monogamous relationship, there appear to be differential effects of sexual activity on psychological and physiological health outcomes. One fascinating study (Brody 2010) found that various sexual activities produce different effects on health outcomes. For example and specifically, penile-vaginal sexual intercourse without a condom was found to be associated with a divergent range of positive psychological and physiological health outcomes. This study also found that other sexual practices, such as anal intercourse or masturbation, were associated with negative psychological and physiological health outcomes.

There is evidence to suggest, however, that the middle path regarding sexual activity may not be associated with one positive health outcome. For example, in a comprehensive Australian study, researchers discovered that 5–7 ejaculations per week significantly reduced the risk of prostate cancer in men (Giles et al. 2003). Although sexual appetites may vary, it seems safe to speculate that this frequency of ejaculation may not fall within the recommendations of moderation suggested by Buddhist practices. It is also interesting to note that, in this line of research, the manner in which a man reaches ejaculation does not matter (i.e., masturbation was just as effective as intercourse in achieving the orgasm). As stated, this is a difficult area to explore, as each Buddhist must decide for himself or herself what a healthy sexual life looks like.

The Fourth Precept: Avoid False Speech

The fourth precept is typically understood as involving two components: being honest and avoiding gossip. There is a surprisingly small amount of research related to the relationship between honesty and health outcomes. Nevertheless, there is some evidence suggesting that being honest has a positive impact on overall health and physical wellness, lowers levels of stress, may decrease the rate of cellular aging, serves to increase longevity, and increases overall psychological health (ten Brinke, Lee, and Carney 2015). In contrast, dishonesty has been found to be associated with elevated heart rate, increase in blood pressure, elevated levels of cortisol, and vasoconstriction (ten Brinke et al. 2015). Thus, we seem to find unequivocal support for a positive relationship between honesty and health outcomes.

The picture is a little different when we turn our attention to the second aspect of this precept, gossip. *Gossip* is defined as communicating negative information about an individual to a third party, in the absence of the person who is the target of the gossip. Research has discovered negative outcomes related to this behavior, including an increase in self-criticism of the gossiper (Cole 2013), and an increase in cynicism toward the work environment (Kuo et al. 2015). However, there are several paradoxically positive health outcomes associated with the practice of gossip. For example,

Feinberg, Willer, and Schultz (2014) suggest that workplace gossip can decrease egotistical behavior on the part of the gossip target. In this way, gossip may serve to reform hostile employees, thwart the exploitation of vulnerable co-workers, and eventually lead to a higher degree of cooperation among group members. In another study, Feinberg et al. (2012) found that gossip served the function of maintaining social order. A concrete health outcome from this study was the observation that when a participant saw a third person behave inappropriately, the participant's heart rate increased, and if the participant then gossiped about this poor behavior, the heartbeat returned to normal. In this way, gossip is suggested to be a form of release from the hostility felt toward the person behaving poorly. These authors called this "prosocial gossip," and suggested that this serves to warn innocent third parties of the possibility of danger from the target of the gossip; in this way, social order is maintained. Gossip here is seen as potentially altruistic. In a creative, qualitative study on the immigration experience for Taiwanese in Canada, Lu (2015) also asserts that gossip can serve a valuable and positive function of buffering the stress of the immigration experience. Specifically, Lu (2015) suggests that gossip eases the process of cultural integration, and reduces impermeable ethnic boundaries for the newly arrived immigrant.

The Fifth Precept: Avoid Intoxicants

This precept serves two goals. First, it reminds that the use of intoxicants may actively interfere with mindfulness. Second, it recognizes that use of intoxicants may increase the likelihood that one will break the other precepts. In this way, intoxication becomes a gateway to the violation of the other precepts. The state of addiction is a powerful metaphor for unhealthy attachment to the physical world. Drug addiction is a universally common phenomenon that results in a wide range of negative health outcomes (e.g., increased risk for lung disease, cardiovascular disease, stroke, cancer, and mental disorders; National Institute on Drug Abuse 2014).

The acceptance of the use of intoxicants varies greatly among Buddhist communities and adherents. Clearly, overuse of alcohol to the point of intoxication is frowned upon, but total abstinence is not typically emphasized except for clergy. Here, we have some of the best empirical support for the middle path. Research suggests that there is a U curve in describing the relationship between alcohol use and cardiovascular disease. Both total abstinence and overuse of alcohol have been linked with increased risk for cardiovascular disease, whereas use of alcohol in moderation (i.e., one or two drinks a day) has been found to serve as a protective factor lowering the risk of cardiovascular disease (Thun et al. 1997).

TEA CONSUMPTION AND BUDDHISM

The role of tea in Buddhism has a long and complicated history. An example of this is my favorite myth regarding the origin of the tea plant. Bodhidharma was a revered patriarch in Buddhist history and the father of Chan Buddhism. The tea origin myth states that Bodhidharma was meditating, and after nine years, he briefly dozed off. Feeling angry at his lapse in mindfulness, he cut off his eyelids and threw them to the ground so that he would not falter in his meditation again. Where his eyelids landed on the ground, the tea plant grew, serving as an aid in maintaining mindfulness to Buddhists for ages to come. There are a few problems with this origin story beyond plants sprouting from discarded human tissue. Bodhidharma was a monk in the 5th–6th century BCE, yet there is historical evidence documenting the consumption of tea for a considerable length of time prior to this, with the earliest origin tale dating its use to 2700 BCE. Thus, consumption of tea predates the Buddha himself (600 BCE). Nevertheless, the myth demonstrates the vital role, importance, and ubiquity of tea consumption in Buddhism.

The behavioral practice in Buddhism that has the strongest correlation with positive physical health outcomes is the consumption of tea. Tea drinking has been suggested to produce a myriad of positive health effects, such as the prevention of cancer (including skin, prostate, lung, and breast cancers); cardiovascular disease, particularly atherosclerosis; and diabetes (Khan and Mukhtar 2013). Apparently, it is the polyphenolic compounds in tea that prevent heart disease. The catechins and theaflavins that are present contribute to the broad array of other positive physical health outcomes.

VIEWS SHARED WITH OTHER TRADITIONS

Within our discussion of Buddhist practices, beliefs, and health outcomes, we can recognize that several commonalities exist between Buddhism and other religious and spiritual traditions. Although a thorough exploration of these shared commonalities is beyond the scope of this chapter, a brief overview is provided in order to highlight similarities among major religious and spiritual traditions (e.g., Hinduism, Christianity, Islam, Judaism). Of course, considering common themes in these traditions is exceedingly difficult without the risk of stereotyping, oversimplifying, and ignoring complex historical and cultural contexts, including within-group diversity. This risk is taken, however, in the hope of situating our discussion of Buddhist views within a larger religious and spiritual context.

We can begin with a unifying definition for what constitutes a religious or spiritual tradition. English and English (1958) submit that these traditions can be viewed as systems of attitudes, practices, rites, ceremonies, and beliefs by means of which individuals or communities put themselves in relation to God or to a supernatural world, and often to each other, and derive a set of values by which to judge events in the natural world. Expanding on this definition, Loewenthal (1995) suggests that most major religious traditions have a number of features in common, including (1) a belief in the existence of a nonmaterial (i.e., spiritual) reality; and (2) the belief that the purpose of life is to increase harmony in the world by doing good and avoiding evil through adherence to guidelines.

The first theme, a shared belief in the existence of a nonmaterial reality, is intimately tied to a religious tradition's fundamental teachings of suffering and freedom from suffering. As previously discussed, according to Buddhist thought, the underlying cause of all forms of suffering involves the ignorance that arises from being attached to the world, its pleasures, and an inherently existing self. Hence, a central aim of Buddhist beliefs and practices is to be liberated from attachment to the material and develop an unwavering understanding of the impermanence of self (Shonin, Van Gordon, and Griffiths 2013). Despite the fact that, within mono- and polytheistic religions, the ultimate goals involve unity with the divine (i.e., God), similar themes of suffering through attachment to the material (turning away from God), and the belief in nonmaterial (unity with God) still arise. For example, in Christian traditions, suffering is the result of sin, which is caused by turning toward the self and to the things of this world and away from God. The belief in unity with God is also a central tenet of Judaism. Misfortune is seen as a warning to the individual to improve through adherence to prescribed lifestyle guidelines, which is done in the service of attaining unity with God. Similarly, the Islamic view of sin is that sin involves forgetfulness of divine unity and is rooted in pride and self-sufficiency. In Hindu traditions, the ultimate goal is infinity (God), and misfortunes are seen as a consequence of harmful actions taken in a previous incarnation (*karma*), which is not unlike the Buddhist concept of kamma, the process of mental proliferation and its consequences discussed earlier in this chapter. An individual can be emancipated from *karma* through adherence to different types of principles (*marga*), including duty, knowledge, and devotion (Loewenthal 2000). Thus, like Buddhism, other major religious and spiritual traditions believe that the path to freedom from suffering leads to some form of nonmaterial existence, and that the path away from this goal involves harmful or self-interested actions and attitudes.

The second theme, the belief that the purpose of life is to increase harmony in the world by doing good and avoiding evil through adherence to guidelines, is also inextricable from a tradition's views of suffering. In the Buddhist tradition, the *Eightfold Path* outlines a guide to freedom from suffering; this path includes the development of ethical discipline, mental discipline, and wisdom. The Five Precepts (i.e., refrain from killing, stealing, lying, sexual misconduct, and misuse of intoxicants) provides the ethical foundation for liberation and freedom (Purser and Milillo 2015). The Abrahamic "Ten Commandments" similarly outline behaviors that are believed to contribute to sin and suffering, such as idol worship, murder, theft, envy, and sexual immorality. The guidelines for the path to salvation include adherence to the commandments and the removal of sin and its effects through penance, confession, absolution, and forgiveness. In addition to these commandments, the path to unity with God in Judaic traditions involves a lifestyle in accordance with prescribed guidelines for proper diet, sexual behavior, work, business ethics, and worship (Loewenthal 2000). In Islamic traditions, the Five Pillars of Islam provide guidance for what constitutes good behavior, including a belief in God and the prophets, frequent prayer, giving away a proportion of personal possessions, fasting during Ramadan, and pilgrimage. Islamic teachings also refer to the importance of caring for family, having concern for the welfare of parents and the elderly, learning, and work. Harmful behaviors include suicide, sexual perversions, crime, and racial discrimination (Husain 1998). In Hindu traditions, a pious life is one of regular prayer, fasting, good thoughts and deeds, pilgrimage, and reverence for elders (Juthani 1998). Thus, we can see common themes regarding guidelines for ethical behaviors across religious traditions that distinguish between paths to suffering and paths to freedom from suffering, such as refraining from bad deeds and doing good deeds.

Buddhist views share some general commonalities with other major religious and spiritual traditions, including the belief that a spiritual reality exists, and that it is important to cultivate an awareness of this through specific practices (e.g., prayer, contemplation, meditation). These traditions also provide guidance as to the right way to live (freedom from suffering), which includes mandates regarding justice, kindness, and sexual morality.

BUDDHIST VALUES AND PRACTICES IN OTHER SOCIAL- AND HEALTH-RELATED CONTEXTS

As we discussed earlier in this chapter, aspects of Buddhist traditions have been increasingly applied to Western conceptualizations of medical and psychological health and well-being (e.g., self-compassion, mindfulness). This integration has given way to the incorporation of secularized Buddhist practices into Western medical and psychological treatment and intervention (e.g., mindful breathing, yoga, MBSR, MBIs). More specifically, the application of Buddhist values of alleviating suffering through the incorporation of compassion and mental training continues to yield positive outcomes within medical, psychological, and broader scientific communities.

Beyond medicine and psychology, Buddhist values have begun to manifest within Western socioeconomic contexts. A central defining feature of economics is the identification and understanding of the patterns of behavior in society that are related to *livelihood*, which in the context of economics is defined as the provision for physical and social needs and wants in the face of scarcity of appropriate resources (Daniels 2005). Several traditional Buddhist values and beliefs have economic implications, such as the moderation of material consumption through the middle path, the renunciation of self-interest discussed in the Eightfold Path, and the concept of Dependent Arising, the belief that all living beings are identified and interconnected with all other living beings (Bodhi 2005). In addition, Buddha's teachings include a discussion of the importance of providing the *Four Requisites* of food, clothing, shelter, and medicine. Poverty is considered to impede the achievement of harmony in an individual's social and natural environment and constrain spiritual progress (Payutto 1993). Therefore, the manifestation of these Buddhist views on day-to-day economic behavior can be identified as the increasing virtue attached to pursuing a middle path and the fundamental concern expressed for the welfare of others. That is, increasing numbers of Western individuals are moving away from capitalist material consumption and toward a middle path of maximum well-being with minimum consumption, attention to the implications for the welfare of others, and action leading toward spiritual development (Daniels 2005).

Within organizational and leadership contexts, Kriger and Seng (2005) discuss the influences of the Buddhist values and practices of impermanence (*anicca*), selflessness (*anatta*), and the four positive states of mind (*Brahmaviharas*). With an understanding of impermanence in Buddhist philosophy, an individual thinks, feels, senses, and observes the changing aspects of the world and the inner contents of the mind. This is seen in organizations in which individuals are encouraged to attend to the dynamic individual and group processes that affect workplace relationships, productivity, and well-being. The Buddha advocated for the absence of essential distinctions between the self and others. In this view, everyone and everything in the world is intimately interconnected. Within more egalitarian organizational structures, the tendency to emphasize these distinctions, particularly in regard to competition with others, is seen less often, as individuals de-emphasize distinctions between leaders and followers. The four positive mind states (love, compassion, heartfelt joy, equanimity) can be observed in workplace contexts that encourage a culture of meeting failure with compassion, not sacrificing productivity and efficiency for the cultivation of joy and love, and work-life balance.

The contributions of traditional Buddhist values and practices to Western medical and psychological contexts have been widely discussed in the existing academic literature. Emerging literature has also identified recent Buddhist contributions to Western socioeconomic and organizational leadership contexts. As components of Buddhist traditions continue to gain popularity and attention, particularly in Western cultures and societies, we will likely continue to see more examples of these values and practices in other social and health contexts.

REFERENCES

Acosta, M. C., J. Manubay, and F. R. Levin. 2008. "Pediatric Obesity: Parallels with Addiction and Treatment Recommendations." *Harvard Review of Psychiatry* 16(2): 80–96.

Analayo, B. 2004. *Sattipatthana: The Direct Path to Realization.* Cambridge, UK: Windhorse Publications.

Bodhi, B. 2005. "In the Buddha's Words." *Scripts Social Networking* 12(40): 73–74.

Bodhi, B. 2011. "What Does Mindfulness Really Mean? A Canonical Perspective." *Contemporary Buddhism* 12: 19–39.

Bohlmeijer, E., R. Prenger, E Taal, and P. Cuijpers. 2010. "The Effects of Mindfulness-Based Stress Reduction Therapy on Mental Health of Adults with a Chronic Medical Disease: A Meta-Analysis." *Journal of Psychosomatic Research* 68: 539–544.

Bond, F. W., S. C. Hayes, R. A. Baer, K. M. Carpenter, N. Guenole, H. K. Orcutt, . . . R. D. Zettle. 2011. "Preliminary Psychometric Properties of the Acceptance and Action Questionnaire–II: A Revised Measure of Psychological Inflexibility and Experiential Avoidance." *Behavior Therapy* 42: 676–688.

Bowen, S., N. Chawla, S. E. Collins, K. Witkiewitz, S. Hsu, J. Grow, . . . M. E. Larimer. 2009. "Mindfulness-Based Relapse Prevention for Substance Use Disorders: A Pilot Efficacy Trial." *Substance Abuse* 30: 295–305.

Brody, S. 2010. "The Relative Health Benefits of Different Sexual Activities." *Journal of Sexual Medicine* 7: 1336–1361.

Christopher, M. S., R. J. Goerling, B. S. Rogers, M. Hunsinger, G. Baron, A. L. Bergman, and D. T. Zava. 2015. "A Pilot Study Evaluating the Effectiveness of a Mindfulness-Based Intervention on Cortisol Awakening Response and Health Outcomes Among Law Enforcement Officers." *Journal of Police and Criminal Psychology* 31: 1–14.

Cole, J. M. 2013. "Short Term Effects of Gossip Behavior on Self-Esteem." *Current Psychology: A Journal for Diverse Perspectives on Diverse Psychological Issues* 32(3): 252–260.

Crocker, J., and A. Canevello. 2008. "Creating and Undermining Social Support in Communal Relationships: The Role of Compassionate and Self-Image Goals." *Journal of Personality and Social Psychology* 95: 555.

Cutler, J., and G. Newland (eds.). 2015. *The Great Treatise on the Stages of the Path to Enlightenment* (vol. 1). Boulder, CO: Shambhala Publications.

Daniels, P. L. 2005. "Economic Systems and the Buddhist World View: The 21st Century Nexus." *Journal of Socio-Economics* 34: 245–268.

Dass, R., and D. Goleman. 1990. *Journey of Awakening: A Meditator's Guidebook.* Newburyport, MA: Bantam.

David, D. 2014. "Some Concerns about the Psychological Implications of Mindfulness: A Critical Analysis." *Journal of Rational-Emotive & Cognitive-Behavior Therapy* 32: 313–324.

Davidson, R. J., A. Harrington, and E. Rosch. 2003. "Visions of Compassion: Western Scientists and Tibetan Buddhists Examine Human Nature." *Contemporary Psychology [APA Review of Books]* 48: 330.

Davidson, R. J., J. Kabat-Zinn, J. Schumacher, M. Rosenkranz, D. Muller, S. F. Santorelli, . . . J. F. Sheridan, 2003. "Alterations in Brain and Immune Function Produced by Mindfulness Meditation." *Psychosomatic Medicine* 65: 564–570.

Desbordes, G., T. Gard, E. A. Hoge, B. K. Hölzel, C. Kerr, S. W. Lazar, . . . D. R. Vago. 2014. "Moving Beyond Mindfulness: Defining Equanimity as an Outcome Measure in Meditation and Contemplative Research." *Mindfulness* 6: 356–372.

Dhargyey, G. N. 1974. *Tibetan Tradition of Mental Development: Oral Teachings of Tibetan Lama.* Gangchen, India: Library of Tibetan Works & Archives.

Domínguez-Rodrigo M, T. R. Pickering, F. Diez-Martín, A. Mabulla, C. Musiba, G. Trancho . . . C. Arriaza. 2012. "Earliest Porotic Hyperostosis on a 1.5-Million-Year-Old Hominin, Olduvai Gorge, Tanzania." *PLoS ONE* 7(10). Retrieved from http://journals.plos.org/plosone/article?id=10.1371/journal.pone.0046414

Dreeben, S. J., M.H. Mamberg, and P. Salmon. 2013. "The MBSR Body Scan in Clinical Practice." *Mindfulness* 4: 394–401.

English, H., and A. C. English. 1958. *A Comprehensive Dictionary of Psychological and Psychoanalytic Terms.* New York: David McKay.

Feinberg, M., R. Willer, and M. Schultz. 2014. "Gossip and Ostracism Promote Cooperation in Groups." *Psychological Science* 25: 656–664. doi:10.1177/0956797613510184

Friedman, N. L. 2002. "Zen Breath Meditation Awareness Improves Heart Rate Variability in Patients with Coronary Artery Disease." *Dissertation Abstracts International: Section B: The Sciences and Engineering* 62(12-B), 5948.

Gard, T., J. J. Noggle, C. L. Park, D. R. Vago, and A. Wilson. 2014. "Potential Self-Regulatory Mechanisms of Yoga for Psychological Health." *Frontiers in Human Neuroscience* 8: 770. doi:10.3389/fnhum.2014.00770

Garland, E. L., B. Froeliger, and M. O. Howard. 2014. "Effects of Mindfulness-Oriented Recovery Enhancement on Reward Responsiveness and Opioid Cue-Reactivity." *Psychopharmacology* 231: 3229–3238.

Giles, G.G., G. Severi, D. R. English, M. R. E. McCredie, R. Borland, P. Boyle, and J. L. Hopper. 2003. "Sexual Factors and Prostate Cancer." *BJU International* 92: 211–216.

Goyal, M., S. Singh, E. M. Sibinga, N. F. Gould, A. Rowland-Seymour, R. Sharma, . . . P. D. Ranasinghe. 2014. "Meditation Programs for Psychological Stress and Well-Being: A Systematic Review and Meta-Analysis." *JAMA Internal Medicine* 174: 357–368.

Gross, C.R., M. J. Kreitzer, M. Reilly-Spong, M. Wall, N. Y. Winbush, R. Patterson, . . . M. Cramer-Bornemann. 2011. "Mindfulness-Based Stress Reduction vs. Pharmacotherapy for Primary Chronic Insomnia: A Pilot Randomized Controlled Clinical Trial." *Explore* 7(2): 76–87.

Grossman, P. 2015. "Mindfulness: Awareness Informed by a Body Ethic." *Mindfulness* 6(1): 17–22.

Grossman, P., U. Tiefenthaler-Gilmer, A. Raysz, and U. Kesper. 2007. "Mindfulness Training as an Intervention for Fibromyalgia: Evidence of Post Intervention and 3-year Follow-Up Benefits in Well-Being." *Psychotherapy and Psychosomatics* 76(4): 226–233.

Halifax, J. 2012. "A Heuristic Model of Enactive Compassion." *Current Opinion in Supportive and Palliative Care* 6: 228–235.

Hayes, S. C., J. Pistorello, and M. E. Levin. 2012. "Acceptance and Commitment Therapy as a Unified Model of Behavior Change." *Counseling Psychologist* 40: 976–1002.

Hayes, S. C., K. G. Wilson, E. V. Gifford, V. M. Follette, and K. Strosahl. 1996. "Experiential Avoidance and Behavioral Disorders: A Functional Dimensional Approach to Diagnosis and Treatment." *Journal of Consulting and Clinical Psychology* 64(6): 1152–1168.

Heron, M., and B. Tejada-Vera. 2009. "Deaths: Leading Causes for 2005. National Vital Statistics Reports: From the Centers for Disease Control and Prevention, National Center for Health Statistics." *National Vital Statistics System* 58(8): 1–97.

Hofmann, S. G., P. Grossman, and D. E. Hinton. 2011. "Loving-Kindness and Compassion Meditation: Potential for Psychological Interventions." *Clinical Psychology Review* 31: 1126–1132.

Hofmann, S. G., A. T. Sawyer, A. A. Witt, and D. Oh. 2010. "The Effect of Mindfulness-Based Therapy on Anxiety and Depression: A Meta-Analytic Review." *Journal of Consulting and Clinical Psychology* 78(2): 169–183. doi:10.1037/a0018555

Hollis-Walker, L., and K. Colosimo. 2011. "Mindfulness, Self-Compassion, and Happiness in Non-Meditators: A Theoretical and Empirical Examination." *Personality and Individual Differences* 50: 222–227.

Husain, S. A. 1998. "Religion and Mental Health from the Muslim Perspective." In H. G. Koenig ed., *Handbook of Religion and Mental Health*, pp. 279–291. San Diego, CA: Academic Press.

Irving, J. A., P. Dobkin, and J. Park. 2009. "Cultivating Mindfulness in Health Care Professionals: A Review of Empirical Studies of Mindfulness-Based Stress Reduction (MBSR)." *Complementary Therapies in Clinical Practice* 15(2): 61–66.

Juthani, N. V. 2004. "Hindus and Buddhists." In A. Josephson and J. Peteet, eds., *Handbook of Spirituality and Worldview in Clinical Practice*, pp. 125–137. Arlington, VA: American Psychiatric Publishing.

Kabat-Zinn, J., L. Lipworth, and R. Burney. 1985. "The Clinical Use of Mindfulness Meditation for the Self-Regulation of Chronic Pain." *Journal of Behavioral Medicine* 8(2): 163–190.

Kabat-Zinn, J., E. Wheeler, T. Light, A. Skillings, M. J. Scharf, T. G. Cropley, . . . J. D. Bernhard. 1998. "Influence of a Mindfulness Meditation-Based Stress Reduction Intervention on Rates of Skin Clearing in Patients with Moderate to Severe Psoriasis Undergoing Photo Therapy (UVB) and Photochemotherapy (PUVA)." *Psychosomatic Medicine* 60: 625–632.

Key, T. J., G. E. Fraser, M. Thorogood, P. N. Appleby, V. Bera, G. Reeves, . . . K. McPherson. 1999. "Mortality in Vegetarians and Nonvegetarians: Detailed Findings from a Collaborative Analysis of 5 Prospective Studies." *American Journal of Clinical Nutrition* 70: 516–524.

Khan, N., and H. Mukhtar. 2013. "Tea and Health: Studies in Humans." *Current Pharmaceutical Design* 19: 6141–6147.

Khoury, B., M. Sharma, S. E. Rush, and C. Fournier. 2015. "Mindfulness-Based Stress Reduction for Healthy Individuals: A Meta-Analysis." *Journal of Psychosomatic Research* 78: 519–528.

Kriger, M., and Y. Seng. 2005. "Leadership with Inner Meaning: A Contingency Theory of Leadership Based on the Worldviews of Five Religions." *Leadership Quarterly* 16: 771–806.

Kristeller, J., R. Q. Wolever, and V. Sheets. 2014. "Mindfulness-Based Eating Awareness Training (MB-EAT) for Binge Eating: A Randomized Clinical Trial." *Mindfulness* 5: 282–297.

Kuo, C. C., I. K. Chang, K. Kingdom, S. Quinton, C. Y. Lu, and I. Lee. 2015. "Gossip in the Workplace and Implications for HR Management: A Study of Gossip and Its Relationship to Employee Cynicism." *International Journal of Human Resources Management* 26: 2288–2307.

Loewenthal, K. 1995. *Mental Health and Religion*. London, UK: Chapman & Hall.

Loewenthal, K. 2000. *Psychology of Religion*. London, UK: Oneworld Publications.

Lu, P. H. 2015. "Gossip Makes Us One: A Qualitative Analysis of the Role of Gossip in Process of Taiwanese Immigrants' Social integration in Canada." *Journal of Asian Pacific Communication* 25: 279–304.

Marlatt, G. A., and J. R. Gordon. 1985. *Relapse Prevention: Maintenance Strategies in Addictive Behavior Change*. New York: Guilford.

Mitchell, J. T., L. Zylowska, and S. H. Kollins. 2015. "Mindfulness Meditation Training for Attention-Deficit/Hyperactivity Disorder in Adulthood: Current

Empirical Support, Treatment Overview, and Future Directions." *Cognitive and Behavioral Practice* 22(2): 172–191.

Monteiro, L. M., R. F. Musten, and J. Compson. 2015. "Traditional and Contemporary Mindfulness: Finding the Middle Path in the Tangle of Concerns." *Mindfulness* 6(1), 1–13.

National Institute on Drug Abuse. 2014. "Drugs, Brains and Behavior: The Science of Addiction." Retrieved February 16, 2017, from https://www .drugabuse.gov/publications/drugs-brains-behavior-science-addiction

Neff, K. D. 2003. "The Development and Validation of a Scale to Measure Self-Compassion." *Self and Identity* 2(3): 223–250.

Neff, K. D., Y. P. Hsieh, and K. Dejitterat. 2005. "Self-Compassion, Achievement Goals, and Coping with Academic Failure." *Self and Identity* 4(3): 263–287.

Neff, K. D., K. L. Kirkpatrick, and S. S. Rude. 2007. "Self-Compassion and Adaptive Psychological Functioning." *Journal of Research in Personality* 41: 139–154.

Neff, K. D., and E. Pommier. 2013. "The Relationship Between Self-Compassion and Other-Focused Concern Among College Undergraduates, Community Adults, and Practicing Meditators." *Self and Identity* 12(2):160–176.

Olendzki, A. 2011. "The Construction of Mindfulness." *Contemporary Buddhism* 12(1): 55–70.

Olson, K., K. J. Kemper, and J. D. Mahan. 2015. "What Factors Promote Resilience and Protect Against Burnout in First-Year Pediatric and Medicine-Pediatric Residents?" *Journal of Evidence-Based Complementary & Alternative Medicine* 20(3): 192–198.

Ong, J., and D. Sholtes. 2010. "A Mindfulness-Based Approach to the Treatment of Insomnia." *Journal of Clinical Psychology* 66: 1175–1184.

Orlich, M. J., P. M. Singh, and J. Sabate. 2013. "Vegetarian Dietary Patterns and Mortality in Adventist Health Study 2." *Internal Medicine* 173: 1230–1238.

Paonil, P., and L. Sringernyuang. 2002. "Buddhist Perspectives on Health and Healing." *Chulalongkorn Journal of Buddhist Studies* 1(2): 93–105.

Park, Y. J., and Y. B. Park. 2012. "Clinical Utility of Paced Breathing as a Concentration Meditation Practice." *Complementary Therapies in Medicine* 20: 393–399. doi:10.1016/j.ctim.2012.07.008

Payutto, B. P. A. 1993. *Good, Evil and Beyond*. Tullera, Australia: Buddha Dharma Education Association.

Perez-De-Albeniz, A., and J. Holmes. 2000. "Meditation: Concepts, Effects and Uses in Therapy." *International Journal of Psychotherapy* 5: 49–58.

Porges, S. W. 1992. "Vagal Tone: A Physiologic Marker of Stress Vulnerability." *Pediatrics* 90: 498–504.

Pradhan, E. K., M. Baumgarten, P. Langenberg, B. Handwerger, A. K. Gilpin, T. Magyari, . . . B. M. Berman. 2007. "Effect of Mindfulness-Based Stress Reduction in Rheumatoid Arthritis Patients." *Arthritis Care & Research* 57(7): 1134–1142.

Prakhinkit, S., S. Suppapitiporn, H. Tanaka, and D. Suksom. 2014. "Effects of Buddhism Walking Meditation on Depression, Functional Fitness, and Endothelium-Dependent Vasodilation in Depressed Elderly." *Journal of Alternative and Complementary Medicine* 20: 411–416.

Purser, R. E., and J. Milillo. 2015. "Mindfulness Revisited a Buddhist-Based Conceptualization." *Journal of Management Inquiry* 24: 3–24.

Rama, S., R. Ballentine, and A. Hymes. 1998. *Science of Breath: A Practical Guide.* Honesdale, PA: Himalayan Institute Press.

Rockliff, H., P. Gilbert, K. McEwan, S. Lightman, and D. Glover. 2008. "A Pilot Exploration of Heart Rate Variability and Salivary Cortisol Responses to Compassion-Focused Imagery." *Journal of Clinical Neuropsychiatry* 5: 132–139.

Rosenkranz, M. A., R. J. Davidson, D. G. MacCoon, J. F. Sheridan, N. H. Kalin, and A. Lutz. 2013. "A Comparison of Mindfulness-Based Stress Reduction and an Active Control in Modulation of Neurogenic Inflammation." *Brain, Behavior, and Immunity* 27: 174–184.

Rosenzweig, S., D. K. Reibel, J. M. Greeson, J. S. Edman, S. Jasser, K. D. McMearty, and B. J. Goldstein. 2007. "Mindfulness-Based Stress Reduction Is Associated with Improved Glycemic Control in Type 2 Diabetes Mellitus: A Pilot Study." *Alternative Therapies in Health and Medicine* 13(5): 36–38.

Ross, A., E. Friedmann, M. Bevans, and S. Thomas. 2013. "National Survey of Yoga Practitioners: Mental and Physical Health Benefits." *Complementary Therapies in Medicine* 21(4): 313–323.

Sayadaw, M. 1994. *The Progress of Insight.* Kandy, Sri Lanka: Buddhist Publication Society.

Schroeder, D. A., E. Stephens, D. Colgan, M. Hunsinger, D. Rubin, and M. S. Christopher. 2016. "A Brief Mindfulness-Based Intervention for Primary Care Physicians: A Pilot Randomized Controlled Trial." *American Journal of Lifestyle Medicine* (February 4, 2016): 1–9. doi:10.1177/1559827616629121

Sethi, S., and S. C. Bhargava. 2003. Relationship of Meditation and Psychosis: Case Studies. Australian and New Zealand." *Journal of Psychiatry* 37: 382–382.

Shennan, C., S. Payne, and D. Fenlon. 2011. "What Is the Evidence for the Use of Mindfulness-Based Interventions in Cancer Care? A Review." *Psycho-Oncology* 20: 681–697.

Shonin, E., W. Van Gordon, and M. D. Griffiths. 2013. "Buddhist Philosophy for the Treatment of Problem Gambling." *Journal of Behavioral Addictions* 2(2): 63–71.

Shonin, E., W. Van Gordon, and M. D. Griffiths. 2014a. "Meditation Awareness Training (MAT) for Improved Psychological Well-Being: A Qualitative Examination of Participant Experiences." *Journal of Religion and Health* 53: 849–863.

Shonin, E., W. Van Gordon, and M. D. Griffiths. 2014b. "Are There Risks Associated with Using Mindfulness in the Treatment of Psychopathology?" *Clinical Practice* 11: 389–392.

Smith, H. 1991. *The World's Religions*. New York: HarperCollins.

ten Brinke, L., J. J. Lee, and D. R. Carney. 2015. "The Physiology of (Dis)Honesty: Does It Impact Health?" *Current Opinions in Psychology* 6: 177–182.

Ṭhānissaro, B. 2012. *Right Mindfulness: Memory & Ardency on the Buddhist Path*. Valley Center, CA: Metta Forest Monastery.

Thich Nat Hanh. 2007. *For a Future to Be Possible: Buddhist Ethics for Everyday Life*. Berkeley, CA: Parallax Press.

Thun, M. J., R. Peto, A. D. Lopez, J. H. Monaco, S. J. Henley, C. W. Heath, and R. Doll. 1997. "Alcohol Consumption and Mortality Among Middle-Aged and Elderly US Adults." *New England Journal of Medicine* 337: 1705–1714.

Van Dam, N. T., S. C. Sheppard, J. P. Forsyth, and M. Earleywine. 2011. "Self-Compassion Is a Better Predictor than Mindfulness of Symptom Severity and Quality of Life in Mixed Anxiety and Depression." *Journal of Anxiety Disorders* 25: 123–130.

Van Dam, R. M., T. Li, D. Spiegelman, O. H. Franco, and F. B. Hu. 2008. "Combined Impact of Lifestyle Factors on Mortality: Prospective Cohort Study in US Women." *British Medical Journal* 337: a1440. Retrieved from http://www.bmj.com/content/337/bmj.a1440

Van Diest, I., K. Verstappen, A. E. Aubert, D. Widjaja, D. Vansteenwegen, and E. Vlemincx. 2014. "Inhalation/Exhalation Ratio Modulates the Effect of Slow Breathing on Heart Rate Variability and Relaxation." *Applied Psychophysiology and Biofeedback* 39(3–4): 171–180. doi:10.1007/s10484-014-9253-x

Wanden-Berghe, R. G., J. Sanz-Valero, and C. Wanden-Berghe. 2010. "The Application of Mindfulness to Eating Disorders Treatment: A Systematic Review." *Eating Disorders* 19: 34–48.

Witkiewitz, R., C. R. Roos, D. D. Colgan, and S. Bowen. 2017. *Mindfulness: Advances in Psychotherapy Evidence-Based Practice* (Vol. 37). Boston, MA: Hogrefe.

Chapter 4

Health, Spirituality, and Chinese Thought

Robert Santee

Within the context of classical Chinese thought there are no categorical distinctions between health, spirituality, religion, lifestyle, and simply living one's life. These are Western distinctions reflective of the abstract, logical, rational, and decontextualized thought of Plato and Aristotle. The Chinese worldview is concrete, practical, and context-oriented. To incorporate this Chinese perspective into an integrated, interdisciplinary approach to health care, both proactive and reactive, it is necessary to find a commonality between the cultures.

EVOLUTION AND CHRONIC STRESS

No matter what culture individuals are from, the underlying commonality is that we are all creatures whose behavior and thought are grounded in a series of survival mechanisms provided to us courtesy of evolution (Buss 2015). One such mechanism, the fight/freeze/flee or stress response, alerted our distant ancestors to acute physical threats in their ever-changing environment and provided them with the appropriate physical and psychological adaptive solutions to resolve them (Benson 2000; McEwen and Lasley 2002; Sapolsky 1998; Selye 1978). Once an adaptive solution resolved the acute adaptive problem of a physical threat, the stress response was turned off (Benson 2000). This evolutionary mechanism has been passed on to us because it kept our distant ancestors alive and thus allowed them to find a mate, reproduce, and maintain their gene pool (Benson 2000; Nesse and Young 2000; Sørensen, Holmstrup, Sarup, and Loeschcke 2010).

Although we have, courtesy of evolution and our DNA, essentially the same brain and body as our distant ancestors, we do not have the same environment as our distant ancestors. Most of the threats we encounter are not physical; rather, they are primarily psychosocial (Benson and Casey 2013; McEwen and Lasley 2002; Sapolsky 1998; Seligman 2006). However, because our brains do not make a distinction between real physical threats and psychosocial threats generated by our thinking, our stress response will be activated in either case (Kabat-Zinn 2005; Seligman 2006; Stuart, Webster, and Wells-Federman 1993). The problem is that in the case of psychosocial threats, the activation of the stress response often does not help to resolve the perceived threats; in fact, it tends to make these situations worse, and is maintained if you continue to think about them.

The stress response did not evolve to be chronically activated or yo-yoed on and off throughout the day. This chronic activation/yo-yoing of your stress response significantly compromises your physical and psychological health and well-being (Benson 2000, Benson and Casey 2013; Koenig 2012; McEwen and Lasley 2002; Sapolsky 1998; Stefano, Fricchione, Slingsby, and Benson 2001). It has been noted and documented by research that the symptoms, physical and psychological, reported during 60% to 90% of all office visits to medical doctors are associated with chronic stress (Avey, Matheny, Robbins, and Jacobs 2003; Benson 1996; 1998; Nerurkar, Bitton, Davis, Phillips, and Yeh 2013; WebMD 2016). No physical cause for the symptoms, which are real, can be found (Benson 1996; Citizens Commission on Human Rights 2016).

Thus, the commonality that will be explored to incorporate this Chinese perspective into an integrated and interdisciplinary approach to health care is that of chronic stress. The *Huangdi Neijing*, Daoism, and Confucianism are the specific focus.

THE *HUANGDI NEIJING*

The *Huangdi Neijing* (*The Yellow Emperor's Classic of Internal Medicine*), believed to be the oldest medical book in China, represents the movement from a shamanistic worldview in which disease, illness, health, and well-being were due to the influence of the spirits, to a worldview in which they were due to lifestyle and behavior. The author or authors are unknown. It consists of two texts: the *Suwen* and the *Lingshu*.

The *Suwen* or *Simple Questions* is the better-known of the two texts. It addresses what we today would call chronic stress and diagnostic methods, and offers a holistic lifestyle approach to preventive medicine/health care. The *Lingshu*, or spiritual pivot, is more clinical in nature, with its major focus on acupuncture, the meridians or channels through which *qi* flows, anatomy, physiology, and various diseases.

Suwen

The structure of both the *Suwen* and the *Lingshu* is a question-and-answer format between the mythological Yellow Emperor and his ministers about various aspects of health and well-being. As the focus of the *Suwen* is on the relationship between lifestyle, interpersonal, physical, and psychological behavior, the environment, and health, it is clearly more immediately relevant to the relationship between spirituality and health. Hence, the focus of this chapter is on this text.

The author or authors of the *Suwen* assume that the reader understands some basic philosophic principles and concepts that are used not only to explain/describe health, well-being, illness, disease, and the physical, psychological, and interpersonal behavior of the individual, but also to explain/describe the workings of the entire universe. These basic concepts and principles are *Dao*, *qi*, *yin* and *yang*, *jing*, and *shen*.

Dao has the meaning of a path, a journey on that path, a way of life, the source of everything, the fundamental principle of/nature of existence (Cheng 2003a; D. Zhang 2002). It can be viewed as dynamic, extended, still-empty space that allows everything to occur without interfering with it. In Part 1, Chapter 5 of the Appendix (*Xici Shang*) to one of the fundamental classic texts of all Chinese thought, the more than 2000-year-old *Book of Changes* (*Yijing* or *Changes of Zhou* (*Zhouyi*), Dao is defined:

The dynamic, symbiotic, continually changing, cyclical process or *yin* and *yang* is called *Dao* (*Zhouyi*).

Qi is the basic building block of everything (Cheng 2003b; Zhang and Rose 2001). It is a life force (D. Zhang 2002). It is breath. It is vital energy. It is what propels movement. If it flows throughout the body through the channels/meridians without any obstruction, then the individual is healthy. If it is excessive, deficient, static, or obstructed, the individual is not healthy. Acupuncture, moxibustion, fire cupping, herbs, and *tuina* (massage and manipulation) are all, in most cases, reactive practices used to remove obstructions and allow *qi* to naturally flow throughout the body; this allows the individual to return to a healthy life.

Yin and *yang* are the very nature of change. They are the consistent, organizational patterns of continual change and transformation. They are the cyclical, reciprocal, interdependent relationship amongst all things. Yin is the female, the receptive, the moon, the dark, the soft, and so on. Yang is the male, the aggressive, the sun, the light, the hard, and so on. Essentially, though, *yin* and *yang* are the form and function of *qi*. There is no *yin* and *yang* apart from *qi* (D. Zhang 2002). While *qi* is the stuff of existence, the interaction of *yin* and *yang* is what shapes *qi* into the various configurations that make up existence.

Jing is essence. It is what allows the body to grow. It is the material component of the body. According to Chapter Four of the *Suwen* and Chapter Four of the *Lingshu:*

Jing is the foundation of the body.

The Yellow Emperor said, "Essence (*jing*) is required at the beginning of life for a person. When essence comes into existence, the brain and marrow begin to grow, the bones become the material of support, the channels-meridians, veins and arteries are built, the tendons and muscles become firm and strong, the flesh become[s] walls, the skin becomes solid, the hair grows, the nutrients enter the stomach, the pathway of the vessels open, connect, and communicate, the blood and *qi* flow (*Huangdi Neijing* n.d.).

Shen has the meaning of spirit in the sense of the charisma, charm, and/or the way you present and express yourself to others. It is also the cognitive processes (Shi and Zhang 2012).

Selections from the *Suwen*

To enhance understanding of the holistic viewpoint of the *Suwen*, this section presents a series of selections from it. In the first chapter, the following conversation takes place between the Yellow Emperor and his minister Qi Bo regarding the natural lifespan:

The Yellow Emperor asked: "I have heard that people during the ancient period all lived well into 100 years old. Furthermore, their actions and movements were not compromised, weak, or feeble. People today live half as long and their actions and movements are compromised, weak, and feeble. What is the difference between these times? What got lost or neglected?"

Qi Bo responded, "People of ancient times understood the pathway [*dao*] and modeled themselves on yin and yang. They were in harmony with the art, skill and assessment of living life. They practiced moderation in eating and drinking. Throughout their daily life their behavior was consistent. They did not overwork.

Thus, their body [*xíng*] and spirit [*shen*] were not fragmented. They completed their natural lifespan of 100 plus years before dying.

Today, people act differently. They drink wine as if it were merely water. They are consistently rash and impulsive in their behavior. They are drunk when they enter the bedroom. Their desires exhaust their essence [*jīng*]. They squander and dissipate what is truly real. They do not know how to maintain satisfaction. They are unable to control their spirit [*shen*]. They devote themselves to instant happiness. Their daily life is without moderation. Thus, at the age of 50 they are feeble and weak." (*Huangdi Neijing* n.d.)

The description provided by Qi Bo regarding the people of his day is a clear description of what is today known as *chronic stress*. Their lifestyle results in physical and psychological damage, known today as *allostatic load*, and early death (McEwen and Lasley 2002). Their behavior was irregular, impulsive, excessive, deficient, and reactive in nature. It was not modeled after yin and yang. They were unable to relax, be happy, or be at peace. They lacked patience. There was no integration of mind/spirit, body and environment. Their overall well-being and health were significantly compromised.

In contrast, the description of the people of ancient times is indicative of being free from chronic stress. They were free from chronic stress because of their holistic lifestyle that was based in modeling their behavior on yin and yang. A fundamental component of that lifestyle is the consistent practice of moderation. As a result, unlike the people of Qi Bo's time, they had healthy and long lives.

Qi Bo further explains, in Chapter One, that the lifestyle required to be free from what we today call chronic stress was handed down from the ancient sages. Of particular importance are the teachings regarding the necessity of having a mind that is not continually agitated by threats and desires, and being aware and acting accordingly in regard to unhealthy influences in the environment. If the path is followed, the individual will be healthy, with a health that is far beyond simply being free from physical and psychological illness and disease.

In ancient times the teachings of the sages were passed down. All of these teachings said that unhealthy influences in the social and physical environment should be avoided at all times. Be without grief and worry. Be tranquil. The inborn *qì* will then follow. Internally protect your mind (essence [*jīng*] and spirit [*shén*]), and you will always be safe against illness. Thus, your will [*zhì*] is not agitated and your desires are few. Your mind is at peace and there are not any threats. The body labors yet it is not drained or weary. The vital energy [*qì*] will flow freely and naturally.

Each followed their desires and all attained that which they desired. Thus they were satisfied with their food and clothing. They enjoyed following the customs. They did not admire the distinctions of superior and inferior. These people were said to be simple and plain. Therefore, sensual desire did not trouble their eyes. Excessiveness and unhealthy influences did not confuse or agitate their mind. Stupid or wise, virtuous or unworthy, they were not threatened by anything. Thus, they were in accord with the Dao. As a result, they were able to live for a hundred years plus. Their movements and actions were not compromised, weak, or feeble. Their internal power [dé] was complete and they were not threatened. (*Huangdi Neijing* n.d.)

In addition to a healthy long life, Qi Bo, in responding to a question from the Yellow Emperor about aging and reproduction in Chapter One, goes on to say that those individuals who follow the pathway Dao can slow the process of aging to the extent that they can reproduce at even 100 years old. Thus, this healthy lifestyle espoused by the *Huangdi Neijing* not only results in a long life, but in a long life that is not compromised by the normal aging process that can significantly hinder psychological and physical well-being, to the extent that the practitioners are able to reproduce. As Chapter One notes,

The Yellow Emperor said, "For all those who follow the Dao and live to 100 or more years, are they able to have children?" Qi Bo responded, "Those who follow the Dao are able to repulse aging. Their physical form is intact. Even though their body has achieved a long life, they are able to produce a child." (*Huangdi Neijing* n.d.)

The role model for putting into practice this holistic lifestyle was the *zhenren* or authentic person. Adding to the practice of moderation, reducing desires, removal of chronic negative and absolute thinking, stilling and emptying the mind of all agitation, and understanding and being guided by yin and yang, this section on the *zhenren* offers a technique on how to actually still and empty the mind, and thus integrate the mind, body, and environment. It is a meditative, standing breathing exercise known today as *Zhan zhuang* or standing like a tree, stake, or post in the ground (Liu 2010). It is the basis of all Chinese martial arts and *qigong*.

The Yellow Emperor said, "I have heard that in ancient times there were the *zhenren* or authentic people. They were guided and supported by the sky and the earth. They firmly grasped the continual changing and transformative processes of yin and yang. Inhaling and exhaling jing and qi, they stood in solitude observing and protecting their spirit [shen] as they integrated and unified it with their body. Thus, they were able to live as long as the sky and the earth without an end. This is the Dao of life (daosheng)." (*Huangdi Neijing* n.d.)

Aside from what has been presented earlier, another area where the Western approach to health and wellness differs significantly from the classical

Chinese holistic approach is in the ever-changing environment. In the West, there is discussion of integrating mind and body or integrating mind, body, and spirit. There is no real mention of or concern regarding the ever-changing environment. This is not the case in the *Huangdi Neijing*. In Chapter Two of the *Suwen*, there is a discussion of the holistic lifestyle approach relative to the qi of each of the four seasons and the appropriate behavior to be healthy and in harmony with each season. In the following selection regarding the Spring, the importance of sleep, physical exercise, and stretching are presented. In addition, the concept of *yangsheng* or nourishing life is introduced. This is an umbrella term covering a wide series of holistic, preventive practices, including meditation, *daoyin/qigong*, physical exercise, diet, sleep, visualization, stretching, interpersonal relations, sexual relations, breathing exercises, and the practice of moderation (Kohn 2008a 2012; Santee and Zhang 2015).

"The three months of Spring are called issue forth and display. The sky and the earth produce life together. All things are thriving. At night lie down and go to sleep. Rise early in the morning, stretch out and take a brisk walk in the courtyard. By issuing energy the body recuperates. This is applying your will [*zhi*] to live and grow. Living and growing you will not weaken. Enjoying life and not punishing yourself. This is responding to the qi of spring. This is the Tao of nourishing life [*Yangsheng*]." (Santee and Zhang 2015, p. 26; also see *Huangdi Neijing*, n.d.)

At the end of Chapter Two and the start of Chapter Five in the *Suwen*, the emphasis on importance of understanding, following, and putting into practice the process of yin and yang regarding one's own health and well-being and the treating of patients is quite salient:

Yin, yang, and the four seasons are the beginning and end of all things. They are the root of life and death. To act contrary to them results in disaster and harms life. Being in accordance with them, severe illness does not arise. This way of self-cultivation [*dao*] was put into practice by the Sages [*shèngrén*]. The ignorant treated it superficially. To follow yin and yang results in life. To act contrary to yin and yang results in death. To follow yin and yang results in well-being, order and peacefulness. To act contrary to yin and yang results in illness, disorder and confusion. To oppose this practice is to act contrary to what is natural. This is called internal resistance.

The Yellow Emperor said, "Yin and Yang is the way [*dao*] of Heaven and Earth. They are the organizational patterns, regulators and guides for all things. They are the father and mother of all change and transformation. They are the root and beginning of life and death. They are the home of spiritual clarity. To treat illness, you must seek their root." (*Huangdi Neijing* n.d.)

Spiritual clarity in the preceding excerpt is used in the sense that it is through understanding the process of yin and yang that the occurrences of life, death, change, and transformation can be grasped. This understanding is the root of treating illness. The bottom line, though, is that the classic Chinese medical doctors were expected to focus on their patients before they became ill. This holistic approach is preventive in nature: Prevent what may lead to illness and disease. The end of Chapter Two clearly indicates this to be the case.

Thus, the Sage did not treat those who were already sick and ill. They treated those who were not yet ill and sick. . . . This is what has been said: To use drugs/medicine with those who have already become sick and ill, is it not like digging a well after you are thirsty, . . . is it not too late! (*Huangdi Neijing* n.d.)

INTERLUDE

The concept of spirituality as found in the *Huangdi Neijing* is considerably different from the Western perspective regarding health and well-being. The focus/paradigm of the medical profession in the West, at least in the United States, is primarily to incorporate spirituality, however the patient defines it, as part of a holistic approach to medical care, especially with patients who are facing life-threatening diseases and/or are terminal. These patients are clearly chronically stressed as they face the greatest threat known to them. Some members of the medical profession clearly recognize that if spirituality will help their patients cope with this ultimate threat, and thus reduce their stress and the suffering associated with it, then it must be incorporated into the treatment. Nonetheless, it is reactive in nature!

The approach in the *Huangdi Neijing* is proactive in nature. Even though it is not overtly mentioned as such, the concept of spirituality is part and parcel of being healthy, physically, psychologically, and interpersonally, and in harmony with the world around one throughout the year. There is no distinct aspect of spirituality separate from body, mind, and environment. Even though the term *shen* is defined in the West as "spirit," it simply does not have the same connotation in the *Huangdi Neijing*. According to the *Huangdi Neijing*, individuals who follow the path (Dao) of self-cultivation will understand and experience the dynamic, symbiotic, continually changing and transforming process of yin and yang, and thus will have a tranquil mind; their *jing*, *qi*, and *shen* will be integrated. They will be in harmony with the world around them. This being the case, they will unintentionally manifest their well-being through their attitude, behavior, and expressions to others. For the *Huangdi Neijing*, this is *shen*.

DAOISM

Like the *Huangdi Neijing*, Daoism arose in a time that reflected the transition from a shamanistic worldview to one based on observing the patterns and symbiotic relationships in an ever-changing environment. It was a period of political unrest, social instability, warfare between feudal states, and spiritual crisis, as belief in the Zhou dynasty (1027–221 BCE) deity Tian and the effectiveness of the sacrificial system was coming under serious doubt (Graham 1995; Schwartz 1985; Wong 1997).

According to tradition, the most fundamental text of Daoism, the *Daodejing*, attributed to Laozi (6th century BCE), was written to address this turmoil by teaching the ruler how to rule and people how to live in harmony with Dao. The primary goal was social harmony. The second major text of Daoism, the *Zhuangzi*, has been attributed, in part, to a man named Zhuang Zhou (4th-3rd century BCE). He simply focused on teaching people how to free themselves from self-imposed and societally imposed restrictions so they could live in harmony with Dao. The third major text, the *Liezi*, is attributed to Lie Yukou (late 5th-4th century BCE) who provided a practical approach to living in harmony with Dao. From a Western perspective, these writings, known in the West as Early Daoism, are viewed as essentially being philosophical in nature (*daojia*). The actual term *daojia* was coined during the late 2nd century BCE (Littlejohn 2016).

From a Western perspective, Daoism is considered to have become an organized religion during the Eastern Han dynasty (25–220 AD), when a man named Zhang Ling, in 142 CE, received a revelation from the deified Laozi (TaiShang Laojun). This revelation resulted in the subsequent creation of the Tianshi or Heavenly Masters sect of Daoism. Over the next thousand years or so, the *Shangqing* or Highest Clarity, *Lingbao* or Numinous Treasure, and *Quanzhen* or Complete Reality schools/sects were created. This grouping has come to be known as Later Daoism or religious Daoism (*daojiao*).

A commonality across this entire field is health and well-being. It is accomplished through simplifying life; *wuwei* or noninterference; *wushi* or not getting entangled in the activities of the world; yielding; noncontention; stilling (*jing*) and emptying (*xu*) the mind; being in harmony with yin and yang; integrating qi, shen, and jing; reducing desires; and practicing moderation. The goal is to achieve a oneness with Dao. Essentially, Daoism is a holistic approach to living life.

From a Chinese perspective, this distinction between philosophy and religion is artificial and does not capture the common thread that runs throughout Daoism. In fact, the Western tendency to separate philosophy, religion, spirituality, and health/well-being into distinct categories is fundamentally inconsistent with the Daoist holistic way of life.

Chronic Stress

Regarding health/well-being within the context of Daoism, the primary concern appears to be removing what we today call chronic stress. The following selection from the *Zhuangzi* provides a very clear picture of chronic stress and the significant negative impact it has on physical and psychological health and well-being:

When people are asleep their spirits are knotted up. When they are awake, their form is scattered. Interacting in the world creates entanglements. Daily their mind/hearts battle: plodding, concealing, and tentative. Their small fears result in apprehensiveness. Their large fears result in being overwhelmed. In their judging of right and wrong their words shoot out as if an arrow was released from a bow. They hold onto their judgments as if they were sacred oaths. Guarding what they call their victory, they are executed like autumn moving into winter. (Q. Guo 1956, 3/2/10-12[1]; Santee 2004)

It is important to note that this selection is not referring to specific individuals. It is essentially a statement about the overall human condition. This human condition is one of chronic stress. The continuous threat-based thinking that gives rise to chronic stress not only is harmful psychologically, it also harms the body.

This focus on threat-based thinking, its generation of chronic stress, and the physical and psychological harm that results from it is still apparent more than 900 years later. The Shangqing Daoist patriarch, Sima Chengzhen (647–735 CE) wrote a fundamental Daoist text called the *Zuowang lun* or *A Discussion on Sitting in Oblivion* (Kohn 2010). The link between threat-based thinking, chronic stress, and illness is described, respectively, in the *Shouxin* section and the *Shūyì* section or appendix of this text:

When you obsessively think about something and hold on to it, the mind/heart is strained. This is not only irrational, it causes the individual to become ill [*bing*]. (Saohua 2007)

If the mind/heart is restrained by excessive distress, the distress will lead to illness [*bìng*]. Frenzied, erratic and unstable breath is symptomatic of this. (Santee 2010)

The description of compromised breathing, shallow and rapid, is symptomatic of chronic stress and is one of the factors that distinguish a person who is chronically stressed from a person who is not. Probably the clearest selection in the *Zhuangzi* that distinguishes being free from chronic stress with being chronically stressed compares the *zhenren* who has a holistic lifestyle with everybody else (Kohn 2011):

The authentic person [*zhenren*] of ancient times slept without dreaming, upon awakening was not chronically stressed [*you*], ate without relishing, and breathed very deeply. The authentic person breathes from the heels. All other people breathe from their throats. Being restricted, their words are like a throat retching. Their desires long standing and deep, their essential nature is shallow. (Q. Guo 1956, 15/6/6-7; Santee 2004).[2]

The zhenren have a restful and undisturbed sleep because they do not dream. This is because they are free from self-imposed and societally imposed threats. They are not chronically stressed. The two most famous commentators to the *Zhuangzi* are Guo Xiang (252–312 CE) and Cheng Xuanying (fl. 631–652 CE). In his commentary regarding the zhenren not dreaming, Guo observes that the "Zhenren do not have any expectations" (Q. Guo 1974, 124; Santee 2008, 116). Cheng's sub-commentary on the same issue states:

Those who dream have vain hopes and unsatisfied wishes. The authentic person is without emotions and has cut off deliberation. Therefore, when they sleep they are anchored in a quiet place and do not dream. (Santee 2008, 116)

Because the zhenren are free from self-imposed and societally imposed restrictions, their minds are calm and at peace. As a result, they naturally breathe from the diaphragm. Thus, their breathing is deep or from their heels. Because other people have chronic unresolved desires, wishes, and expectations—in other words, self-imposed and societally imposed restrictions—their thinking is essentially threat based. Thus, their minds are continually agitated. This being the case, their fight/freeze/flight response is chronically activated. This has a direct impact on breathing, resulting in the shallow breathing that is a symptom of chronic stress. Thus, they are chronically stressed. Their physical and psychological health and well-being are compromised.

A Daoist Solution

According to the *Shūyì* section of or appendix to the *Zuowanglun*, there are three guidelines that practitioners must follow if they plan to merge with the Dao. To do so requires the elimination of chronic stress. Though listed as three separate guidelines, they are in fact all part of an interrelated, holistic, reciprocal process:

If you intend to return to the Dao, a deep and vivified faith [*xin*] must first receive three guidelines. . . . The first one is simplifying your circumstances. The second one is to be without desires, and the third one is to still the mind/heart. (Santee 2010, p. 13)

Individuals must have faith that the path they will be following will eliminate their chronic stress and allow them to return to the Dao. An intense and lively faith is necessary to receive and implement the three guidelines.

Simplifying your circumstances is both cognitive and behavioral in nature. The following three passages from the *Zhuangzi*, the first two from Chapter Four and the last one from Chapter Five, make this crystal clear:

Take responsibility for your own mind/heart so that sorrow and joy do not easily affect you. Knowing what you cannot resolve, and being at peace with it by adapting to destiny, is the perfection of power. As a subject and a son, there is that which you cannot avoid. Forget about your ego and deal with the situation.

Reside in the world by letting your mind/heart flow without any obstructions. Accepting what you cannot avoid as well as nourishing what is within is perfection. What more can be said?

To know what you cannot resolve and to be at peace with it by adapting to destiny, only the person of power can do this. (Santee 2011, p. 50)

For the Daoist, simplifying your circumstances is known as *wuwei*. *Wuwei* means not interfering with yourself and not trying to coerce others to do something for you for your own benefit. Given that in your life there is that which you cannot resolve and that which you cannot avoid, do not interfere with yourself psychologically and physically by wasting energy stressing yourself out trying to resolve that which you cannot resolve and avoiding that which you cannot avoid. Examine your lifestyle. Determine what is essential and healthy and what is not. Eliminate that which is not healthy and not essential.

A major occurrence that cannot be avoided is that of death. For the Daoist, death is merely another change. Stop wasting energy worrying about it and trying to figure out what will happen. Simplify your circumstances by dynamically acknowledging this change, and adapt to your destiny.

Death and life are destiny. They are as ordinary as night and day. They are natural. They cannot be interfered with by people. They are the circumstances of all things. (Q. Guo 1956, 16/6/2021; Santee 2004, p. 6)

Being without desires means not having excessive desires. It is not letting your senses and thoughts control and chronically stress you. It is not getting entangled (*wushi*) in the activities of the world. It is not letting the activities of the world control and chronically stress you. Thus, the *Daodejing* says:

The greatest calamity is not knowing when enough is enough. The greatest fault is the desire [*yu*] for purely self-benefit and gain. (Yang 1972, ch. 46)

Those who maintain this Dao, do not desire [*bu yu*] excessiveness. (Yang 1972, ch. 15)

See the plain, maintain simplicity [*po*]. Eliminate selfishness, have few desires [*yu*]. (Yang 1972, ch. 19)

Essentially, both simplifying your circumstances and reducing your desires consist of practicing wuwei, wushi, and moderation. This is the mind-based, cognitive, investigative, behavioral, and intentional perspective for the elimination of chronic stress. The specific focus is on addressing agitation and threat-based thinking. This is made quite clear in Chapters 48 and 67, respectively, of the *Daodejing* and Chapter 29 of the *Zhuangzi*.

Through the practice of wuwei there is nothing that cannot be accomplished. To obtain the world, don't get entangled with the activities of the world [wushi]. (Santee 2007, p. 154)

I have three treasures which I preserve and protect. The first is compassion [*ci*]. The second is moderation [*jian*]. The third is not daring to be prior to the world. (K. Wang 1993, p. 67)

Moderation is happiness. Excessiveness is harmful. There is no activity in life where this is not so! (Q. Guo 1956, 84/29/92-93)

Stilling your mind/heart is naturally emptying it of all the self-induced and societally induced agitation. This perspective is body-based, experiential, and nonintentional. It is essentially meditation. There is no focus on agitation or threat-based thinking. There are no judgments. It is essentially being completely in the present, letting the mind/heart naturally still and empty. In the *Shouxin* section of the *Zuowanglun*, the practice of the meditative technique *zuowang* is described:

When you begin to study the Dao, it is essential to sit peacefully, focus your attention, let go of all concerns, and not dwell on anything. Because you are not dwelling on anything, you are not affected by a single thing. You will naturally enter emptiness. The mind/heart merges with Dao. (Santee 2010, p. 11)

The implementation of these three guidelines is common across all manifestations of Daoism. For the practitioner, following this path (*Dao*) not only results in the removal of chronic stress and the establishment of optimal health and well-being, it allows the practitioner to merge with Dao. In this sense, even though the Daoist would not make such a distinction, health, well-being, and spirituality are intimately intertwined.

CONFUCIANISM

Confucius (551-479 BCE) lived in a time of social and political instability. Authenticity, trust, respect, and empathy between individuals were problematic, as self-centeredness and personal gain appeared to dominate interpersonal behavior. The goal of Confucius and subsequent Confucians throughout its extensive history was to teach rulers and government officials how to govern and live their lives for the purpose of establishing social harmony. The methodology was that of teaching moral self-cultivation. The expectation was that the morally correct behavior of the officials would serve as a role model and, being observed by others, it would be dutifully assimilated and put into practice. Confucius looked back to the ancients for role models of appropriate moral interpersonal behavior and the ideal government. His teachings were compiled by his followers in the *Lunyu* (the *Analects*).

For Confucius, however, the fundamental foundation for all his teachings was the family. It is in a healthy family dynamic where one first learns to positively interact with others in an authentic, loving, respectful, trusting, and empathetic manner. As a society in social harmony was the goal of the Confucians at the macro level, it is the harmony of the family, not the individual, that is of primary importance at the micro level.

Confucianism is clearly not an organized, formal religion (Adler 2014). The Dao for Confucius was a moral Dao. On the surface, the teachings of Confucius do not appear to be oriented toward spirituality or anything that would fall within the realm of the sacred:

Li Lu asked about the affairs of supernatural beings [*guishen*]. The Master (Confucius) said, "You do not know of the affairs of people, how can you ask about the affairs of the supernatural beings?" "May I venture to ask about death?" The Master said, "You do not know about life. How can you know about death?" (Santee 2007, p. 260; *Analects* n.d., Book XI)

Confucius overlooking a flowing river said, "Everything passes away like this! Not stopping day or night." (*Analects* n.d., Book IX)

Confucius did not address or discuss the spirits and the afterlife because such a discussion was simply not relevant; for him, cultivating and living a moral life in the present and establishing social harmony was most important. His concern was the positive and respectful interaction between people, with the common goal of establishing social harmony. Nevertheless, from a Western perspective, his focus on the ideal, authentic, trusting, respectful, and empathetic interaction between individuals for the purpose of establishing social harmony appears to border on that of spirituality and sacredness (Fingarette 1972).

Chronic Stress

Confucius makes a clear distinction between his role model for appropriate behavior, the morally integrated person or *junzi*, and the morally fragmented person or *xiaoren*. The junzi practice moderation while the xiaoren are excessive and/or deficient in their behavior. It is quite apparent from the descriptions that the junzi are concerned for the common good and are free from chronic stress. The xiaoren, in contrast, are concerned for self-benefit and are chronically stressed.

Confucius said, "If one's primitive stuff/physicality [*zhi*] overwhelms refinement/cultural patterns of behavior [*wen*], then there is unruliness. If refinement/culture patterns of behavior overwhelm one's primitive stuff/physicality, then there is a parading of one's learning. Refinement/culture patterns of behavior and the primitive stuff/physicality must be equally distributed. Then there is the *junzi*." (Santee 2007, p. 195; *Analects* n.d., Book VI)

The Master said, "The *junzi* is composed and at peace. The *xiaoren* is chronically agitated and distressed." (Santee 2007, p. 205; *Analects* n.d., Book XII)

The Master said, "The *junzi* is calm and not arrogant, the *xiaoren* is arrogant and not calm." (Santee 2007, p. 205; *Analects* n.d., Book XIII)

The Master said, "The *junzi* is guided by appropriate contextual moral choice, the xiaoren is guided by personal gain." (Santee 2007, p. 197; *Analects* n.d., Book IV)

Si Maniu (a disciple of Confucius) asked about the *junzi*. The Master replied, "The *junzi* is not chronically stressed [*bu you*] nor fearful [*buju*]. Si Maniu said, "If a person is not chronically stressed and not fearful, it then can be said the person is a *junzi*? The Master said, "Finding neither fault nor illness within himself, why should he be chronically stressed or fearful?" (Santee 2007, p. 50; *Analects* n.d., Book XII)

Solution

To establish social harmony, individuals needed to move from the perspective of the xiaoren to that of the junzi. It required a move from being unhealthy to being healthy. To do so obviously necessitated a change in behavior.

For Confucius, there are several fundamental concepts that guide one's behavior. *Li* is appropriate, contextual moral behavior. For Confucius, depending upon the context and the individuals within it, there is a pre-scribed morally acceptable way to behave. This behavior manifests authenticity, trust, respect, and empathy. *Yi* or appropriate, contextual moral choice refers to correctly choosing, based on the context and individuals within it, the appropriate, contextual moral behavior or li. Both li and yi are directed toward the benefit of all those involved and ultimately the benefit of society. It is not for personal benefit or self-gain. The initial context for learning li and yi is in the family.

The highest virtue for Confucius is that of interpersonal, selfless love or *ren*. *Ren* exists only in the relationship between people. It is not a characteristic of the individual. It manifests during an interaction. It is intimately intertwined with li and yi. Ren cannot occur if chronic stress is present.

Yan Yuan (a disciple of Confucius) asked about interpersonal selfless love [*ren*]. The Master said, "Overcoming your self-centeredness and returning to appropriate, contextual moral behavior [*li*] is *ren*. If for one day people overcame their self-centeredness and returned to *li*, then the whole world would come together in *ren*. This is because *ren* is due to the relationship between yourself and other people" Yan Yuan said, "May I ask about what this entails?" The Master said, "If it is not appropriate contextual behavior [*li*] do not look. If it is not li, do not listen. If it is not li, do not speak. Do not do anything contrary to li." Yan Yuan said, "Although I am not very smart, I will engage in what you have said." (Santee 2007, p. 197; *Analects* n.d., Book XII)

Fan Chi asked about *ren*. Confucius said "Love the people." He asked about *zhi*. The Master said, "Recognize the difference between good and bad behavior." (Santee 2007, p. 198; *Analects* n.d., Book XII)

For the Confucian, moral self-cultivation is a continuous process of self-cultivation in which individuals are always monitoring, examining, correcting, and improving their thinking and behavior. The purpose of this process of self-cultivation is twofold. The first is for the elimination of self-centeredness, narcissism, desire for self-gain and self-benefit, and the removal of any other inappropriate thinking and behavior. The removal of this negative thinking behavior results in the elimination of chronic stress and the physical and psychological damage associated with it. The second is for the development of authenticity, trust, respect, and empathy. It results in the wisdom of yi, li, and ren. It also results in the positive physical and psychological health and well-being of the junzi.

Cengzi [a disciple of Confucius] said, "I daily examine myself in three areas. In working for other people, have I not done my best/been authentic [*zhong*]? In interacting with my friends have I not been trustworthy [*xin*]? Have I not practiced what has been passed on to me?" (Santee 2007, p. 194; *Analects* n.d., Book I)

The Master said, "When traveling with 3 people, I will certainly have teachers. I will select that which is good and follow it. That which is not good, I will change it in myself." (Santee 2007, p. 194; *Analects* n.d., Book VII)

Confucius said, "Zeng [a disciple of Confucius]! My *Dao* uses a single thread." Zengzi said, "So it does." The Master left. The disciples asked, "What did he mean?" Zengzi said, "The way of the Master is doing your best, being authentic [*zhong*] and being empathic [*shu*]. That's it!" (Santee 2007, p. 201; *Analects* n.d., Book IV)

"What you do not desire, do not impose on others." (Santee 2007, p. 202; *Analects* n.d., Book XV)

Fan Chi [a disciple of Confucius] asked about *ren*. The Master said, "In your home be respectful [*gong*], in managing your affairs be attentive [*jing*], and when interacting with others do your best/be authentic [*zhong*]. Even if you were amongst the barbarian tribes, it is not possible to abandon these." (Santee 2007, p. 203; *Analects* n.d., 3 Book XIII)

From the perspective of Confucius, health and well-being are intimately intertwined with appropriate moral behavior, which is interpersonal in nature. In the West, health and well-being are something found in the individual. For Confucius, true health and well-being are found in the relationship between people: a relationship that expresses trust, sincerity, authenticity, empathy, and respect among the participants. A fundamental component of this relationship is the practice of moderation.

Confucius said, "The 300 odes in the *Shijing* [Book of Songs], can be summed up in single phrase." He said, "Your thinking and behavior remain healthy by not going astray." (Santee 2007, p. 191; *Analects* n.d., Book II)

Confucius said, "Practicing moderation [*zhongyong*] is supreme moral excellence [*de*]. It has been rarely seen amongst the people for a long time." (Santee 2007, p. 207; *Analects* n.d., Book VI)

From a Western perspective, the question is whether this process of moral self-cultivation represents spirituality. From a Confucian perspective, the question is not relevant. The question is what constitutes the path to being truly human.

Confucius said, "The path [*Dao*] of the *Junzi* has three aspects of which I am incapable: Regarding *ren*, the *Junzi* is not chronically stressed [*you*]. Regarding knowing [*zhi*], the Junzi is not perplexed [*huo*]. Regarding courage [*yong*], the *Junzi* is not fearful [*ju*]." Zi Gong [a disciple of Confucius] said, "Master. This is your path!" (Santee 2007, p. 51; *Analects* n.d., Book XIV)

RESEARCH

The domain of Western medicine, and the science in which it is based, is extremely conservative. If the claims that are made about the occurrence of natural events, such as "acupuncture eliminated my pain," cannot be demonstrated in methodically sound, randomized controlled trials (RCTs), where the variables are operationalized, measured, statistically analyzed, and subject to replication and eventual meta-analysis, then for all intents and purposes the claims are not valid. Such is a conclusion about the benefits of acupuncture (Colquhoun and Novella 2013). This focus on the scientific method and evidence-based research certainly has been an argument against Traditional Chinese Medicine (TCM) and its most fundamental components such as jing, qi, the internal meridians through which qi flows, shen, yin and yang, and Dao (Novella 2012).

There are certainly no such studies regarding the overall effect of Daoism and Confucianism, with or without the context of religion and/or spirituality, on health and well-being. There are several articles advocating the importance of including Confucian moral philosophy, concepts, sense of family, and personhood as a framework to assist health professionals in understanding East Asian/Chinese patients' beliefs regarding health and illness, address and explore issues in bioethics, determine resource allocations, and in approaching and interacting with these patients (Fan 2002; Park and Chesla 2007; Z. Guo 1995; Shih 1996; Tsai 2001, 2005). These are, however, theory-focused articles, not evidence-based research.

The Daoist-related practices such as taijiquan and qigong are primarily oriented to health and well-being. Both practices focus on diaphragmatic breathing, slow movements, and focused, nonjudgmental awareness of the present. They both are, in one sense, forms of moving meditation. The major difference is that taijiquan is also a martial art. There is no real downside to practicing taijiquan and qigong. The basic concepts from both the *Huangdi Neijing* and Daoism, such as the continual process of change, yin and yang, qi, shen, jing, Dao, stilling and emptying the mind, deep diaphragmatic breathing, being in harmony, and moderation are clearly present.

The results of research, using the Western scientific method, into the benefits of taijiquan and qigong are mixed. The major issues concern methodology, sample sizes, issues with control groups, randomization, and design, with the primary concern being the necessity for more randomized controlled trials. Some of the research suggests positive benefits for balance, bone health, sleep, cardiovascular fitness, quality of life, certain physical functioning, self-efficacy, exercising for the elderly, exercising for those who are recovering from or at risk for coronary heart disease, stress management, enhancing the immune system, lowering blood pressure with hypertensive patients, and psychological well-being (Dalusung-Angosta 2011; Jahnke, Larkey, Rogers, Etnier, and Lin 2010; Lee, Pittler, Guo, and Ernst 2007; Liu 2010; Ng and Tsang 2009; C. Wang et al. 2010; Wayne and Furst 2013).

There is no question that meditation practices such as mindfulness and the relaxation response are significantly beneficial for physical and psychological health and well-being (Benson 2000; Kabat-Zinn 2005; Kohn 2008b; Santee 2005a, 2005b, 2008; Walsh and Shapiro 2006). An integral aspect of Daoism is meditation. However, there appears to be no RCTs of specific Daoist meditation practices such as sitting in oblivion (*zuowang*). This being the case, according to the standards of the scientific community, no claims can be made about the physical and psychological benefits of practicing zuowang until it has undergone a strict scientific analysis.

This barrier would also seem to apply to a holistic lifestyle approach oriented toward eliminating chronic stress which integrated diet, exercise, meditation, interpersonal interactions, sleep, the simplifying of psychological and behavioral circumstances, moderation, and the reduction of desires, such as found in the approach of the *Huangdi Neijing*, Daoism, and Confucianism. There certainly appears to be no downside to following a holistic lifestyle, with moderation being front and center. However, is following a holistic lifestyle only beneficial if the scientific community has RCT results that say it is?

CONCLUSION

Across the *Huangdi Neijing*, Daoism, and Confucianism, the common solution for enhancing health and well-being is the removal of what we call chronic stress. This is accomplished by accepting change as fundamental, practicing a holistic lifestyle, following the three Daoist guidelines, and practicing moderation. Although these approaches are certainly relevant for addressing illness and disease, they are fundamentally preventive in nature. As far as the relationship, within the context of Chinese thought, among religion, spirituality, health, and well-being is concerned, this is a decision each person must make.

NOTES

1. The format of 3/2/10-12, for citation of the original Chinese text, indicates the page/chapter/lines in the Harvard-Yenching Institute Sinological Index Series (HYSIS) Supplement 20, *A Concordance to Chuang Tzu* (Q. Guo 1956).

2. The character *you* has the meaning of worry, sorrow, anxiety, sadness, melancholy, suffering, etc.; thus the interpretation/translation as chronic stress.

REFERENCES

Adler, J. A. 2014. *Confucianism as a Religious Tradition: Linguistic and Methodological Problems.* Paper presented at the Institute for Advanced Studies in Humanities and Social Sciences, National Taiwan University (Taipei) and the Department of Philosophy, Tunghai University (Taichung).

Analects. n.d. Retrieved from http://www.chineseclassic.com/13jing/LeungYu/LeungYu01.htm

Avey, H., K. B. Matheny, A. Robbins, and T. A. Jacobson. 2003. "Health Care Providers' Training, Perceptions, and Practices Regarding Stress and Health Outcomes. *Journal of the National Medical Association* 95: 836–845.

Benson, H. 1996. *Timeless Healing: The Power and Biology of Belief.* New York: Scribner.

Benson, H. 1998, September 22. Testimony of Herbert Benson Regarding Mind/Body Interventions, Healthcare and Mind/Body Medical Centers Before the United States Senate Appropriations Subcommittee on Labor/HHS & Education, Senator Arlen Specter, Chairman. Senate Hearing 105-875. Washington, DC: U.S. Government Printing Office. Retrieved from https://www.gpo.gov/fdsys/pkg/CHRG-105shrg54619/pdf/CHRG-105shrg54619.pdfg

Benson, H. 2000. *The Relaxation Response.* New York: Harper.

Benson, H., and A. Casey. (Eds.) 2013. *A Harvard Medical School Special Report: Stress Management.* Boston: Harvard Medical School.

Buss, D. M. 2015. *Evolutionary Psychology: The New Science of the Mind.* Boston: Pearson.

Cheng, C.-Y. 2003a. "Dao (Tao): The Way." In A. S. Cua, ed., *Encyclopedia of Chinese Philosophy,* pp. 202–206. New York: Routledge.

Cheng, C.-Y. 2003b. "Qi (Ch'i): Vital Force." In A. S. Cua, ed., *Encyclopedia of Chinese Philosophy,* pp. 615–617. New York: Routledge.

Citizens Commission on Human Rights (CCHR). 2016. "Real Disease vs. Mental "Disorder." Retrieved from August 10, 2016, from http://www.cchr.org/quick-facts/real-disease-vs-mental-disorder.html

Colquhoun, D., and S. P. Novella. 2013. "Acupuncture Is Theatrical Placebo." *Anesthesia & Analgesia* 116: 1360–1363.

Dalusung-Angosta, A. 2011. "The Impact of Tai Chi Exercise on Coronary Heart Disease: A Systematic Review." *Journal of the American Academy of Nurse Practitioners* 23: 376–381.

Fan, R. 2002. "Reconstructionist Confucianism and Health Care: An Asian Moral Account of Health Care Allocation." *Journal of Medicine and Philosophy* 27: 675–682.

Fingarette, H. 1972. *Confucius: The Secular as Sacred.* New York: Harper Torchbooks.

Graham, A. C. 1995. *Disputers of the Dao: Philosophical Argument in Ancient China.* Chicago: Open Court.

Guo, Q. 1956. *A Concordance to Chuang Tzu* (HYSIS 20). Cambridge, MA: Harvard University Press.

Guo, Q. 1974. *Zhuangzi Jishi* (2 vols.). Taipei: Chung Hwa Book.

Guo, Z. 1995. "Chinese Confucian Culture and the Medical Ethical Tradition." *Journal of Medical Ethics* 21: 239–246.

Huangdi Neijing. n.d. Retrieved from http://ctext.org/huangdi-neijing/zh and http://www.teachingfromtheroots.com/texts/Huang_Di_Nei_Jing.html

Jahnke, R., L. Larkey, C. Rogers, J. Etnier, and F. Lin. 2010. "A Comprehensive Review of Health Benefits of Qigong and Tai Chi." *American Journal of Health Promotion* 24: e1-e25. doi:10.4278/ajhp.081013-LIT-248. Retrieved from https://www.ncbi.nlm.nih.gov/pmc/articles/PMC3085832/?tool

Kabat-Zinn, J. 2005. *Full Catastrophe Living: Using the Wisdom of Your Body and Mind to Face Stress, Pain, and Illness.* New York: Random House.

Koenig, H. G. 2012. "Religion, Spirituality and Health: The Research and Clinical Implications." *ISRN Psychiatry* 2012: 1–33. Retrieved from https://www.ncbi.nlm.nih.gov/pmc/articles/PMC3671693/

Kohn, L. 2008a. *Chinese Healing Exercises: The Tradition of Daoyin.* Honolulu: University of Hawaii Press.

Kohn, L. 2008b. *Meditation Works: In the Hindu, Buddhist and Daoist Traditions.* St. Petersburg, FL: Three Pines Press.

Kohn, L. 2010. *Sitting in Oblivion: The Heart of Daoist Meditation.* Petersburg, FL: Three Pines Press.

Kohn, L. 2012. *A Source Book in Chinese Longevity.* Petersburg, FL: Three Pines Press.

Lee, M. S., M. H. Pittler, R. Guo, and E. Ernst. 2007. "Qigong for Hypertension: A Systematic Review of Randomized Clinical Trials." *Journal of Hypertension* 25: 1525–1532.

Littlejohn, R. 2016. "Daoist Philosophy." In *The Internet Encyclopedia of Philosophy.* Retrieved from http://www.iep.utm.edu/daoism/

Liu, T. ed. 2010. *Chinese Medical Qigong.* London: Singing Dragon.

McEwen, B., and E. N. Lasley. 2002. *The End of Stress as We Know It.* Washington, DC: Joseph Henry Press.

Nerurkar, A., A. Bitton, R. B. Davis, R. S. Phillips, and G. Yeh. 2013. "When Physicians Counsel About Stress: Results of a National Study." *JAMA Internal Medicine* 173: 76–77.

Nesse, R. N., and E. A. Young. 2000. "Evolutionary Origins and Functions of the Stress Response." Retrieved from http://www-personal.umich.edu/~nesse/Articles/Stress&Evolution-2000.PDF

Ng, B. H. P., and H. W. H. Tsang. 2009. "Psychophysiological Outcome of Health Qigong for Chronic Conditions: A Systematic Review." *Psychophysiology* 46: 257–269.

Novella, S. 2012. "What Is Traditional Chinese Medicine." Retrieved from https://www.sciencebasedmedicine.org/what-is-traditional-chinese-medicine/

Park, M., and C. Chesla. 2007. "Revisiting Confucianism as a Conceptual Framework for Asian Family Study." *Journal of Family Nursing* 13(3): 293–311.

Santee, R. 2004. *A Daoist and an Existential Psychotherapist: A Comparative Study.* Paper presented at the 1st World Hong Ming Philosophy Conference, Chaminade University of Honolulu, July 22.

Santee, R. 2005a. *Cultivating Emptiness: The Practice of Xinzhai, An Ancient Daoist Solution for the Problem of Chronic Stress.* Paper presented at the International Conference of Daoist Cultivation and Its Modern Value, Sichuan University, Chengdu, China, October 11–15.

Santee, R. 2005b. "Wandering through the Dao, While the Dao Wanders through All: The Dao of the Daodejing." *Empty Vessel: The Journal of Taoist Philosophy and Practice* 12: 16–21.

Santee, R. 2007. *An Integrative Approach to Counseling: Bridging Chinese Thought, Evolutionary Theory, and Stress Management.* Thousand Oaks, CA: Sage.

Santee, R. 2008. "Stress Management and the Zhuangzi." *Journal of Daoist Studies* 1: 93–123.

Santee, R. 2010. *Sitting in Forgetfulness and the Relaxation Response: An Inquiry into Managing the Physical and Psychological Symptoms of Chronic Stress.* Paper presented at The 6th International Daoist Studies Conference: "Daoism Today: Science, Health and Ecology," Los Angeles, California, June 2–6.

Santee, R. 2011. "The Zhuangzi: A Holistic Approach to Healthcare and Well-Being." In L. Kohn, ed., *Living Authentically: Daoist Contributions to Modern Psychology*, pp. 39–58. Petersburg, FL: Three Pines Press.

Santee, R., and X. Zhang. 2015. "Yangsheng and the Yin Style Baguazhang of Wang Fu and Wang Shangzhi." *Empty Vessel: The Journal of Taoist Philosophy and Practice* 22: 24–30.

Saohua. 2007. "Zuowanglun." Retrieved from http://www.saohua.com/shuku/zongjiao/daojiao/011.htm

Sapolsky, R. M. 1998. *Why Zebras Don't Get Ulcers: An Updated Guide to Stress, Stress-Related Diseases, and Coping.* New York: W. H. Freeman.

Schwartz, B. I. 1985. *The World of Thought in Ancient China.* Cambridge, MA: Belknap Press.

Seligman, M. 2006. *Learned Optimism: How to Change Your Mind and Your Life.* New York: Random House.

Selye, H. 1978. *The Stress of Life.* New York: McGraw-Hill.

Shi, L., and C. Zhang. 2012. "Spirituality in Traditional Chinese Medicine." *Pastoral Psychology* 61 (5–6): 959–974.

Shih, F.-J. 1996. "Concepts Related to Chinese Patients' Perceptions of Health, Illness, and Person: Issues of Conceptual Clarity." *Accident and Emergency Nursing* 4: 208–215.

Sørensen, J. G., M. Holmstrup, P. Sarup, and V. Loeschcke. 2010. "Evolutionary Theory and Studies of Model Organisms Predict a Cautiously Positive Perspective on the Therapeutic Use of Hormesis for Healthy Aging in Humans." *Dose-Response: An International Journal* 8(1): art. 12. Retrieved from http://scholarworks.umass.edu/dose_response/vol8/iss1/12

Stefano, G. B., G. L. Fricchione, B. T. Slingsby, and H. Benson. 2001. "The Placebo Effect and Relaxation Response: Neural Processes and Their Coupling to Constitutive Nitric Oxide." *Brain Research Reviews* 35: 1–19

Stuart, E. M., A. Webster, and C. L. Wells-Federman. 1993. "Managing Stress." In H. Benson and E. Stuart, eds., *The Wellness Book: The Comprehensive Guide to Maintaining Health and Treating Stress Related Illness*, pp. 177–188. New York: Simon & Schuster.

Tsai, D. F.-C. 2001. "How Should Doctors Approach Patients? A Confucian Reflection on Personhood." *Journal of Medical Ethics* 27: 44–50.

Tsai, D. F.-C. 2005. "The Bioethical Principles and Confucius' Moral Philosophy." *Journal of Medical Ethics* 31: 159–163.

Walsh, R., and S. Shapiro. 2006. "The Meeting of Meditative Disciplines and Western Psychology." *American Psychologist* 61: 227–239.

Wang, C., R. Bannuru, J. Ramel, B. Kupelnick, T. Scott, and C. H. Schmid. 2010. "Tai Chi on Psychological Well-Being: Systematic Review and Meta-Analysis." *Complementary and Alternative Medicine* 10: 1–16. Retrieved from https://www.ncbi.nlm.nih.gov/pmc/articles/PMC2893078/

Wang, K. 1993. *Laozi Daodejing He Shanggong Zhangju*. Beijing: Zhonghua Shuju.

Wayne, P. M., and M. L. Furst. 2013. *The Harvard Medical School Guide to Tai Chi: 12 Weeks to a Healthy Body, Strong Heart & Sharp Mind*. Boston: Shambala.

WebMD. 2016. "How Does Stress Affect Health?" Retrieved from http://www.webmd.com/balance/stress-management/effects-of-stress-on-your-body

Wong, E. 1997. *Taoism: An Essential Guide*. Boston: Shambhala.

Yang, J. (Zhubian). 1972. *Laozi Benyi, Laozi Xin Kao Shu Lue*. Taibei: Shi Jie Shu Ju.

Zhang, D. 2002. *Key Concepts in Chinese Philosophy* (E. Ryden, trans.). New Haven: Yale University Press.

Zhang, Y. H., and K. Rose. 2001. *A Brief History of Qi*. Brookline, MA: Paradigm.

Zhouyi [Book of Changes]. n.d. J. Legge, trans. Retrieved from http://ctext.org/book-of-changes/xi-ci-shang/zh

Chapter 5

Ways of Healing and the Roles of Harmony, Purity, and Violent Rhetoric in Japanese Shinto and Shamanism

Carl Olson

The importance of healing in Japanese culture is evident from ancient times based on documentary evidence of some ancient texts. The *Kojiki* (Record of Ancient Matters), a text compiled and edited in 712 CE by the courtier Ō no Yasumaro during the Heian period, is very suggestive because it demonstrates a concern with the interior of the body. For example, following his deceased spouse into the underworld, a husband spies his wife and, with the help of a torch to light the scene, perceives squirming maggots slithering in and out of her body, and equates various parts of her body with different types of thunder (Heldt 2014, pp. 14–15). This scenario enables us to make a close connection between divine beings or spirits (*kami*) and elements of nature, as well as witness a somatic focus, especially impure maggots in this case. This grotesque scene suggests that impurity is associated with death and disorder, and points to the importance of purity and order that are equated with harmony in the world. Within the narrative context of its creation myth, the *Kojiki* also relates the creation of various spirits (*kami*) from the bodily waste of the goddess, such as Kneading Clay Lady from her excrement, Water Gushing Woman from her urine, and Metal

Mountain Lad from her vomit (Heldt 2014, p. 13). In another part of the narrative, Lady Great Sustenance was asked for food by Rushing Raging Man and produced it from her nose, mouth, and buttocks. The male *kami* thought that she fouled the food before offering it to him, which outraged him and caused him to slay her (Heldt 2014, p. 25). This narrative indicates the importance of maintaining purity as it is related to edible food. It is safe to say that the origins of the food from the interior of the body gives the impression in this case of its being impure, with dire consequences for the producer. The tale implies a connection between food, impurity, and illness.

In the *Nihongishoki* (Chronicles of Japan, also known as the *Nihongi*) that was composed in 720 CE by a committee of scholars with the purpose of countering Ō no's excessive emphasis on the imperial Yamato clan appearing in the *Kojiki*, the imperial family stresses the singular nature of the imperial way and directs its soldiers to destroy traitors and get citizens to accept a political oath of loyalty. If subjects break the oath, they risk being punished by a plague sent from heaven (Ashton 2008, p. 38). The possibility of plagues in ancient Japan was a constant concern of the populace as it was in other parts of the globe, and connected the emperor with the health and well-being of his subjects. Later in the text, the composers justify the emperor by linking him to the Sun goddess, Amaterasu, and attributing direct descent by the emperor from the goddess (Ashton 2008, pp. 59–60). This suggests that the emperor is the son of the goddess, and therefore fit to rule because of his divine status.

Around 760 CE, another ancient text was compiled that was called the *Manyōshū* (Collection of 10,000 Leaves), comprising a vast anthology of Japanese poetry on subjects such as religion, myth, and secular themes. The collection contains classical Japanese verses called *tankas* and longer poems called *choka* that focus on the imperial family. These poems also refer to issues related to illness and health. Awareness of the impermanent nature of the body and a wish for long lifespan is expressed in the following poem:

> I know well this body of mine
> Is insubstantial as foam;
> Even so, how I wish
> For a life of a thousand years! (Shinkōkai 1965, p. 180)

Another poem stresses the connection between old age, illness, pain, and suffering:

> So long as lasts the span of life,
> We wish for peace and comfort

With no evil and no mourning,
But life is hard and painful.
As the common saying has it,
Bitter salt is poured into the smarting wound,
Or the burdened horse is packed with an upper load,
Illness shakes my old body with pain. (Shinkōkai 1965, p. 208)

The poet continues by referring to breathing grief, sighing at night, lingering illness, groaning at the pain, and wishing to die, but he is unable to leave his children, implying the importance of social relations and that his suffering will continue into the future.

In the ancient texts, further evidence about the importance of health is provided by the *Nihon ryōiki* (The Record of Miraculous Events in Japan), an initial collection of anecdotal literature in Japanese literary history composed around 822 CE. The Japanese term for anecdotes (*setsuwa*) means "spoken story," which suggests an oral narrative tradition that was eventually written down by Keikai or Kyōkai. This text includes Buddhist figures and the influence of the law of karma (cause and effect). The author claims to be a self-ordained priest, with just such a priest named Gyōgi (668–749) playing a leading role in the text. After gaining a sizable popular following, Gyōgi was prosecuted by the government, but was later asked to build a large statue of the Buddha at the Tōdaiji temple in 794. In contrast to earlier chronicles previously mentioned, in which disease was treated by communal means and cleansing by purification, in the *Nihon ryōiki* disease is the punishment for moral/ethical failures or transgressions during the course of previous modes of existence, according to the irrevocable working of the law of karma that follows one through one's former and current life times like an unshakable shadow. In one tale, a pious female named Hōni, a daughter of a nun, was collecting herbs in the mountains when she saw a snake swallowing a frog. Attempting to save the frog's life, she agreed to marry the snake if it released the frog. Before the snake arrived at her house on the agreed seventh day, she barred herself inside while the snake pounded on the walls. The next day she escaped to Gyōgi in the mountains, but he told her that she could not reject her agreement with the snake. On the way home, she encountered a man with a crab that she exchanged for her skirt and then set it free. When the snake gained entry into her house on the eighth day, through her roof, she was very frightened, but heard a noise on her bed. The next day she saw that the crab had chopped the snake into bits as an act of gratitude for her saving its life (Watson 2013, pp. 79–80).

The *Nihon ryōiki* also contains narratives more directly related to illness. For example, a monk named Azumahito practiced Buddhist doctrine and prayed for good fortune to the bodhisattva Kannon. The virgin daughter of a court official became very ill, without any hope of a cure. Her father asked for help, and Azumahito healed her by chanting spells. The daughter fell in love with him, they married despite her family's objections, and he assumed care of the families' wealth (Watson 2013, pp. 53–54). In another episode, a woman is attacked by a large snake, but she survives after being treated by drugs (Watson 2013, pp. 124). Another narrative relates the tale of a fox killed in a previous life taking revenge on a man who arrives at the temple to ask the monk Yōgō to help him. The monk chanted sacred *mantras* (sacred language formulas) that improved the man's condition, but the man's health would regress when the monk stopped chanting. The fox spirit revealed itself to the monk, and told him that his chanting was useless because the victim had killed the fox in a previous life and the inflicted illness was recompense for that evil act. After the victim died, he returned as a dog and killed the fox (Watson 2013, pp. 137–138). The text also contains tales of adhering faithfully to one's religion and gaining a cure for an illness. With a heavy Buddhist influence, this text demonstrates the interconnection between the law of karma, illness as a form of punishment, and regaining health using religious means.

The purpose of briefly reviewing these ancient texts was to demonstrate that Japanese concerns about health, and its restoration after being lost, were fundamental to its culture, which is a concern that extends from ancient times to more recent history. In order to grasp this thread in Japanese culture, this chapter focuses on Shinto, an indigenous religion, and shamanism, which shows evidence of influence from inner Asian practice. What role did health and healing play in these religious ways of life? How did Shinto and shamanism attempt to deal with and restore health? Shinto and its practices are examined first, before we turn to a consideration of shamanism. Both of them have had a long history in Japan. In addition, they have to some extent become intertwined in Japanese culture with each other and Buddhism.

To answer the types of questions raised in the previous paragraph, this chapter begins by discussing the nature of Shinto, the intertwining of Shinto and Buddhism, and the relationship between Shinto, the Japanese islands, and the way of the *kami*. Within Shintoism, concerns are expressed for health, illness, and healing that are interconnected with notions such as harmony, pollution, purification, and the conception of the human body. In the following section, attention is paid not only to these issues, but also to the wide variety of ways for dealing with illness. Other topics include the relationship between divine beings, disease, and healing; the ancient connection between pilgrimage and healing; and the popular use of practices intended to prevent or restore health by using amulets and visiting temples. To provide a broader view of healing in Japan, the role of shamanism in healing is examined. Finally, this chapter touches briefly on the relation between healing and violence, because restoring health is often conceived as a battle, with violent and military overtones.

THE WAY OF SHINTO

Scholars have called attention to a vagueness that surrounds the term *Shinto* that makes it difficult to accurately define. Within the context of discussing the Emperor Yōmei (ruled 585–587 CE), the *Nihongishoki* records the first use of the term when it mentions the emperor's faith in Buddhism and Shinto and his role as a deity. During its early usage, the term Shinto was used as a synonym for Japan's native deities or *kami* (Nobutaka 2003, p. 1). But the term was not used to indicate an indigenous religion, which did not occur until Yoshida Kanetomo (1435–1511 CE) applied the term to a coherent or independent religious system (Naumann 2000, p. 64). This development occurred gradually during the medieval period, as people conceived of Shinto with an increasing awareness of their ethnic self-identity. Instead of designating an identifiable religion, the term Shinto was used primarily to refer to "the *kami* way" (Teeuwen and Sheid 2002, p. 199; *see also* Teeuwen 2002). Moreover, Shinto, a synonym for *kami*, began to assume a more sectarian identity during the medieval period in reaction to the introduction of Buddhism into Japan.

The interaction of Shinto, an indigenous tradition, with Buddhism, a foreign religious tradition from Korea and China, sparked an amalgamation of the two traditions that was called *Shinbutsu shūgō* (meaning *shin* or *kami*, *butsu* or buddhas, and *shūgō* or amalgamation). Beginning in the Nara period (710–940 CE), *kami* and buddhas began to merge, with the development culminating in the late Heian period (794–1192 CE). The rationale for this syncretic movement specified that *kami* were emanations of Buddhist divine beings left on Japan, implying that Buddhism constituted the original source of the *kami* (Satoshi 2003, p. 68). The theory also claimed that these buddhas manifested themselves as *kami* in order to bring salvation to the Japanese, an assertion called *honji suijaku* that literally means "leaving a trace" such as a footprint (Satoshi 2003, p. 69). This development stands in sharp contrast to the attempt by the court to establish an organized (*ritsuryō*) system of *kami* worship. These historical developments ushered into existence the splitting apart of *kami* cults into diverse directions, depending on political and social agendas of the adherents.

Along with the syncretism of *kami* and buddha figures, Buddhism introduced into Japan a new cosmology, ontology, and theoretical rationale. As evident in narratives of the *Nihon ryōiki* referred to previously, the doctrine of karma was used to explain illness and the status of local *kami*, which were conceived as sentient beings needing salvation (Havens 2006, p. 23). None-theless, the *kami* had to be honored, venerated, and thanked by the people with the purpose of maintaining a balanced, harmonious, and productive relationship that would benefit both the natural order and its inhabitants. From the perspective of ordinary people, it was essential for their welfare to direct the energy of the *kami* toward creative and beneficial ends rather than destructive directions. Although such actions were essential for a good life, it was recognized that there was a continuity between humans and *kami*. In fact, some humans could become *kami* (Reader 1991, p. 25).

The path of Shinto, the Japanese islands, and the way of the *kami* are synonymous from the perspective of the Japanese people, even though the ancient *kami* were considered unpredictable. For example, Japan was called *shinkoku*, or "the land of the *kami*." The *kami* were believed to inhabit specific natural locations such as a rock, a spring, a river, a mountain, or a tree. With the advent of Buddhism, *kami* also began to be enshrined in specific locations and human structures. Although ancient *kami* were conceived as being unpredictable, they later became associated with compassion, which may reflect a Buddhist influence on the indigenous religion. From ancient times, the Japanese conceived of the *kami* as associated with epidemics, disease, floods, and drought that were examples of their malevolent nature when offended by humans, which necessitated worshipping and thus placating them to protect vulnerable humans.

Due to the multiplicity of *kami* in nature, Shintoism reflects a sensitivity, respect, mutual sympathy, and awe toward nature, as evident in the following poem of Yamabé Akahito in *The Manyōshū* about Mount Fuji, which was an active volcano at the time of composition:

Even since heaven and earth were parted,
It has towered lofty, noble, divine,
Mount Fuji in Suruga!
When we look up to the plains of heaven,
The light of the sky-traversing sun is shaded,
The gleam of the shining moon is not seen,
White clouds dare not cross it,
And forever it snows.
We shall tell of it from mouth to mouth,
O the lofty mountain of Fuji! (Shinkōkai 1965, pp. 87–88)

Not only are phenomena of nature, such as Mount Fuji, divine, but nature and the *kami* are interdependent and interwoven together into a sacred totality. When a *kami* enters a natural object, it infuses that object with a spiritual power (*tama*). Kasulis observes, "To sum up: for Shinto the relation between the spiritual and the material may be external, internal, or both; but the material never exists without some relation to the spiritual" (Kasulis 2004, p. 16).

The naturalism characteristic of Shinto suggests a cosmic orientation to a scholar such as Joseph Kitagawa. What Kitagawa means by the cosmic orientation of Shinto is that "no object or human act has autonomous intrinsic value" (Kitagawa 1966, p. 16). This implies that a person is an integral part of the cosmos and shares in the sacred *kami* nature. People are not divorced from the cosmos and the rhythm of nature. There is thus a deep and abiding kinship between humans and nature, which entails that humans must not attempt to coerce, control, or conquer nature, but should rather cooperate with it and flow with its rhythms. This scenario is also indicative of a harmonious correspondence between humans and *kami*. In addition, there is also a vitalism that characterizes Shinto, as evident by the conception of a vital force (*ki*) that is both spiritual and physical and is present in matter and within humans as a life-giving and nourishing power.

Besides its intimate relation and sensitivity to nature, Shinto embodies a strong folk element (which will become evident as we proceed), an emphasis on simplicity, a value that derives from its naturalism, stress on maintaining purity, and a commitment to communal solidarity via ethnic identity. The folk element is represented by practices such as divination, use of magical instruments such as amulets to protect oneself, and embrace of shamanistic expertise. The emphasis on simplicity is associated with the stress on naturalness. At Shinto shrines, for example, there are no artifacts on the altars, unspiced rice is offered, chopsticks are unmarked, and rice bowls are of a simple design. The simplicity of things allows the natural to express itself (Kasulis 2004, p. 84). Another example of this phenomenon is the *torii* (entrance arch to temples and sacred places that distinguish the outside profane space from the sacred space of the interior) that is not painted, with the consequence of exposing the natural grain of the wood.

If a person is to have a relationship to a *kami*, he or she must become pure. In other words, pollution and defilement (*tsumi*) must be avoided by purifying oneself with water, salt, or fire. Water is the most common means of purification; it is a way to protect oneself from defilement that could potentially pollute a *kami* and motivate it to cause an impure person harm, such as an illness of some kind. Salt is white, a color associated with purity, and evokes emotions connected to the sea and life in general. The ethnic and communal aspects of Shinto manifest a separateness from other cultures, fostering internal relations that bind people together into a community; Shinto is grounded in an intimate relationship between the people, *kami*, and the land. This implies that a person's individual identity is intrinsically social.

Within the context of adhering to Shinto, a person's life represents a combination of personal spirituality, practice of folk religion, being a member of a state religion, sharing a national ideology, being part of a religious organization, and participating in a civil institution (Kasulis 2004, p. 54). Overall, Shinto is world-affirming and celebrates life, which sets it apart from the world-negating aspects of Buddhism. Despite such an attitude, those practicing Shinto over the centuries have been deeply concerned with health, illness, and healing. Shinto practitioners have devised a wide variety of religious means to combat illness.

WAYS OF COPING WITH ILLNESS

The maintenance of cleanliness has been an important aspect of Japanese culture from ancient times to the present. The cultural emphasis on cleanliness is grounded in the ancient opposition between pure and impure, embodied in a narrative contained in the ancient *Kojiki* that tells of the major deities being born out of a purification rite. However, the deity Izanagi is defiled after seeing the corpse of his wife, Izanami, in the underworld covered with maggots. In this theogony, he attempts to cleanse himself by washing his left eye, which gives birth to Amaterasu, Sun goddess, whereas her brother is born when Izanami washes his nose. This *Kojiki* myth lucidly distinguishes between pure and impure. As the narrative suggests, the distinction between purity and impurity is also related to the opposition between life and death, above and below, health and sickness. It is clearly implied that any association with death, handling of corpses, and illness is associated with impurity.

Practices associated with maintaining cleanliness are connected to a conception of the human body along with spatial and temporal classifications. The human body, for instance, is arranged in a hierarchical manner, with the upper half of the body being pure, while the lower half is defiled, with the feet being considered the most impure. The intestinal or stomach area represents the center of the body that serves as the seat of the soul. This basic conceptualization of the human body forms the foundation for cultural practices such as removing footgear before entering a house. When doing laundry, it is essential not to mix clothing from the upper and lower parts of the body. Washing hands, gargling with water (a purifying agent), brushing one's hair, or washing one's feet are everyday ways of maintaining personal hygiene, cleanliness, and beyond them purity. During the transition period of moving from night time to daylight, a person folds the mattress (futon) and stores it in a closet; it is also often hung outside to dry it of bodily moisture accumulated during sleep. In addition to the importance of the pattern of the body, there is a strong distinction between the inside and the outside of the house. The general rule is that the area inside of a home is clean, whereas the outside is considered dirty, which implies that one must not bring dirt from outside into a home and defile it (Ohnuki-Tierney 1989, p. 61).

The Japanese make a distinction between two notions of illness: *taishitsu* and *jibyō*. The former type of illness is basically the constitution that a person inherits from birth, which can differ according to strength or weakness. Examples of this type would include someone who is healthy and ordinary, weak and nonenergetic, having inborn weakness, or being extra sensitive. The latter type (*jibyō*) is an illness that a person carries with him or her throughout life; in short, it is "my" illness. This type might include such malaise as constipation, low blood pressure, headaches, dizziness, menstrual cramps, hemorrhoids, and allergies. These notions of illness suggest that illness is something that a person must live with and endure (Ohnuki-Tierney 1989, pp. 62–63). From a related perspective, life alternates between health and illness, which in a religious sense is conceptualized as fluctuating between good and evil.

Although today modern biomedicine exists along with traditional forms of medicine in Japan, the traditional institutional form of medicine is called *kampō*, which assumes a number of different forms that can include herbal and animal medicine and acupuncture. Having been introduced to Japan from China, *kampō* does not recognize ordinary classifications of illness because it is more concerned with the totality of symptoms, which are called *shōkōgun*. This method measures a patient's gender, age, bodily constitution, and climate in which the patient lives before deciding on a prescription. In *kampō*, there are four means of making a diagnosis: close observation of the color and texture of the skin, external parts of the body, tongue, and excreta; listening to a patient's voice, breathing, and coughing, along with the smell of excreta and body odor; questioning a patient about the history of the disease; and touching diagnosis that involves reading a patient's pulse, touching the stomach area, and examining other parts of the body (Ohnuki-Tierney 1984, p. 93). The periodic change of seasons is, for instance, potentially harmful to a person's health because of the danger of creating a humoral imbalance. The anthropologist Ohnuki-Tierney discovers a cultural contradiction at this point: "The Japanese meticulously avoid the climatic and extreme humoral elements, but they also use the same elements for preventive and healing purposes" (Ohnuki-Tierney 1984, p. 33). This *kampō* method renders each illness of a patient unique, which calls for an equally distinctive set of personalized treatments (Ohnuki-Tierney 1984, p. 64). The *kampō* treatments do not include surgery because that would increase the bodily imbalance. In sharp contrast to surgery, herbal medicines operate on the whole bodily system. An example of *kampō* is moxibustion, a treatment that takes young mugwort leaves and burns them on the body to stimulate heat and thus healing. *Kampō* treatment should be viewed as a treatment that is natural and seeks to restore balance to a patient's body.

DEITIES, DISEASE, AND HEALING

The Japanese Shinto/Buddhist pantheon is populated with divine beings who are intimately associated with various types of diseases and physical/mental aliments. The religio-cultural situation is somewhat unique in the sense that Japanese citizens have commonly practiced two religions—Shinto and Buddhism—simultaneously for centuries. In the popular imagination, Buddhism is associated with death, corpses, and funerals, whereas Shinto-ism is connected to the normal life cycle of birth, growth, and life. This means that when a person dies, he or she is disposed ritually by Buddhist priests, whereas one is married, for instance, by Shinto priests. When ill, a person might turn to either a Buddhist divine figure or a Shinto deity, because among their benevolent functions (*goriyaku*) is the ability to cure illness.

Whether they are primarily Shinto or Buddhist, deities tend to assume an occupational specialization, although the Japanese do not draw sharp distinctions between supernatural figures. In fact, deities tend to overlap in their medical functions of curing illness. A patient can choose, for example, either one of an overlapping Shinto deity or Buddhist divine figure or choose both of them (Ohnuki-Tierney 1984, p. 69). Among some of the common Shinto/Buddhist divine figures associated with illness, there are the following: Kōjin-sama (Kitchen God), related to general illness; Iboishi-sama (Wart-Store Deity), concerned with illness of the face; Mekura-gami (Deity of the Blind), associated with eye illness; Kawaya-no-kami (Deity of the Toilet), connected to illness of the teeth; Hōso-shin (Deity of Smallpox and contagious diseases in general); Odok-sama (Deity of Dirt and Poison), related to childhood forms of illness; and Hōki-no-kami (Deity of the Broom), associated with pregnancy and childbirth.

As examples, we highlight a few of these figures. The Kitchen God is a fierce deity who protects the home and represents the entire household itself. The Deity of the Toilet is depicted as androgynous, and is said to have originated from the excretion and urine of Izamani, Goddess of the Under-world. In general, the Deity of the Toilet is endowed with the power to heal illness of the eyes, teeth, and gynecological problems. Another interesting figure is Sai-no-kami (Deity of the Boundary), who is often represented by a large rock at the edge of a village. The term *sai* means to block, suggest-ing that it obstructs evil spirits and devils at the boundaries of the village.

The Deity of the Boundary is associated with male and female sexual organs in the sense of representing the meeting place of the two sexes in the area of the genitalia. Thus, it is connected to problems related to reproduction and illness associated with the sexual organs. As with other divine figures, these three highlighted deities can be both benevolent and fierce.

Two popular Buddhist figures are Jizō, a deity associated with boundaries between this world and the next; and Kannon, a bodhisattva of infinite compassion. Jizō's statue is often located at boundaries because these places are considered dangerous. During the middle ages in Japan, six Jizō statues were placed at the seven major entrances to the city of Kyoto to ward off epidemics and other dangerous influences (Glassman 2015, pp. 129–130). Jizō's cult was associated with pacifying restless spirits. His cult included worship with ecstatic dances performed by *miko* (shrine maidens, shamans) and *yūjo* (prostitutes) (Glassman 2015, pp. 102–103). There are many subtypes of Jizō, such as Roped Jizō who overlaps with the Kitchen God, Lifting Jizō who overlaps with Wart-Stone Deity, Jizō of Easy Childbirth who overlaps with the Deity of the Broom, and several others. To obtain a cure from one of these figures, a sick person might, for example, tie a statue of Roped Jizō with ropes to convey to the deity the kind of pain being endured by the patient, who also prays for a cure. When the person is cured, he or she frees the statue by unbinding the ropes.

Kannon is also very popular with Shinto adherents and Buddhists. In India, Kannon is known as Avalokiteśvara (literally, "The Lord who Looks Down"), implying that he sees the suffering of humankind and responds with compassion by helping and healing the afflicted. Around the tenth century CE in China, this bodhisattva was transformed into Guanyin, a female figure and giver of children (Yü 2001). In addition to Kannon and Jizō, Konnyaku Emma represents a heavenly Buddha who governs a person's longevity.

In addition to these supernatural figures, mention should also be made of ancestors. Those individuals who have recently died are equivalent to germs, which makes them dangerous. They are marginal figures existing in the underworld between the world of the living and the dead and residing between nature and culture. The dead are considered very dangerous, especially if one died young, suffered an injustice during life, or died tragically; hence, they must be transformed into less harmful ancestors and reintroduced into the family. From August 13 to 15, priests perform the *bon* rituals, or rites for the deceased. These rites are intended to arrange the return of the deceased to their earthly home as ancestral spirits with a stake in the ongoing welfare of the family (Smith 1974). When these rites transform and welcome the departed back into the family, there is an expectation that the ancestor will assist family members either to regain or to maintain their health, assuming that family members continue to fulfill their religious duties.

PURIFICATION, PILGRIMAGE, AND HEALING

From ancient Japanese culture to the present, there has been a close inter-relationship between healing, purification, and pilgrimage. For instance, during the Nara period (710–781 CE), the Ministry of Kami Affairs performed public purification rites in an attempt to avert epidemics and keep them from afflicting the populace. At the midpoint of the Heian period (781–1191 CE), the Bureau of Yin and Yang also sponsored another purification rite to avoid the threat of an epidemic (Satoshi 2003, p. 98). These rites are evidence of the importance of government support and intervention in illness prevention. It was a common belief that epidemics were caused by demonic beings, who had to be thwarted and defeated, suggesting a situation of justified violence on the part of the people threatened by an epidemic.

When people are in an impure condition, they are a danger to others and themselves, which creates a precarious social situation. A person can become impure by touching bodily waste products, coming into contact with an impure person, or having contact with dead animals or humans. Impure heavenly *tsumi* (defilements) can cause mischief by destroying rice paddy dikes, filling in ditches designed to control flooding, or scattering excrement, whereas earthly *tsumi* cause skin cuts, leukoderma, sexual transgressions, and death to livestock. Skin diseases are informative because they are viewed as a form of defilement, functioning as a visible sign of a divine curse for everyone to witness (Naumann 2000, p. 61). In order not to offend these demonic spirits, persons must restore themselves by means of purification, which can be achieved by means of water, throwing salt, or lighting a fire and embracing its smoke. Within the context of the distinction between pure and impure, illnesses of various kinds are conceived to be dirt or polluting substances. Being in a state of purification is a prerequisite for going on pilgrimage to sacred places.

The term for pilgrimage in the Japanese language is *junrei*, which combines the notion of "going around" (*jun*) and "worshipping" (*rei*), suggesting a journey to a destination. Another Japanese term used to refer to pilgrimage is *henro*, constructed of two ideograms consisting of *hen* meaning "everywhere" and *ro* meaning "route" or "road." The circuit structure of the *henro* suggests being encompassed (Reader 2005, p. 33). Pilgrimage is also a means of transforming oneself and a way to self-discovery (Reader 2015, pp. 21–22, 28). The phenomenon of pilgrimage thus entails travel to some destination, usually a place of destination that is considered very special or sacred, and some type of veneration. These features of pilgrimage indicate that it is not an errant or aimless type of wandering, even though the individual pilgrim may be restless (Reader 2015, p. 27). Pilgrims are convinced that where they are going is a location with structures (which can be natural or made by humans) that possess power. By journeying there, pilgrims can share and participate in that place's power. Pilgrims believe that one of the powers is the ability to heal a person from illness or some other type of malaise. By going on pilgrimage, a person can cure himself or herself or another person who is unable to make the journey.

An especially interesting and popular Japanese pilgrimage site, for centuries, has been Shikoku, because it involves a journey that encompasses 88 temples that must theoretically be visited by the pilgrim. These numerous temples are laid out to form the pilgrimage circuit. The Shikoku pilgrimage was begun by monks in the 12th century, seeking relief from general suffering and particular diseases. This origin of the pilgrimage combined the site of Shikoku with the promise of healing. The path of the Shikoku pilgrimage is closely associated with a monk named Kōbō Daishi, a renowned miracle worker. This was a posthumous title granted to the Buddhist monk named Kūkai (774–835 CE), who established the Shingon sect in Japan, was born at the location of Shikoku, and was believed to have transcended death there. Thus, pilgrims literally walk in the footsteps of this famous monk, known for his ability to heal the infirm, to protect them, and to empower them. At each temple along the route, Kōbō Daishi is ubiquitously present, which hints at his powerful abilities to help others.

The symbols worn by pilgrims are especially informative about the event. Pilgrims don a white shirt, a paradoxical symbol of both purity and death that implies the ability to accomplish their journey, which is popularly called "two people, one practice." The shirt is tied in reverse order from a normal shirt, which usually done when dressing a corpse. In this way, it symbolizes the pilgrim's burial shroud. Because everyone is wearing a white shirt, this gives pilgrims the distinct impression that they are part of a community. Many pilgrims also carry a staff that symbolizes the body of Kōbō Daishi and the pilgrim's gravestone. The typical pilgrim wears a bamboo hat inscribed with words from a poem concerning the transient nature of life that is normally engraved on coffins, suggesting that the hat represents the pilgrim's coffin. The symbolic association with death continues with some pilgrims carving their posthumous name (*kaimyō*), which is the name by which one will be known in the afterlife (Reader 2005, p. 63; Reader 2015, p. 25).

When pilgrims reach a temple, it is common practice for them to chant a song associated with just that particular temple. A stop at a temple also involves getting the temple seal imprinted on a book, scroll, or shirt, which makes these items more valuable and prized by pilgrims. This popular act is a manifestation of a pilgrim's religious merit. The temple stamp (*nōkyō*) also functions as a passport to the Pure Land after death (Reader 2005, pp. 22–23). It has become common practice for pilgrims, while on the journey, to pray for protection against senility in their old age. Pilgrimages are not merely for protection against illness, but are also intend to heal those already suffering from some disease or handicap.

POPULAR MEASURES TO PREVENT ILLNESS OR RESTORE HEALTH

The use of amulets, and visits to shrines and temples, are popular and common ways to protect oneself against illness or to heal oneself. Amulets are intended to ward off evil spirits and misfortunes associated with illness, and to protect a person against dangers. While on a pilgrimage, it is possible for a pilgrim to acquire amulets at shrines and temples. By making the pilgrimage to the Grand Shrine at Ise, for example, a pilgrim can purchase an amulet that embodies the power of the deities of this shrine and take it back to his or her village with the purpose of thereby protecting the home and community, and ensuring a bountiful harvest. There are amulets that are purchased at shrines and then wrapped in white paper and rubbed against the afflicted part of a person's body (Ohnuki-Tierney 1989, p. 78). Besides amulets obtained at shrines, a person can also construct charms, consisting, for instance, of a ritual stick and wooden swords that are placed at the entrance to a home. Or one can hang a plant at the upper corner of a doorway: the strong smell of the plant is intended to repel demons (Ohnuki-Tierney 1984, p. 64).

Shinto followers also use talismans identified as *fuda* and *o-manari* to bring good fortune and protection against illness. In a home, an area is made sacred, which is the *fuda*. On a flat piece of wood, an inscription is carved that might include the name of a temple/shrine and its *kami*. These items are wrapped in white paper and tied with a bow of colored string. The name of a temple or shrine is written on an *o-manari*, a small brocade bag with drawstrings that is intended to protect a particular person. These types of amulets are placed before an image of Fudō, a fierce-looking divine figure surrounded by fire, to allow his power to be transferred into the object. However, the power embodied in these amulets is ephemeral and thus must be recharged periodically (Reader 1991, p. 178). At some shrines, there are shops that sell porcelain figures of badgers, frogs, monkeys, and other animals. Badgers are used to exorcise evil such as disease, whereas frogs are believed to bring good luck. The Japanese term for frog is *kaeru*, which can also mean return. This suggests that the frog signifies returning home safely from a journey or returning to health (Reader 1991, p. 178).

Fudō is an especially interesting figure because he was brought to Japan by esoteric monks during the early Heian period. He can be traced back to India where he was called Acala, who was originally a Hindu figure adopted by Buddhists as one of the five wisdom kings, emanations of primordial wisdom. Fudō was originally adopted to function as a youthful servant of the Buddha. Fudō is described as ugly, a feature that is related to his Tantric background and its belief that in order to combat frightening demons successfully one must assume the appearance of the demons (Faure 2015, p. 131). Within his shrines, his worship included possession in the sense that he protected people from possession, although he also was known to possess children. In addition to his association with possession, Fudō protected ascetics by burning away obstacles to their gaining wisdom, which is symbolized by the ring of fire that surrounds his icon and purifies humans from defilements (Faure 2015, pp. 117, 135). His upward- and downward-pointed fangs had a sexually symbolic significance, which along with his chthonian association and being a symbol of the center, connected him with *nāgas* (serpent figures), rain, and fertility. In the popular imagination, he was thus associated with embryonic development and birth (Faure 2016, p. 145). His popularity in medieval Japan was reflected by many miracle narratives and healing powers associated with him.

Shrines and temples are places of healing in the Japanese religious imagination. A shrine visited by Ohnuki-Tierney keeps symbols—a sharp sword and an arrow—of two *kami* related to the Sun goddess (Amaterasu). Representing the bodies of the *kami*, these symbols evoke notions about cutting hard things, and thus signify curing tumors by cutting them out (Ohnuki-Tierney 1989, p. 74). A sick person can also buy packages of rice at a shrine or temple. The ill are instructed to swallow a single grain of this rice every morning with their initial drink of water (Ohnuki-Tierney 1989, p. 78). At the Ishikiri Shrine, people practice *ohyakudo* (which literally means "one hundred times"), a practice that involves a pilgrim making 100 journeys or visits to a shrine or temple with the intention of regaining health. Directly in front of the main shrine, there are two cylindrical stones located about 10 meters apart. The practice involves people walking rapidly back and forth between the two stones, touching each stone as they journey between them, for a grand total of 100 times (Ohnuki-Tierney 1981, p. 23). Similar practices are evident at other temples around Japan.

Pregnant women will visit the Nakayama Temple, wearing a traditional long white sash (*iwata obi*) over their stomach on which a priest writes a sacred verse (Ohnuki-Tierney 1989, p. 81). This practice is intended to assist the pregnant woman to deliver a healthy baby without too much pain. This scenario suggests an association between obstetrics, gynecology, pediatrics, and temples. Another temple practice related to healing is manifested by people purchasing bundles of incense, lighting the sticks of incense, and placing them in the burner. As the smoke from the burning incense rises, the person uses the hands to scoop up the smoke and place it on the ailing part of the body, with the intention of using the healing power of the smoke from the burning incense to effect a cure (Ohnuki-Tierney 1989, p. 81).

In addition to the roles played by amulets, shrines, and temples in healing, there is additionally a role for statues. The relationship between a practitioner and a statue can become very intimate because people decorate, touch, pray to, and make offerings to the statues. For instance, someone who is suffering from some bodily malaise may rub a part of the statue that directly corresponds to the afflicted part of the person's body. This type of healing touch can be executed in reverse by rubbing oneself before touching the statute. By this reverse procedure, the practitioner is attempting to evoke the compassion of the deity to absorb the pain or illness into itself and relieve the human sufferer (Reader 1991, p. 172).

Statues play a different role for women who have had abortions, a miscarriage, or a stillborn infant. In a culture that exalts motherhood as the ideal role for women, these types of health misfortunes are a direct cause of guilty feelings, even though the woman might not be at fault (as in the case of a miscarriage). These unfortunate women can, however, turn to their religion and memorial rites called *mizuko kuryō* (nourishing a water child) for some comfort and heal themselves mentally. The rite involves a memorial service at which offerings of light, food, flowers, incense, and prayers are directed to Jizō. The observance includes the bereaved couple buying a sculpted stone statue about two feet high that resembles a Buddhist monk, or more accurately a child-monk. These statues are left within the temple by the bereaved couple and given a posthumous name, which is inscribed on a mortuary tablet that can either be taken home or left at the temple (LaFleur 1992).

JAPANESE SHAMANISM AND HEALING

There is a long history of shamanism in Japanese cultural history that has existed along with Shinto and Buddhism. In the 14th chapter of the ancient *Kojiki*, there is a description of the fury of Amaterasu, Sun goddess, which symbolizes a shaman possessed by the goddess, serving as an early example of a person being divinely possessed by a higher power. Traditionally, shamans have been intimately involved in healing. Many of the Japanese shamans have been women, especially blind women. Whether male or female, a shaman can be defined as an expert in ecstatic trance states (Eliade 1964, p. 4). These trance states enable the shaman to converse with supernatural and ancestral spirits, and travel to unimagined places to find lost souls, retrieve them, and restore them into the body of the afflicted person suffering from soul loss.

According to the anthropologist Ichiro Hori, there are two types of Japanese shamans: (1) *kan-nagi*, which includes the *miko* (female shaman) that belonged to the imperial court and Shinto shrines; and (2) *kuchiyose*, which those who live in villages or migrate from one village to another, making use of trance states to practice telepathy, mediumship, divination, and fortune telling. There is also a more magical shamanistic system served by the magician (*jussha*) or *gyōja* practitioner (Hori 1968, pp. 182–183). In her study of Japanese shamanism, Blacker identifies two types: the *miko* (medium), and what she calls the ascetic, a figure that is mostly a healer with the power to leave the body and to banish malevolent spirits (Blacker 1982, p. 22). According to Blacker, the ascetic shaman figure has the power to heal by means of an innate power, and does not necessarily have to rely on the aid of spirits (Blacker 1982, p. 180).

When a Japanese shaman goes into an ecstatic trance, it is common to witness symptoms such as violent shaking of the hands, roaring, strenuous breathing, and levitating of the body from a sitting posture (Blacker 1982, p. 220). The shaman is assisted by a drum that induces a trance state, summons spirits, and serves as a charm against spirits (Ohnuki-Tierney 1981, p. 75). The Ainu shamans of Sakhalin, Japan, use a catalpa bow—a single hempen-stringed instrument—to summon spirits, which can trigger a lament from a ghost causing illness when striking it with a bamboo rod. In order to become a shaman, a person must be initiated, which symbolically involves the death and rebirth of the shaman in a violent scenario of being killed, transformed, and reborn into a new status that is associated with the power to heal. After initiation is successfully concluded, the shaman has the ability to leave the body and travel to other regions inaccessible to ordinary mortals.

It is ironic that shamans suffer from sickness related to their profession, exhibiting symptoms such as physical pains, headaches, vomiting, and joint and back pains before they are initiated. More hysterical behavior is also evident when shamans wander aimlessly in the forest, suddenly fall asleep, or hide from light, suggesting possible mental illness. However, these types of medical malaise leave the shamans at the conclusion of their initiation, after they have been reduced to a mere skeleton, which is symbolic of their death (Blacker 1982, p. 24). With their newfound powers, the shamans have clairvoyant vision that enables them to see which spiritual beings are responsible for a particular sickness and to take remedial measures to counteract the evil spirits. In the case of sickness due to the loss of one's soul, the shaman goes into an ecstatic trance, leaves the body, travels to the underworld, retrieves the soul of the sick person, and restores the patient to health.

HEALING WITHIN A VIOLENT CONTEXT

Sometimes disease is caused by polluting a *kami* by means of menstrual or birth blood, death, or impure substances. Becoming defiled causes the *kami* to act decisively to punish the polluter, who is always in the wrong. Whether it is a *kami*, ancestral spirit, or demonic being afflicting a person, the context of the affliction becomes a battlefield evoking images of violence. It is believed that when people become sick, they have been invaded by more powerful forces, which reflects a discourse of violence. Shinto *kami* that are normally irenic can quickly inflict harm in the form of diseases. Yet they can, paradoxically, be propitiated by offerings and prayers to come to the aid of sick persons and heal them.

Despite its traditional advocacy of nonviolence as a central teaching, aspects of Buddhism evoke images of violence associated with the discourse pertaining to healing (Olson 2015, pp. 85–86). Buddhist guardian deities are depicted as fierce, angry, and fiery figures. In Japan, there are the Five Great Buddhist Kings (Godai Myōō), who are conceived as emanations of the primordial Buddha, functioning as his agents and messengers on earth. Each of the Kings rules over a geographical direction, with the center area dominated by Fudō, who is portrayed in colors of blue, red, or black with one eye gazing downward and the other directed upward. His twisted mouth manifests an upper tooth grasping his lower lip and a lone lower tooth grasping his upper lip. Long hair hangs over his shoulder. In his right and left hands, he holds (respectively) a sword and a rope, while standing surrounded by a ring of fire. He also is associated with the opposite of fire: namely, water. This portrait suggests that he represents a coincidence of opposites and an absolute paradox. His fierce appearance can be attributed to his role as the protector against illness, implying that he has the power to frighten away harmful diseases. Moreover, he serves as the guardian spirit for many shamans.

Ancient Shinto myths depict images and episodes of violence and healings. After the separation of heaven and earth in primordial times and several generations of deities, Izanagi (male principle) and Izanami (female principle) were born and created the Japanese islands by dipping their spears into the ocean and bringing up mud to the surface. This brother-and-sister tandem proceeded to have the sexual relations that created nature and *kami* (deities). After committing a ritual error by speaking first, Izanami was punished by giving birth to a leech. A more auspicious result is achieved when the male Izanagi speaks first, but Izanami tragically dies. This episode is indicative of the dangers associated with giving birth.

After the death of his wife/sister, Izanagi creates the Sun goddess, Amaterasu, after washing his left eye, whereas the cleansing of his right eye produces the Moon god, Tsukiyomi. When Izanagi cleans his nose, the hot, fiery deity Susano-o is created, who proceeds to act counter to the creative activity of Amaterasu by polluting the earth and threatening crops. A series of polluting actions causes Amaterasu to escape to a cave, but she is finally induced to emerge from her seclusion. Her brother is punished by being banished to the underworld, a place of impurity and violence.

The violent discourse associated with mythical narratives is reflected in everyday life. The treatment of diseases, especially epidemics that afflict many people and threaten their existence, occurs within an imaginary context of violence. If a disease represents a hostile invading army of demonic beings, it is they who must be destroyed before they destroy the patient. The Japanese shaman has filled this role for centuries.

The traditional violent rhetoric surrounding disease in Japan is basically situational. Although the context of violence is important, violence is intertwined with fear, anger, and excitement. The association of these types of phenomena with violence suggest that violence is dynamic because it begins with confrontational tension and fear (Collins 2008, p. 10). In contrast to the theory of René Girard, Collins offers some constructive criticism from a microsociological perspective: "Violence is not primordial, and civilization does not tame it; the opposite is much nearer the truth" (Collins 2008, p. 10). This type of position depicts violence as a situational process that is also dynamic because it begins with confrontation and the threat of violence.

CONCLUSION

The narratives recounted to introduce this chapter were intended to set it within a dialectical contextualism that also considers the religious beliefs and modes of behavior about healing, which are interdependent, interpenetrating, and internally connected with each other. This approach has drawn from both the verbal (e.g., grounded in textual evidence) and the nonverbal (e.g., observable behavior). We have seen evidence that Shinto and shamanistic systems demonstrate the complex and multiple interconnected levels of meaning for an individual and the society with respect to beliefs about healing. This intertwining has occurred to such a cultural extent that the advent of secularism and its accompanying materialistic proclivities in Japan have not dwarfed or eliminated traditional religiously based attitudes toward healing.

In summary, amulets, shrines, temples, and statues all assist with the process of healing for followers of both Shinto and Buddhism. This is made possible by the Japanese tendency not to construct rigid distinctions between the two major religions and their supernatural figures, who often overlap as to the diseases that they specialize in curing. Because some supernatural figures perform the same functions, people are free to choose between them or to use both of them.

In a cultural worldview in which there are a ubiquitous number of *kami*, buddhas, and ancestral spirits available to heal a person, the cause of illness can be traced to human beings: for instance, a person may have offended a supernatural spirit by neglecting it, by breaking moral or social codes, or by becoming defiled by some form of pollution. Because these types of behavior cause social disruptions and subvert the human/divine relationship, they give rise to disharmony and potential social disorder (Ohnuki-Tierney 1984, p. 80). This scenario suggests that illness in Japanese culture is directly connected to spiritual well-being and represents a disharmony between the sick person and the universe. Shamans, priests, and holy figures attempt to correct cosmic and social disharmony.

The Japanese evidence indicates an intimate connection between healing and religion, which implies that illness is socially defined, that sickness has a culture-specific nature, and that it can be treated naturally by herbal remedies and not by invasive surgery. Within the Japanese cultural context, a path is provided for people to conceptualize illness, to have certain expectations that various kinds of treatment will be successful, and to deal with different forms of sickness. This suggests that a shaman, for example, can be successful because the patients bring certain assumptions with them to the treatment about the possibilities of being healed. It is only within a shared worldview that the shaman can successfully treat a member of the same culture and assign meaning to an illness. Just as the shaman is a liminal figure during the initiation rite, a sick person resides in a liminal phase of life between life and death.

No matter how a person enters a liminal period, it is a time of danger and uncertainty that can evoke a discourse of violence. In other words, the restoration of health is akin to a battle between opposing forces, with one side attempting to retrieve harmony and the other party pulling toward disorder. Rhetoric about demonic beings possessing a person or inflicting harm on them describes a dire situation in which shamans and other healers can come to the rescue. In some instances, an ill person can turn to more magical means, such as using amulets and statues. It is also possible to go on pilgrimage to find healing or simply to visit a shrine or temple located nearby. Currently, these traditional forms of healing exist alongside of modern biomedicine, which traces illness to the onset of germs.

On the one hand, traditional Japanese religio-cultural ways of responding to illness have been accepted for centuries. On the other hand, these old methods of treatment now encounter modern biomedicine, with its more secularized and scientific methodological presuppositions that clash sharply with traditional cultural ways of treating illness. Does this mean that modern medicine will completely replace traditional methods of dealing with illness? There is evidence that current clinical practitioners remain interested in psychosomatic forms of medicine (Nakao and Ohara 2014, pp. 46–55). There is, of course, a danger that modern medicine will subvert the ancient Shinto and shamanistic connection with health restoration with a more secular and scientific agenda. This medical drama will unfold into the foreseeable future.

REFERENCES

Ashton, W. G. Trans. 2008. *The Nihongi*. Middletown, DE: Biblio Bazaar.

Blacker, C. 1982. *The Catalpa Bow: A Study of Shamanistic Practices in Japan*. London: Routledge Curzon.

Collins, R. 2008. *Violence: A Micro-Sociological Theory*. Princeton, NJ: Princeton University Press.

Eliade, M. 1964. *Shamanism: Archaic Techniques of Ecstasy* (Bollingen Series LXXVI). Translated by W. R. Trask. New York: Pantheon Books.

Faure, B. 2015. *Gods of Medieval Japan. Vol. 1: The Fluid Pantheon*. Honolulu: University of Hawaii Press.

Glassman, H. 2015. *The Face of Jizō: Image and Cult in Medieval Japanese Buddhism*. Honolulu: University of Hawaii Press.

Havens, N. 2006. "Shinto." In P. L. Swanson and C. Ghilson, eds., *Nanzan Guide to Japanese Religions*, pp. 14–37. Honolulu: University of Hawaii Press.

Heldt, G. 2014. *The Kojiki: An Account of Ancient Masters*. New York: Columbia University Press.

Hori, I. 1968. *Folk Religion in Japan: Continuity and Change*. Chicago: University of Chicago Press.

Kasulis, T. P. 2004. *Shinto: The Way Home*. Honolulu: University of Hawaii Press.

Kitagawa, J. M. 1966. *Religion in Japanese History*. New York: Columbia University Press.

LaFleur, W. R. 1992. *Liquid Life: Abortion and Buddhism in Japan*. Princeton, NJ: Princeton University Press.

Nakao, M. and C. Ohara. 2014. "The Perspective of Psychosomatic Medicine on the Effect of Religion on the Mind-Body Relationship in Japan." *Journal of Religion and Health* 53(1): 46–55.

Naumann, N. 2000. "The State Cult of the Nara and Early Heian Periods." In J. Breen and M. Teeuwen, eds., *Shinto in History: Ways of the Kami*, pp. 47–67. Honolulu: University of Hawaii Press.

Nobutaka, I. 2003. "What Is Shinto?" In *Shinto: A Short History*, pp. 1–13. Translated by M. Teeuwen and J. Breen. London: Routledge Curzon.

Ohnuki-Tierney, E. 1981. *Illness and Healing among the Sakalin Ainu: A Symbolic Interpretation*. Cambridge, UK: Cambridge University Press.

Ohnuki-Tierney, E. 1984. *Illness and Culture in Contemporary Japan: An Anthropological View*. Cambridge, UK: Cambridge University Press.

Ohnuki-Tierney, E. 1989. "Health Care in Contemporary Japanese Religions." In L. E. Sullivan, ed., *Healing and Restoring: Health and Medicine in the World's Religious Traditions*, pp. 59–87. New York: Macmillan.

Olson, C. 2015. *Indian Asceticism: Power, Violence, and Play*. New York: Oxford University Press.

Reader, I. 1991. *Religion in Contemporary Japan*. Honolulu: University of Hawaii Press.

Reader, I. 2005. *Making Pilgrimage: Meaning and Practice in Shikoku*. Honolulu: University of Hawaii Press.

Reader, I. 2015. *Pilgrimage: A Very Short Introduction*. Oxford, UK: Oxford University Press.

Satoshi, I. 2003. "The Medieval Period: The Kami Merge with Buddhism." In *Shinto: A Short History*, pp. 63–107. Translated by M. Teeuwen and J. Breen. London: Routledge Curzon.

Shinkōkai, N. G. 1965. *The Manyōshū*. New York: Columbia University Press.

Smith, R. J. 1974. *Ancestor Worship in Contemporary Japan*. Palo Alto, CA: Stanford University Press.

Teeuwen, M. 2002. "From Jindō to Shinto." *Japanese Journal of Religious Studies* 29: 233–263.

Teeuwen, M., and B. Scheid. 2002. "Tracing Shinto in the History of Kami Worship: Editors' Introduction." *Japanese Journal of Religious Studies* 29(3/4): 195–207.

Watson, B., trans. 2013. *Record of Miraculous Events in Japan: The Nihon ryōiki*. New York: Columbia University Press.

Yü, C.-F. 2001. *Kuan-yin: The Chinese Transformation of Avalokiteśvara*. New York: Columbia University Press.

Chapter 6

Judaism and Health

Miriam Korbman, Moses Appel,
and David H. Rosmarin

INTRODUCTION

According to a Pew Research study (Pew Research Center 2015a), Jews make up roughly 1.8% of the U.S. population, and only 0.2% of the population worldwide. Though representing a small percentage of the populace, Judaism is currently the most common non-Christian religion in the United States, with approximately 44% of the world's Jews living in North America (Pew Research Center 2015a). Additionally, Jews bear an estimated 2.3 children per family; the Jewish total fertility rate exceeds that which is typically necessary to maintain stable population growth (Pew Research Center 2015a). Thus, despite a relatively small population size, encountering Jewish patients in a healthcare setting is not unlikely. The burgeoning literature on religion and health indicates that religious beliefs and customs can impact healthcare practices, as well as mental and physical well-being, in both positive and negative ways (Koenig, King, and Carson 2012; Rumun 2014). It is therefore critical to explore and understand the customs and values of this unique minority as they pertain to healthcare practices and outcomes.

In the last decade, several empirical studies have directly explored relationships between spiritual/religious observance and health in the Jewish population. Specific investigations have found favorable effects of faith and trust in God on mental health, such as lower levels of anxiety and depression (e.g., Rosmarin, Pirutinsky, Pargament, and Krumrei 2009a; Rosmarin, Pargament, and Mahoney 2009). Similarly, research has pointed to significant positive correlations between levels of Jewish religious observance, as well as synagogue membership, attendance, and involvement, and self-rated health conditions (Levin 2011). Other studies have found Jewish communal religious involvement to be associated with health benefits such as lower occurrence of chronic pain (Kabat-Zinn, Lipworth, and Burney 1985), and even lower mortality rates (McCullough, Hoyt, Larson, Koenig, and Thoresen 2000; Kark et al. 1996; Strawbridge, Cohen, Shema, and Kaplan 1997). Another area of study has found that religious coping—the process of turning to spirituality/religion when coping with distress—is very common in the Jewish community (Rosmarin, Pargament, Krumrei, and Flannelly 2009), and the use of positive strategies is associated with better mental health outcomes in the context of life stress (Pirutinsky, Rosmarin, Pargament, and Midlarsky 2011).

However, just as religion can be beneficial for both physical and mental health among Jews, negative effects have also been identified and explored. One area that has garnered recent attention is spiritual struggles, which involve psychologically maladaptive beliefs or attitudes of a spiritual/religious nature (e.g., feeling unjustly punished or abandoned by God, feeling excessively guilty for transgressions, or having a sense of being unworthy of spiritual blessing). Not surprisingly, spiritual struggles are associated with lower levels of physical and mental health for Jews as a whole (Rosmarin, Pargament, and Flannelly 2009). It is therefore critical to understand the values, beliefs, and practices inherent to the Jewish faith in order to ascertain how best to help members of this population. To this end, the present chapter provides an overview of the orienting worldviews, core beliefs, and general religious practices within Judaism, and discusses how each of these facets may influence physical and mental health in this population.

JEWISH ORIENTING WORLDVIEWS

Prior to discussing the influence of Jewish religious practices on Jewish life, health, and well-being, we must first understand what Judaism is, upon which tenets of faith this religion is based, and how it is practiced. Judaism is a monotheistic religion dating back to approximately 1,500 BCE. Over the course of Jewish history, several different sects have developed within traditional Judaism, and today Judaism encompasses a spectrum of religious beliefs and practices. Broadly speaking, the Jewish community comprises two major groups, Orthodox and non-Orthodox Jews, distinguished by differences in levels of faith and observance.

The term *Orthodox* signifies "conforming to established doctrine especially in religion" (*Merriam-Webster Collegiate Dictionary* 2003). Orthodox Jews believe in the divine origin of both the Written Torah (e.g., the Five Books of Moses) as well as the Oral Torah (e.g., the Talmud), and practice these laws in their daily lives. Minimally, Orthodox Jews can be differentiated from non-Orthodox Jews through their strict adherence to the core laws of Orthodox Jewish life, including Sabbath observance, Kashrut (dietary restrictions), and Taharat HaMishpacha (laws of family purity) (Liebman 1965; Huppert, Siev, and Kushner 2007). The term *non-Orthodox* refers to Jews who identify religiously and ethnically as Jewish, and whose religious practices reflect some significant changes in, and additions to, Jewish tradition (Don-Yihya 2005). Additionally, the obligation to observe the Mitzvot (religious laws/commandments) is central to Orthodox Judaism. Non-Orthodox Jews do not emphasize traditional doctrine as heavily (Liebman 1965).

The distinction between Orthodox and non-Orthodox Jews dates back to the early 19th century, following the emancipation of European Jews; at that time, Reform Judaism, first in Germany and then in the United States, began to take root, followed by the birth of Conservative Judaism in late 19th-century America (Don-Yihya 2005; Gillman 1993; Meyer 1995). Today, the Orthodox Jewish community includes Jews from both Ashkenazic (European) as well as Sephardic (Spanish) descent who maintain strict adherence to the core of Jewish law and practice (Bank 2002). There are also Hassidic and other ultra-Orthodox groups who maintain an even stricter level of observance (Huppert et al. 2007). According to a 2015 survey of American Jews, about 10% of all American Jewish adults are Orthodox (Pew Research Center 2015b); however, in some geographic locales, such as Baltimore and parts of New York, upwards of 20% of local Jewish communities affiliate with Orthodoxy. The non-Orthodox Jewish community comprises Reform (35%) and Conservative (18%) Judaism, as well as other sects including Reconstructionist, Progressive, and Open Orthodox Judaism (36%) (Israel and Judaism Studies 2016; Pew Research Center 2015b).

In exploring the influence of religion and culture on health practices among Jews, it is also critical to understand the variations in faith and practice across the Jewish community and the impact of those differences. For example, research indicates that Orthodox Jews tend to experience greater physical and mental health benefits than non-Orthodox Jews (Levin 2011). Therefore, it is important to identify and differentiate between the salient features among Orthodox Jews and the noteworthy qualities among non-Orthodox Jews. Although some areas of Jewish faith and practice are similar across sects, differences in ideology, practice, and culture do exist, and distinctions are noted where applicable regarding the impact of religious practice, observance, and culture on health. For the purposes of this chapter, the term *Orthodox* describes all groups of Orthodox and/or ultra-Orthodox Jews, while the term *non-Orthodox* refers to all other sects.

This chapter explores three main features of Judaism that are related to health among Jews: (1) Jewish religious practice, including the laws, rituals, and commandments observed by both Orthodox and non-Orthodox Jews (and the differences therein); (2) Jewish ideology, the beliefs and principles of faith to which Jews of different sects ascribe and that influence Jewish attitudes toward areas of living such as health practices; and (3) Jewish culture, which refers to other ideas, perceptions, and traditions specific to Judaism and Jewish life irrespective of Jewish Law. There is some overlap among these three domains, and this intersectionality contributes to Jewish attitudes toward health, seeking or use of medical or psychological treatment, and overall health outcomes.

JEWISH RELIGIOUS PRACTICE

Judaism is a religion characterized by practices and rituals, although the precise customs differ between sects and communities (Huppert et al. 2007). These practices are rooted in more than 3,000 years of tradition, and, especially among Orthodox Jews, must be understood through the prism of many detailed laws and bylaws. The primary text that informs religious practice and from which all Jewish laws and traditions originate is called the Torah. The Torah, or Written Law, comprises 24 books, with 5 main volumes containing history and law as well as 19 additional books of prophecy and history called *Neviim* (prophets) and *K'tuvim* (writings). The Talmud, also known as the Oral Law, is a secondary text often used to inform Jewish law.

For generations, the Oral Law was passed down from teacher to student and father to son until it was written down and published between the years 200 and 500 CE (Spiro 2001). The Talmud is made up of two parts: the Mishna, the laws; and the Gemara, the rabbinic commentary on and practical application of the laws (Spiro 2001). The Torah and Talmud combined constitute the main repository of knowledge about Judaism that has been passed down throughout the generations. Together, they delineate all of the Torahitic as well as rabbinic laws and traditions, and specify Jewish religious beliefs and commandments that are at the crux of the faith (Kaplan and Sutton 1992). It should be noted, however, that while the Torah remains the focal point of Jewish religious belief and practice, practical applications and interpretations of the laws differ among the various sects within Judaism; typically, the exact understanding of a specific law derived from either the Torah or Talmud will depend upon an individual Jew's personal rabbi or teacher, or the tradition that his or her family or community follows (Huppert et al. 2007; Kaplan and Sutton 1992).

Tertiary holy texts within Judaism include the rabbinic *Responsa*, a vast collection of writings by preeminent Jewish scholars over the ages, which delve into both the Torah and Talmud to explain their applications and address specific issues within Jewish law (Goldsand, Rosenberg, and Gordon 2001). One foundational tenet of Judaism is the learning of Jewish texts, to provide its constituents with an understanding of the commandments and laws contained therein, as well as the interpretation of these laws by Jewish scholars over the ages.

Although the exact interpretations and applications of these texts may differ across sects, the importance of learning about Jewish history as well as tradition is a global Jewish idea. Exploring how the laws of daily living permeate Jewish life, and Orthodox Jewish life in particular, is one prerequisite to understanding how religion influences other aspects of a Jew's daily life. Many derivations of these laws, as indicated by the texts just discussed, have implications for religious practice across the different sects of Judaism. Orthodox Jews tend to engage in the most practice, including weekly Sabbath observance, synagogue attendance, and other rituals, but 70% of all American Jews attended a Passover Seder (traditional holiday meal with many accompanying rituals) in 2012 (Pew Research Center 2015b).

Some influential Halachic (Jewish law) aspects of Jewish life include (though are not limited to): dietary restrictions (*Kashrut*); laws of family purity (*Taharat HaMishpacha*), including sexuality and marriage; observance of the Sabbath and other holidays; consultation with rabbis and other spiritual leaders with regard to physical or psychological maladies and general distress; and medical ethics through the lens of Jewish law.

JEWISH IDEOLOGY

It is important to recognize the centrality of the Torah and its dictates to the daily life and practices of observant and nonobservant Jews alike; however, it is also critical to understand the role of Jewish values and beliefs in shaping the worldview of Jews across various levels of religious observance. There are certain foundational tenets of faith within the Jewish tradition that influence the Jewish worldview. Primary among these is the belief that God exists, that God created the world from nothing, and that God continues to sustain the world and every particle and creature within it, day in and day out (Kelemen 1990). Today, only 72% of all American Jewish adults believe in God (Pew Research Center 2015b). In addition, an oft-cited list of some of the basic tenets of Judaism is attributed to Maimonides, Rabbi Moshe ben Maimon, also known as the Rambam, who delineated

Table 6.1 Maimonides' 13 Principles of Faith

1. God exists.
2. God is One and God is unique in the world.
3. God has no physical body or characteristics.
4. God is eternal.
5. Prayer should be directed only to God.
6. The words of the prophets are true.
7. Moses was the greatest of the prophets, and his words are true.
8. Moses received both the Written and the Oral Law from God.
9. There will be no other Torah.
10. God is all-knowing and knows the thoughts and actions of all humankind.
11. God will reward those who do good and punish the wicked.
12. The Messiah (Final Redemption) will come.
13. The dead will be resurrected.

13 Principles of Faith, as listed in Table 6.1 (Bank 2002). At the core of Jewish faith, these principles provide insight for how Jews relate to God.

Another fundamental belief in Jewish faith and tradition is that God is omnipotent and omniscient, at the center of the universe and in control of all living things. According to Jewish thought, nothing exists without God's willful, purposeful design and desire, including both inanimate objects as well as all living things (Kaplan and Sutton 1992). Judaism encourages fervent trust in God and belief that God orchestrates the daily events of each and every individual creature, person, and country worldwide; Judaism posits that God created and continues to sustain the world, and that God can and does provide for the needs of every living thing (Bank 2002; Kelemen 1990; Rosmarin, Pargament, and Mahoney 2009). Additionally, it is a fundamental Jewish belief that God created the world in order to give to humankind, and that God desires to give to His creations and shower us with good (Kaplan 2001). Although Jews believe that God is benevolent, God is also known to allot rewards and punishments, and Jews are commanded both to fear and to love Him, as part of six constant commandments (Mitzvot Temidiot) that Jews are responsible for keeping (observing) at all times (Simmons 2014). These seemingly dichotomous beliefs may contribute to Jewish attitudes toward suffering, sickness, healing, and life's purpose.

An additional core Jewish belief is that, while parents are responsible for the biological creation of human beings, God provides every person with a divine soul (Bank 2002). Many Jews view God as the ultimate healer, and believe that while God is the source of all suffering, He is also the source of healing and recovery (Kaplan and Sutton 1992). It is important to note as well that although viewing God as the omnipotent and ultimate healer, Jews also have a religious imperative to take care of their bodies, as it is written, *"Guard carefully your souls"* (Deuteronomy 4:15). Thus, while Judaism firmly adheres to the belief that God can heal any malady, Jews are also obligated to maintain their physical and psychological well-being, and to seek help in this process from doctors and other professionals (Clarfield, Gordon, Markwell, and Alibhai 2003). Rabbis, Jewish religious and spiritual leaders, are often consulted for advice and guidance in lieu of, or prior to, consulting a professional on matters pertaining both to medical and to psychological health concerns (*see* Dancyger et al. 2002; Goodman and Witztum 2002; Greenberg and Shefler 2002; Huppert et al. 2007; Mark and Roberts 1993; Mittman, Bowie, and Maman 2007). This concept sheds light on another important value within the Jewish worldview: the primacy and inherent value of human life. Judaism so highly values life that Jews are obligated to do their utmost to save a life, a tenet that has many implications for medical and health care (Clarfield et al. 2003). Some areas in which this particular value becomes especially important include abortion, fatal illness and euthanasia, and assessment of medical risk (Goldsand et al. 2001). The extent to which these beliefs are upheld by and influence different Jews depends heavily upon the individual's educational background, as well as the specific religious sect and community of which he or she is a part.

JEWISH CULTURE

Jewish culture includes traditions, attitudes, and values not otherwise included in practice or ideology, though with overlap therein, and is perhaps the most salient aspect of Jewish life for Jews of various backgrounds and levels of religious observance. This may be evidenced by the 70% of American Jews who attend a Passover Seder, in contrast with the roughly 25% who believe in God (Pew Research Center 2015b). Even though not identifying as a practicing or Orthodox Jew, many Jews still participate in various rituals and Jewish community events because of a cultural attachment to the religion.

One fundamental aspect of Jewish culture is the importance of family and the role of the family in the life of a Jew (Krieger 2010; Schlossberger and Hecker 1998). This idea is seen in law as well, such as in the commandment for a man to have children, the obligations of husbands to wives and vice versa as delineated in the Talmud, and the commandment for children to fear and honor their parents (Feldman 1992). The emphasis Judaism places on family life, marriage, child rearing, and familial relationships means that all have a unique impact on Jewish health and living (*see* Krieger

2010; Pirutinsky, Schechter, Kor, and Rosmarin 2015; Schlossberger and Hecker 1998).

Another pivotal cultural aspect of Jewish life found among Jews of various backgrounds is the importance of having religious and spiritual leaders and teachers. Conservative, Reform, and Orthodox Judaism alike emphasize the pivotal role of a rabbi in teaching, guiding, advising, and counseling Jewish congregants (Gillman 1993; Kestenbaum 1988; Meyer 1995). This unique relationship between Jews and their rabbis is influential in many areas of Jewish life, including and perhaps especially regarding medical and mental health concerns (Goodman and Witztum 2002; Huppert et al. 2007; Keshet and Liberman 2014).

Research has shown that the social support and community involvement inherent in religious participation is one of the most beneficial aspects of religious life, with many favorable mental health outcomes, including decreased depression and increased positive religious coping (Ellison and George 1994; Krause, Ellison, Shaw, Marcum, and Boardman 2001; Nooney and Woodrum 2002; Harrison, Koenig, Hays, Eme-Akwari, and Pargament 2001). Recent studies expanding the existing literature to include the Jewish community yield similar findings (Lazar and Bjorck 2008; Pirutinsky, Rosmarin, Holt et al. 2011). Often, church attendance and membership are most closely related to this social support. Similarly, Jewish social support is derived from the close-knit communities created around the synagogue or temple in which most community members attend services (Huppert et al. 2007). Additionally, many Orthodox as well as non-Orthodox Jews are affiliated with a synagogue or temple, with nearly 25% of all American Jews reporting either weekly or monthly attendance at Jewish religious services. Synagogue membership is arguably one of the most important aspects of Orthodox Jewish life in modern America (Pew Research Center 2015b; Liebman 1965).

Aside from the social support garnered by affiliation with a house of worship or community, a unique sense of communal responsibility is part and parcel of the Jewish cultural landscape. In fact, 63% of all Jews and 92% of Orthodox Jews report feeling a special responsibility to care for fellow Jews in need (Pew Research Center 2015b). The extent to which Jews help, support, and take care of one another is almost unparalleled, and is an essential part of Jewish living. This communal responsibility and social support has major consequences for Jewish health and well-being as well.

Some of the core cultural considerations in Judaism and health may differ by community, level of religious observance, or country of origin. It is critical to explore the prevalence of, importance of, and research surrounding some of these cultural components, including: level of education within the community; average expected income and allocation of funds in families, including financial constraints such as high tuition costs, which may affect availability of quality insurance for medical care; stigma against treatment for specific mental health disorders and/or physical or medical complaints; communal and familial support; and the role of prayer in healing and anxiety, to name a few. The following sections of this chapter highlight some of the most salient areas of Jewish practice, ideology, and culture that may influence Jewish medical and mental health today.

JUDAISM AND HEALTH

Dietary and Digestive Health

The Jewish dietary restrictions, or Kashrut laws, are one of the many characteristic aspects of Judaism and Jewish culture. Aside from the laws pertaining to what an observant Jew can or cannot eat, there are also many cultural components of Judaism related to food and digestive health that must be explored and understood in the context of treating Jewish patients. Although there are differences in Kashrut observance across sects, this section highlights a few key factors to keep in mind about Jewish law, as well as Jewish cultural tradition, with regard to food intake and other dietary matters.

Laws of Kosher Food

The laws of Kosher food (Kashrut) determine which foods can and cannot be consumed by a Jew who is observing Kashrut (Regenstein, Chaudry, and Regenstein 2003). Although these laws are not considered health laws, and are followed as part of God's ordinances within Jewish law, there are various health considerations related to Kashrut that should be considered in dealing with Jewish patients in different contexts (Regenstein 1994). The three primary areas of Kashrut observance are: (1) prohibited animals; (2) the prohibition against consuming animal blood; and (3) mixing milk and meat together, a prohibition that includes using separate utensils for milk and meat and adhering to a specified waiting period between consumption of milk after meat (Lamm 1973; Regenstein et al. 2003; Orthodox Union 2017). With regard to prohibited animals, the Torah lists all of the animals that a Jew may or may not eat; the Sages elaborate on this further in the Talmud.

In accordance with these laws, Jews are forbidden to eat pork, a rule that has important ramifications for Jewish health, including the near-immunity of Jews to trichinosis, a potentially fatal disease caused by eating infected pigs (Gorwitz 1962). Kosher meat is also watched meticulously, from before the animal is even slaughtered to the end of the sales chain. It is forbidden for Kosher meat to come from a diseased animal: a law that subsequently provides an added measure of protection against food poisoning and other food-related illnesses (Barrow 2010). Additionally, there are specific obligations regarding ways to prepare meats after ritual slaughter, including salting even after the blood has been drained from the meat in order to guarantee that as little blood as possible is consumed. Salting meat in this way may make it less likely for consumers to be exposed to salmonella or E. coli bacteria (Barrow 2010). Given these strictures, medical personnel should be aware that Jewish patients might already adhere to specific diets that render them immune to some diseases, though exposure to certain diseases is still possible.

Dietary restrictions are an important consideration for health professionals working with Jewish patients. In America today, Jewish patients can request Kosher foods from outside institutions to be brought into hospitals or outpatient settings, and some hospitals in areas with larger Jewish populations have Kosher food options more readily available (Noble, Rom, Newsome-Wicks, Engelhardt, and Woloski-Wruble 2009; Selekman 2003). Medical personnel in these settings should always defer to the patient and ascertain whether the food provided is in line with his or her Kashrut standards, or whether outside food must be brought in to accommodate the patient's needs (Noble et al. 2009).

It is additionally important for doctors and health professionals to consider Jewish dietary restrictions when making nutrition-related health recommendations, such as change in diet or prescription of nutritional supplements. Generally, there are many vitamins and dietary supplements available with Kosher certification, though some specific vitamins may not require certification (see Blech 2009; Orthodox Union 2017). Health professionals prescribing vitamins or other similar natural health supplements should check with their patients regarding availability of Kosher items, or consult a comprehensive list such as those on KosherVitamins.com or on the Orthodox Union (OU) website.

Ritualized Eating/Feasting

Kashrut laws have some profound health benefits, as noted earlier, such as near elimination of the risk of trichinosis and a significantly lower risk of exposure to salmonella and E. coli (Barrow 2010). However, there are also potential health risks related to Jewish dietary laws and customs. Specifically, Sabbath-observant Jews commemorate the Sabbath each week with three ritual meals, which typically constitute a caloric intake significantly higher than the amount consumed on a regular weekday. For example, a typical Ashkenazi Orthodox Jewish Shabbat meal might include challah (a special braided bread eaten on Sabbath and Jewish holidays), wine, chicken soup and/or gefilte fish (a kind of fish made from a poached mixture of ground fish such as carp, whitefish, or pike), chicken and/or meat, and multiple side dishes, plus dessert (Bank 2002). This may contribute to issues with obesity and weight problems in the American Orthodox Jewish community (Rosenberg, Swencionis, and Segal-Isaacson 2015). Although the data are inconclusive regarding whether Jews, and Orthodox Jews in particular, are more susceptible to obesity or weight-related health issues, some studies have concluded that obesity in the Jewish community is comparable to overall obesity rates in the United States, while others emphasize Jewish proclivity toward obesity (Benjamins, Rhodes, Carp, and Whitman 2006).

In addition to obesity concerns, doctors and mental health professionals alike should consider these cultural components when treating Jewish patients for eating disorders. The emphasis on eating various foods on the Sabbath and festivals constitutes an important and unique factor for Jews with eating disorders. Some research shows that adolescent Jewish females are more susceptible to eating-disordered thoughts, attitudes, and behaviors (e.g., Dancyger et al. 2002; Pinhas, Heinmaa, Bryden, Bradley, and Toner 2008). Other studies conclude that religious and spiritual factors may contribute to positive outcomes in treatment for eating disorders (Miller and Pumariega 2001; Smith, Hardman, Richards, and Fischer 2003; Homan and Boyatzis 2010). All of these factors should be weighed when treating Jewish patients for eating-related health issues.

Fasting from Food/Drink

Though Jews may be vulnerable to obesity as a result of high caloric intake on the Sabbath and festivals, Jews also face another unique dietary challenge in the form of multiple fasts throughout the year. Six fast days are commemorated in the Jewish calendar. Four of these are considered "minor fasts," but two, Yom Kippur and Tisha B'Av, are considered "major fasts," and the stringency of the laws governing these days differs accordingly (Melamed 2001). Typically, about 53% of all Jews fast all or at least part of the Yom Kippur fast, while the other fasts are more often observed by mostly Orthodox Jews (Pew Research Center 2013). Observance of fast days has several health ramifications. The effects of fasting on the body can range from weight loss to hormone changes to severe headaches; however, observance of Jewish fast days more typically leads to the latter, as fasting is not sustained long enough to contribute to the former (Fazel 1998). Doctors should be aware of these fast days and should speak with their patients regarding the Halachic parameters of fasting, as exceptions and leniencies do exist for many patients, particularly for postpartum and/or nursing mothers; diabetics and individuals with other pre-existing medical conditions; patients with gastrointestinal complaints or eating-disorder histories; children; and the elderly (Melamed 2001; Dancyger et al. 2002).

Consumption of Alcohol

In addition to higher-than-average caloric intake, Jews are also more likely to imbibe more alcohol as part of cultural traditions related to the Sabbath and festivals. According to Jewish law, every Sabbath and festival must be consecrated through Kiddush, a Jewish ritual and blessing made over wine (Bank 2002). Additionally, there is a Mitzvah, or positive commandment, to drink alcohol on Purim, a rabbinically ordained holiday observed a month before Passover (Bank 2002; Loewenthal 2014). Alcohol consumption is also a compulsory part of festive occasions such as engagements and weddings. Although there are many places throughout the Torah and books of Jewish Law where excessive imbibing is frowned upon or even condemned, alcohol is still a central part of many Jewish rituals (Loewenthal 2014).

Despite the inclusion of wine in many Jewish traditions and rituals, however, medical records in the United States for most of the 20th century show that Jews tend to succumb to chronic alcoholism far less frequently than non-Jews, and many studies show that Jewish youth tend to be *less* susceptible to alcoholism than non-Jewish youth (Gorwitz 1962; Hanson 1974; Glassner and Berg 1980; Perkins 1985; Yeung and Greenwald 1992). Some more recent research has reinforced the idea that Jewish males, specifically, are less vulnerable to alcoholism than non-Jewish males (Levav, Kohn, Golding, and Weissman 1997; Monteiro and Schuckit 1989). It should be noted, though, that the inclusion of wine in many family events as part of Jewish tradition may make adolescents and young adults more susceptible to underage drinking. In fact, though there are reportedly lower rates of alcoholism among Jews, this does not entirely preclude either Jewish teens or adults from developing alcoholism (Loewenthal 2014).

Therefore, it is critical for doctors and mental health professionals alike to be aware of the centrality of alcohol consumption in many aspects of Jewish religious observance, so that they can sensitively assist Jewish patients who may be suffering from substance abuse or addiction. Additionally, there are some rehabilitation centers, help lines, and Alcoholics Anonymous (AA) support groups that cater to Jews. Although the outcomes for Jews in most rehab centers or AA programs are comparable to those among non-Jewish patients, issues such as obtaining Kosher food, maintaining access to communal prayer services, getting Halachic consultation with rabbinic authorities with regards to future alcohol consumption for religious rituals, and dealing with other cultural sensitivities are best addressed in Jewish centers (Loewenthal 2014). Recommendations for treatment of Jewish patients should include consideration of the particular religious needs of the patient, in addition to his or her particular medical needs; consultation with patients' rabbis may help with these important decisions.

Socioeconomic Status and Financial Issues

Turning our attention away from food, research has projected a negative relationship between socioeconomic status or class and mental health issues, and there is also evidence to suggest that poor health may contribute to financial strain (Kessler and Cleary 1980; Lyons and Yilmazer 2005). As with many cultural and religious groups, there is financial and economic diversity within the Jewish community: 44% of American Jews report an average income of $100,000 or more, but 31% report an average income of $50,000 or less (Pew Research Center 2014). These discrepancies should be considered when exploring common financial issues that are unique to Jewish culture and religion, as they may impact the degree to which these financial issues affect access to, pursuit of, and compliance with health care among Jews.

There are several financial issues that are specific to Jewish families, including the importance of community living and consequent real estate expenses, costs of Kosher food (for observant families), expenses for holidays and the Sabbath, private school or additional Hebrew school tuition for families interested in Jewish education, the moral and religious imperative to give to charity and help those in need, and the effect of family size on many of these variables. The cost of living may therefore be considerably higher for the average Jew, depending on his or her level of observance and the allocation of funds toward these ends; in fact, the average Orthodox family of five may spend anywhere from $50,000 to $110,000 each year in order to maintain a Jewish lifestyle (Wertheimer 2010).

One of the fundamental and important aspects of Jewish religion and culture is community involvement (Rosmarin, Pargament, Krumrei, and Flannelly 2009). Given the constraints of Sabbath observance, which preclude observant Jews from traveling in a car on the Sabbath, many Orthodox Jews live close together, usually surrounding the synagogue of the town (Huppert et al. 2007). Most Orthodox Jews, and often non-Orthodox Jews as well, tend to live in close-knit and somewhat segregated communities (Diamond 2000). For many Jews, therefore, buying homes is not simply a matter of finding a property that fits the family's needs and doesn't break the bank; the importance of living close to a synagogue in a thriving

Jewish community can sometimes cause considerable financial strain for Jewish families. Even among non-Orthodox Jews, who may not choose to live within walking distance of a synagogue, 39% of all Jewish families report that at least one member of the household has synagogue membership (Pew Research Center 2013). Synagogue membership can cost anywhere from a few hundred to well over several thousand dollars a year, depending on the size of the congregation, the location, and the expenses of the synagogue or community (Wertheimer 2010). This, too, is an extra expense that Jews face, which may cause financial strain.

Significant expenses associated with observance of the Sabbath and holidays also contribute to Jews' yearly, monthly, and weekly financial outflow. Because of the expenses of Kosher slaughter for meat and proper watching, checking, and production costs of other food items, Kosher foods typically cost more than comparable nonkosher items (Orthodox Union 2017). In addition, observance of the Sabbath calls for some amount of meat, fish, wine, and bread to be purchased each week, as each of these food items is specifically identified in Jewish tradition as being an important part of celebrating the Sabbath. Thus, Sabbath-observant Jews must allocate weekly funds in order to honor the Sabbath; in addition, many Orthodox as well as non-Orthodox Jews celebrate several holidays year-round that require similar levels of festivity and celebration, replete with food and drink. For example, Passover, a springtime holiday commemorating the Jewish exodus from Egypt, is celebrated by 70% of all American Jews (Pew Research Center 2014). Passover alone requires each individual celebrator to consume four cups of wine each of the first two nights of the holiday, and includes at least eight formal holiday meals. Each food item must be Kosher for Passover, as leavened bread and related ingredients are forbidden during these days, making the food purchased for Passover even more expensive than usual (Bank 2002).

Another important expense for many Jews—perhaps the greatest financial expense of all—is that of private or Hebrew school tuition. According to Jewish law, children should be taught principles of the faith and portions of the Torah and Talmud from an early age. While many non-Orthodox families may send their children to public schools or secular private schools, these families may still send their children to Hebrew schools as well, to supplement their Jewish education. Most Orthodox families send their children to private Orthodox schools where children receive a dual education in both secular and religious studies. Tuition costs for Orthodox private schools can range from $15,000 to $20,000 per child on average, though there are schools that charge even more (Wertheimer 2010).

In addition to the costs of living a Halachic or even cultural Jewish lifestyle, many Jews also uphold the cultural tradition to give charity to the poor as much as possible. There is a specific Torah mandate to give charity to a fellow Jew in need, as well as a cultural and ethical principle of giving charity (Cohen 2009). As such, Jewish philanthropy is quite common across a wide range of Jews, both Orthodox and non-Orthodox (Kosmin and Ritterband 1991). Though there is research supporting the idea that charity and charitable giving have inherent psychological value and can positively affect a person's mental health, allocating funds for charitable causes may be yet another financial strain in the life of the average Jew (Choi and Kim 2011; Kosmin and Ritterband 1991).

Besides the mandate to support other Jews and needy individuals monetarily, Jews also have a specific commandment to love and take care of their fellow Jews as much as possible. This has historically accounted for the characteristically charitable and giving nature of the Jewish people as a whole—a trait that positively affects the entire community through its many and varied nonprofit organizations dedicated to helping the poor and to supporting those in need of many different services (Kelemen 1990). This social support plays a critical role in Jewish culture across Jewish sects, which is especially important given the research evidence supporting the positive impact that this can have on members of a religious community (Ellison and George 1994; Krause et al. 2001; Pirutinsky, Rosmarin, Holt, et al. 2011). Many Orthodox Jewish communities have organizations dedicated to multiple forms of charity; support for domestic violence, infertility, special needs individuals, and hospitalized patients; and volunteer ambulance services, and most of these organizations cater to all Jews, no matter what the person's level of observance or affiliation.

For all of these reasons, many Orthodox and non-Orthodox Jews alike often have more expenses than one would expect, in some cases reducing the impact of the $150,000 income that 25% of all American Jewish families earn (Pew Research Center 2014). Many of these unique financial constraints may contribute to poorer access to care or lower quality of health care, so Jews may be more susceptible to lack of treatment follow-through in cases where treatment recommendations come at a higher cost. For example, studies show that Orthodox Jews report less access to dental care than non-Orthodox Jews (Lazarus, Pirutinsky, Korbman, and Rosmarin 2015). In addition to religious observance and related increases in cost of living for Orthodox Jews, Orthodox families also tend to be larger than non-Orthodox families, which may create still more of a financial burden. It is critical to note, however, that research examining the effects of family size on Jews revealed that larger family size does not predict poorer mental health outcomes, such as anxiety, depression, or family functioning; or parenting stress, indicating that Jewish families typically cope quite well regardless of family size (Pirutinsky et al. 2015).

The Jewish Family

Along these lines, it is important to understand the centrality of family to Jewish life. Family is a focal point of Judaism both in its role within Halacha as well as regarding cultural components of Judaism. According to Halacha, Jewish status is passed down through the mother, but many if not most of the customs practiced by a Jewish family come from the father (Aish HaTorah 2016). Family thus dictates not only an individual's Jewish status, but also how a Jew practices and incorporates Jewish concepts, ideas, and practices into his or her life.

Family life for many Jews begins with marriage, a state that is looked upon as uniquely holy, and which is itself a great Mitzvah (positive commandment; D. Feldman 1998). Marriage is looked upon as ideal in many ways, and a goal toward which many single Jewish men and women aspire throughout their adolescent and young adult years (Bank 2002; Rockman 1994). Procreation is one of the primary foci of marriage according to Jewish thought, as God commanded man to "be fruitful and multiply" (Genesis 1:28; *see also* Bank 2002; D. Feldman 1998). Once children are born, Jewish law and culture place special emphasis on the value of *Chinuch*, raising children and teaching them Jewish precepts and values in order to pass on Jewish tradition to the next generation (Pirutinsky, Schechter, et al. 2015). However, Jewish tradition dictates that this is not the only reason that men and women should marry. The Torah writes that God created Eve, the first woman, as a helpmate for Adam, the first man, because "it is not good for man to be alone," indicating that a Jewish marriage should be predicated on companionship as well as procreation (Genesis 2:18).

For these reasons, many Jewish young adults are faced with the daunting yet critical task of finding a partner in order to fulfill these important and meaningful commandments so central to Jewish culture; this may in turn create social and religious pressures for single Jewish men and women to marry (Rockman 1994; Bank 2002; Schechter 2012). The process of getting married may involve unique expectations for Jewish men and women of both Orthodox and non-Orthodox affiliations, though typically this pressure is felt more keenly among Orthodox Jews, where the expected age for marriage is lower, and pressure to date, marry, and have children may be greater (Kahn 2000; Schechter 2012).

As a result of the focus on children and family in Judaism, Orthodox Jews tend to have more children, which may contribute to greater stress in the home. However, as mentioned earlier, research shows that having a large family does not significantly impact mental health variables such as increases in stress, anxiety, and depression, despite the additional financial constraints facing larger religious families (Pirutinsky, Schechter, et al. 2015). The core value of family and children in Judaism may be a protective factor in this regard. Children and families are also a source of enjoyment and happiness in Jewish life. Family time is often a focal point of the holidays for many Jews, and family is central to the death and mourning process in Judaism, as discussed later in this chapter.

Because of the emphasis on family and childrearing in Jewish culture in general and Orthodox Jewish circles in particular, infertility may be an especially painful ordeal. Infertility can be devastating for any couple, but religious Jewish couples may experience additional difficulties due to the emotional stress and social stigma involved. Many Jewish women who struggle with infertility view their struggle as a kind of disability, excluding them from the social norms of their community and from the special Mitzvah of raising and educating Jewish children (Remennick 2000). Infertility also bars Jewish fathers from fulfilling their obligation to have children and to give a son a *Brit Milah* (ritual circumcision), as well as other important religious imperatives related to having children.

Despite these potential pressures, marriage in Judaism is regarded as sacred, special, and idealized in many regards (Bank 2002; Schechter 2012). Specifically, according to Jewish rabbinic law, a man may marry only one wife (Fleischman 2015). When a Jewish couple marries, a marriage contract, called a *ketubah*, is written, delineating the husband's financial, emotional, and physical responsibilities toward his wife (Epstein 1927). Regarding marital intimacy, Judaism views sex as not only a prerequisite for procreation, but also as part of the husband's obligations toward his wife. In fact, according to Jewish law, a man has an obligation to have children, but it is also his duty to see to it that his wife is sexually satisfied, regardless of whether or not she conceives (Feldman 1998). Furthermore, the Talmud dictates that despite a Jewish man's obligation to do his utmost to have children, he is still allowed to engage in sexual intercourse with his wife even if she is older, barren, or pregnant—that is, even if procreation will not be accomplished—because of this duty to her (Feldman 1998). This perspective on marriage and sexual intimacy between husband and wife stands in stark contrast to other views of marriage and is critical in understanding some of the issues that Jewish couples may face. Specific questions regarding a couple's individual situation should be addressed to their personal rabbi, and any professional who is helping a couple with issues related to marriage, sex, or conception should bear this in mind.

It is important to note that among Orthodox and ultra-Orthodox Jews, education about sex may not fully address the range of issues and concerns that can arise in a marriage, either in terms of Jewish law or as to intimacy in general (Friedman, Labinsky, Rosenbaum, Schmeidler, and Yehuda 2009). This may be an especially critical consideration for doctors and mental health practitioners specializing in couples counseling or treatment of sexual disorders. Given the emphasis on modesty and premarital chastity in Jewish law and thought, many Orthodox Jewish couples may not be comfortable discussing certain intimate details of their relationship, may lack the sexual education to properly cope with such issues, and may struggle to discuss these problems with each other as well (Friedman et al. 2009). It may be helpful to enlist the help of competent and knowledgeable rabbinic authorities in such cases, and, as always, to exercise sensitivity and caution in helping these couples through their struggles.

Another area of Jewish married life that requires specific attention is in the observation of the laws of family purity known as *Taharat HaMishpacha*. The laws of Taharat HaMishpacha constitute an important realm of Jewish life and are widely observed by Orthodox, and some non-Orthodox, Jewish couples (Friedman et al. 2009). Taharat HaMishpacha prohibits any physical contact between the couple during the wife's menstrual cycle and dictates that married women bathe in a ritual bath (*mikvah*) on the seventh clean day following the end of their menstruation before they can resume physical contact with their husbands (Noble et al. 2009; Friedman et al. 2009). There is a special Mitzvah to be intimate on the night that the wife immerses in the Mikvah, when an observant couple might try to conceive (D. Feldman 1998).

These laws can impact various health issues, and dealing with observant couples requires special sensitivity. For example, when an observant couple has a baby, the birth process itself renders the mother ritually impure, precluding the husband from being able to touch his wife throughout or after the labor and delivery (Noble et al. 2009). There are also occasions when a couple struggling with infertility may realize that the wife will ovulate before seven clean days have passed since the end of her period; in such instances, the couple may consult a rabbi to determine whether the wife can go to the mikvah earlier and thus increase the likelihood of the couple being able to conceive (Wasserfall 2015). It is important to exercise special sensitivity in these situations, and, of course, to be willing to consult with a couple's rabbi should any questions arise.

The laws of Taharat HaMishpacha are an important element of peace and harmony within Jewish marriages. While precluding the couple from physical intimacy for an average of 2 weeks out of every month, these laws preserve the novelty of the intimate relationship between husband and wife (Friedman et al. 2009). Many Jewish women appreciate these laws and feel that their sexual lives are improved because of them, whereas other women feel that the experience of going to the mikvah is uncomfortable and inconvenient, and have difficulty adhering to the laws (Friedman et al. 2009; Wasserfall 2015). Both attitudes are found throughout the

Jewish community, and reflect the importance and centrality of these laws to the marriages and lives of observant couples.

The Jewish perspective on sex and marriage becomes particularly important when dealing with contraception and abortion. Although a husband's obligations to his wife may permit intimacy in the absence of procreative intention, this does not necessarily allow an observant couple to use contraceptives (D. Feldman 1998). Many contemporary Orthodox rabbis discuss the issue of contraception at length. There are manifold approaches to this issue across the spectrum of Orthodox Judaism. Some Halachic authorities permit the use of oral contraceptives should a couple be deemed unfit to have children, in order to permit the couple to engage in marital relations to promote peace and harmony in the home, and to enable the husband to fulfill his obligations toward his wife (D. Feldman 1998). Other rabbis, however, do not allow couples to use any sort of contraceptives unless pregnancy or childbirth would cause physical harm to the mother or unborn child. In every case, a couple should consult with their individual rabbi to determine what approach is best.

In terms of abortion, there is similar discrepancy among rabbis when it comes to performing an abortion under certain circumstances. According to Halacha, a fetus has the status of a life from conception, and so abortion at any stage becomes a complicated process in that it is essentially destroying a life (D. Feldman 1998). Of course, there are extenuating circumstances under which abortion is allowed, such as when the unborn fetus puts the mother in fatal danger (D. Feldman 1998).

Mental Health

Jewish beliefs, values, and practices are particularly salient with regard to mental health among Jews. Though there is still a paucity of research pertaining specifically to Jews, the manner in which spirituality and religion influence Jewish mental health is a topic that is gaining traction in the literature. As is the case with many religions, religion and spirituality can have both negative and positive impacts on mental health among Jews (Rosmarin, Pirutinsky, Pargament, and Krumrei 2009). Regarding the potential psychological benefits of religio-spiritual factors for Jews, religious practices, such as prayer, synagogue attendance, community involvement, charity, and observing holidays and other positive commandments (Mitzvot), are related to lower anxiety and depression, and overall psychological distress is negatively correlated with religiosity among Jews (Rosmarin, Pargament, and Mahoney 2009; Rosmarin, Pirutinsky, Pargament, and Krumrei 2009; Rosmarin, Krumrei, and Andersson 2009; Rosmarin, Pirutinsky, Auerbach et al. 2011; Rosmarin, Pirutinksy, Cohen et al. 2011; Krumrei, Pirutinsky, and Rosmarin 2013).

In addition to religiosity, other mechanisms contribute to mental health outcomes for Jews as well. Some of these mechanisms include trust and mistrust in God, particularly in relation to intolerance of uncertainty, gratitude, religious coping, and spiritual struggles. As noted earlier, trust in God—operationally defined as the degree to which an individual Jew trusts that God is benevolent, in control of his or her life, and looking out for his or her best interests—is one of the core foundational beliefs of Judaism. In a series of studies examining Judaism and mental health, Rosmarin and colleagues found that trust and mistrust in God are important underlying mechanisms in understanding both anxiety and depression among both Orthodox and non-Orthodox Jews; specifically, trust in God is related to lower anxiety and depression, whereas mistrust in God is related to greater depression among Jews (Rosmarin, Pargament, and Mahoney 2009; Rosmarin, Pirutinsky, Pargament, and Krumrei 2009; Rosmarin, Pirutinsky, Auerbach, et al. 2011; Rosmarin, Pirutinksy, Cohen, et al. 2011). Of course, trust and mistrust in God may affect individuals who believe in God across a range of religions and levels of religious affiliation; however, Judaism emphasizes trust in God as one of its primary tenets of faith, making it particularly salient for Jews. It is therefore critical for mental health professionals to consider the implications of trust and mistrust in God for Jewish patients and to explore the degree to which an individual's beliefs about God affect his or her mental health.

Intolerance of uncertainty is explored throughout clinical psychology literature, particularly regarding its contribution to anxiety and related disorders (Dugas, Buhr, and Ladouceur 2004; Tolin, Abramowitz, Brigidi, and Foa 2003). Treatment of many anxiety and related disorders thus includes an orientation to the concept of tolerance of uncertainty and being able to cope with the unpredictability of life. This may resonate deeply for God-fearing Jews, as it is a fundamental part of Jewish ideology and practice. To that end, however, it must be noted that a fundamental belief and/or trust in God and God's omnipotence does not necessarily render any Jew immune to anxiety or other mental health issues. Rather, contemporary research is exploring the ways in which salient spirituality constructs and ideas can be effectively integrated into empirically based treatments for these disorders among Jews (e.g., Rosmarin, Pargament, Pirutinsky, and Mahoney 2010).

Gratitude is another important factor contributing to positive mental health outcomes among Jews and non-Jews alike. Religious gratitude includes feeling thankful and appreciative toward God and recognizing His love and benevolence. Being grateful to God and to others is central to religious and spiritual growth in Judaism, and may therefore be especially important to a Jew's mental health. Specifically, gratitude and spirituality may be important components of coping with trauma and loss for Jews

(Rosmarin, Krumrei, and Pargament 2010). Furthermore, religious gratitude (i.e., specific attitudes of appreciation for and directed toward God) may itself be a mediating variable contributing to gratitude for religious Jews, as Judaism emphasizes gratitude and provides opportunities to practice gratitude toward others as well as toward God (Rosmarin, Pirutinsky, Cohen, Galler, and Krumrei 2011). Gratitude may also contribute toward greater positive religious coping, which in turn contributes to positive mental health outcomes in the face of distress among Jews (Rosmarin, Pirutinsky, Greer, and Korbman 2016). It is important to consider all of these factors when counseling Jewish individuals.

Religious coping, or the degree to which individuals turn to religion to cope with stressful life events, is quite prevalent in the general population, and contributes tremendously to psychological and physical well-being in the face of life stressors (Pargament, Smith, Koenig, and Perez 1998). Studies on religious coping among Jews led to the development of a Judaism-specific measure of religious coping called the JCOPE (Rosmarin, Pargament, Krumrei, and Flannelly 2009). Research using the JCOPE shows that among Jews, positive religious coping is related to decreased self-reported anxiety and depression, whereas negative religious coping may contribute to poorer mental health outcomes such as increased depression, and is identified as a causal factor in depression in Orthodox Jews, specifically. Therefore, treatment for depression in this population should target negative religious coping and spiritual struggles more broadly (Pirutinsky, Rosmarin, Pargament, et al. 2011).

Spiritual struggles can be defined as difficulty or tension within oneself, with others, or with God in relation to spirituality (Pargament, Murray-Swank, Magyar, and Ano 2005). Rosmarin, Pargament, and Flannelly (2009) note that spiritual struggles contribute to many mental as well as physical health difficulties for religious and spiritual individuals, including Jews; these authors also found, however, that while spiritual struggles were related to decreased psychological and physical well-being among non-Orthodox Jews, Orthodox Jews' mental and physical health increased with higher levels of spiritual struggle. This may indicate that Orthodox Jews experience growth above and beyond non-Orthodox Jews in the face of significant spiritual struggles or adversity.

Similarly, though religious practice typically correlates with lower anxiety, religious practice is sometimes related to increased anxiety among Orthodox and ultra-Orthodox Jews (Rosmarin, Pargament, and Mahoney 2009). Those observant Jews whose dedication to and level of adherence to Halacha is markedly greater than that of non-Orthodox Jews may experience significant distress when dealing with fulfillment of everyday commandments or in preparing for holidays and other religious rituals. In general, many Orthodox and ultra-Orthodox Jews pay careful attention to the details of many Mitzvot, but there is a fine line between piety and scrupulosity, a religion-based obsessive-compulsive disorder (OCD; Huppert et al. 2007). It should also be noted that among Jews, and perhaps among Jewish practitioners, there is less of an understanding about the clinical presentation of religious OCD among non-Orthodox Jews (Rosmarin, Pirutinsky, and Siev 2010). Psychoeducation regarding scrupulosity is therefore a critical component of diagnosis and treatment for individuals with OCD. Additionally, as noted previously, sensitive treatment of religious OCD should include working with rabbinic authorities and with a patient's own designated rabbi in order to maintain proper adherence to both Torah law and dictates of empirically supported treatments for OCD (such as exposure and response prevention), as treatment may mandate what appears to the patient to be laxity in observance or purposeful violation of Jewish law (Huppert et al. 2007).

There are a few other issues to consider with regard to mental health among Jews, including prayer, community and social support, stigma, and use of medication. Prayer is a significant part of Judaism. Jewish law dictates that men should pray three times daily in a congregation consisting of at least 10 men called a *minyan*, and most Ashkenazi rabbinic authorities hold that Jewish women should pray twice daily, though they do not require a minyan to pray (Bank 2002). In general, the literature is still largely inconclusive as to whether prayer serves a protective function in mental health. Although some studies show that there is no significant correlation between prayer and mental health factors like anxiety, Jewish thought encourages Jews to pray to God specifically in times of distress, which might in turn mitigate anxiety under stressful situations (Ellison, Bradshaw, Flannelly, and Galek 2014; Kaplan and Sutton 1992). Additionally, Jews have specific prayers that are said in connection with particular life situations, including illness, financial difficulties, infertility, and other struggles; in many Jewish congregations, special prayers are said to entreat God on behalf of the sick and in commemoration of the dead (Cutter 2008). It is thus conceivable that Jewish individuals who engage in prayer may do so in order to alleviate anxiety or cope with grief, though the exact nature of this relationship requires further exploration. To these ends, it is important to consult contemporary research on the impact of prayer on mental health, and to examine the role of prayer in patients' lives.

As mentioned earlier, the social and community support afforded by religious involvement are frequently cited as having particular health benefits (e.g., Ellison and George 1994). In Judaism in particular, the importance of community and the subsequent social support afforded by strong communal ties may have a significant impact on Jewish mental health, such as mitigating the effects of depression in Jews with physical illnesses (Pirutinsky, Rosmarin, Holt, et al. 2011). Even among non-Jews, social support, religious involvement, and community involvement are all related to decreased risk for and resiliency in the face of depression (McCullough and Larson 1999). It thus stands to reason that Jews, and perhaps especially Orthodox Jews, reap many benefits from the various social and community organizations catering to the needs of the Jewish community. Mental health practitioners should become familiar with the organizations that may be of service to their patients, as this added support may contribute to better treatment outcomes.

A significant mental health stigma still exists among Orthodox Jews, specifically, and this may deter Jewish patients from seeking mental health treatment (Rosen, Greenberg, Schmeidler, and Shefler 2008). Given Judaism's family-oriented emphasis, mental illness is also perceived as a risk for the family as a whole, and is therefore even more highly stigmatized (Pirutinsky, Rosen, Safran, and Rosmarin 2010). Although medication use for mental disorders is becoming increasingly widespread, it may be even more stigmatized in Jewish communities, as a medical model of mental illness creates greater concerns about individual and family health as well as concerns about genetic contributions to disorders and the implications of these concerns for marriage (Pirutinsky et al. 2010). Work is being done to destigmatize mental illness in the Jewish community, but practitioners should be aware of Jewish patients' attitudes toward mental health treatment and exercise sensitivity in dealing with Jewish patients and their families.

End-of-Life Issues

Many volumes have been written to address the Jewish perspective on medical ethics with regard to terminal illness, death, and mourning. Indeed, the depth and breadth of these issues warrants volumes, and cannot be fully encompassed by a mere subsection of this chapter; thus, we briefly address some of the more common questions that arise. It is important first to review the Jewish ideological perspective on illness and death and its implications. As was mentioned previously, Judaism is a life-oriented religion. So strong is the value of human life in Judaism that one is often obligated to commit a major sin, like breaking Shabbat, for the sake of saving a life (Dorff 1998). This fundamental value of life in Judaism has many implications for dealing with end-of-life issues (Clarfield et al. 2003). Specifically, Jewish law dictates that a person on the brink of death has the exact same status as that of a perfectly healthy, living person, and thus nothing can or should be done to hasten his or her death, as every moment of life is precious in Jewish thought and law (Baeke, Wils, and Broeckaert 2011).

Jewish perspectives on euthanasia and practically all other end-of-life issues relate to this central idea.

Contemporary Jewish Halachic authorities have not yet reached a consensus regarding euthanasia. Generally speaking, Orthodox Judaism stands in staunch opposition, and while there are some Conservative authorities who advocate for euthanasia, there are also many rabbis within both the Conservative and Reform movements who insist that man's body belongs to God, not to man, and thus man has no right to do anything that brings on premature death (see Baeke et al. 2011, and Dorff 1998 for a detailed review of these issues). Because of the complexities involved in determining the Halacha, and given the social and ethical issues surrounding euthanasia, making decisions regarding the care of a terminally ill loved one can be difficult and painful for a Jewish family. It is important to treat these issues with sensitivity, and to work closely with a Jewish family's religious leader to act in the best interests of a patient and his or her family.

Another salient aspect of Jewish faith with regard to death is the belief in the afterlife, known as Olam HaBa, the World to Come (M. Lamm 1969). This belief is a core motivator for fulfillment of the commandments during one's lifetime, and it is also a critical part of understanding Jewish perspectives on death and mourning. Although the precise nature of the World to Come is not entirely clear from the Jewish texts, belief in the afterlife means the complete faith that, while there is reward and punishment in this world as well, humans reap the true reward for their deeds after they pass away (M. Lamm 1969). Thus, one understanding of the World to Come is that when a man dies, his spiritual soul leaves his physical body. It is the World to Come that greets a person's soul after he or she dies, and it is there that one receives one's final reckoning from God.

One can also understand the World to Come in Jewish teachings as referring to the resurrection of the dead, another fundamental tenet of Jewish faith (M. Lamm 1969). Many Jews believe both in life after death for an individual soul and in the eventual resurrection of the dead, which will occur in the times of the Messiah, as God promises throughout the 24 books of Tanach (M. Lamm 1969). Thus, when a person dies, his or her time on this earth as a physical, tangible being ceases; Jewish thought teaches, however, that the soul is eternal, and thus, in mourning, one mourns the absence of the loved one while also striving to elevate the departed soul and provide it with extra merits for its divine judgment (M. Lamm 1969). Many of the customs surrounding the funeral, burial, and mourning process relate to this idea.

In preparation for the funeral, there are specific laws that must be followed in order to respect the body of the deceased as well as to prepare the soul for its journey to the World to Come. These customs and related issues in Jewish law are discussed at length in Maurice Lamm's critical book, *The*

Jewish Way in Death and Mourning (1969). Upon the death of a loved one, immediate family members enter a seven-day mourning period called Shiva (from the Hebrew word *sheva*, which means seven), during which the mourners sit on low chairs, and abide by specific laws to avoid physical pleasure, such as not wearing leather shoes and refraining from marital intimacy (M. Lamm 1969). During Shiva, there is a special Mitzvah for friends and family to visit the mourners in their home, to talk about and honor the deceased and to have a special space to comfort those who are grieving (M. Lamm 1969; Slochower 1993). This seven-day period can be especially therapeutic and beneficial for the mourners, as it allows them time to grieve appropriately and not have to return to work or everyday life without first confronting the pain of their loss (Slochower 1993). The added Mitzvah for others in the family and community to provide support, bring food to the house, and sit with the mourners is an especially important component of the Shiva process (Casariego 2016).

CONCLUSION

Judaism has many unique characteristics. There are multiple sects within Judaism, and thus various ways of practicing the religion, but Judaism's unique outlook on life, health, family, illness, and death is felt and shared on some level by Jews worldwide. Jewish thought, culture, and law have many implications for physical and mental health, and there are benefits, complexities, and potential obstacles that Jews may face as a result of their beliefs and practices. Hence, it is important to be culturally competent and to be as informed as possible when treating Jewish patients across the spectrum of medical and mental health fields. At the same time, given the differences of opinion and interpretation of Halacha across sects, and due to individual differences among Jews even from the same family or background, it is imperative that professionals speak directly with their Jewish clients to ascertain their personal level of observance, as well as to understand how their beliefs and practices uniquely affect their lives. Last, it is always helpful to consult with Jewish patients' rabbis or other religious leaders, so as to be able to best help them in a culturally sensitive manner.

REFERENCES

Aish HaTorah. 2016. "Half-Jewish." Retrieved from http://www.aish.com/atr/Half-Jewish.html

Baeke, G., J.-P. Wils, and B. Broeckaert. 2011. "'There Is a Time to be Born and a Time to Die' (Ecclesiastes 3: 2a): Jewish Perspectives on Euthanasia." *Journal of Religion and Health* 50(4): 778–795.

Bank, R. D. 2002. *The Everything Judaism Book: A Complete Primer to the Jewish Faith—From Holidays and Rituals to Traditions and Culture.* Avon, MA: Adams Media.

Barrow, K. 2010. "More People Choosing Kosher for Health." *New York Times.* Retrieved from http://well.blogs.nytimes.com/2010/04/13/more-people -choosing-kosher-for-health/?_r=2

Benjamins, M. R., D. M. Rhodes, J. M. Carp, and S. Whitman. 2006. "A Local Community Health Survey: Findings from a Population-Based Survey of the Largest Jewish Community in Chicago." *Journal of Community Health* 31(6): 479–495.

Blech, Z. Y. 2009. *Kosher Food Production.* Hoboken, NJ: John Wiley & Sons.

Casariego, J. I. 2016. "What Is Shiva?" *Shiva.com.* Retrieved from http://www.shiva. com/learning-center/understanding/shiva/

Choi, N. G., and J. Kim. 2011. "The Effect of Time Volunteering and Charitable Donations in Later Life on Psychological Wellbeing." *Ageing and Society* 31(4): 590–610.

Clarfield, A. M., M. Gordon, H. Markwell, and S. M. H. Alibhai. 2003. "Ethical Issues in End-of-Life Geriatric Care: The Approach of Three Monotheistic Religions—Judaism, Catholicism, and Islam." *Journal of the American Geriatrics Society* 51(8): 1149–1154.

Cohen, M. R. 2009. *Poverty and Charity in the Jewish Community of Medieval Egypt.* Princeton, NJ: Princeton University Press.

Cutter, W. 2008. *Healing and the Jewish Imagination: Spiritual and Practical Perspectives on Judaism and Health.* Nashville, TN: Jewish Lights.

Dancyger, I., V. Fornari, M. Fisher, M. Schneider, S. Frank, W. Wisotsky, . . . M. Charitou. 2002. "Cultural Factors in Orthodox Jewish Adolescents Treated in a Day Program for Eating Disorders." *International Journal of Adolescent Medicine and Health* 14(4): 317–328.

Diamond, E. 2000. *And I Will Dwell in Their Midst: Orthodox Jews in Suburbia.* Chapel Hill: University of North Carolina Press.

Don-Yihya, E. 2005. "Orthodox Jewry in Israel and in North America." *Israel Studies* 10(1): 157–187.

Dorff, E. N. 1998. *Matters of Life and Death.* Philadelphia, PA: Jewish Publication Society.

Dugas, M. J., K. Buhr, and R. Ladouceur. 2004. "The Role of Intolerance of Uncertainty in Etiology and Maintenance." In R. G. Heimberg, C. L. Turk, and D. S. Mennin, eds., *Generalized Anxiety Disorder: Advances in Research and Practice,* pp. 143–163. New York: Guilford Press.

Ellison, C. G., M. Bradshaw, K. J. Flannelly, and K. C. Galek. 2014. "Prayer, Attachment to God, and Symptoms of Anxiety-Related Disorders among US Adults." *Sociology of Religion* 75(2): 208–233.

Ellison, C. G., and L. K. George. 1994. "Religious Involvement, Social Ties, and Social Support in a Southeastern Community." *Journal for the Scientific Study of Religion* 33(1): 46–61.

Epstein, L. M. 1927. *The Jewish Marriage Contract: A Study in the Status of the Woman in Jewish Law*. New York: The Lawbook Exchange.

Fazel, M. 1998. "Medical Implications of Controlled Fasting." *Journal of the Royal Society of Medicine* 91(5): 260–263.

Feldman, D. M. 1998. *Birth Control in Jewish Law: Marital Relations, Contraception, and Abortion as Set forth in the Classic Texts of Jewish Law*. Lanham, MD: Jason Aronson.

Feldman, P. 1992. "Sexuality, Birth Control and Childbirth in Orthodox Jewish Tradition." *CMAJ: Canadian Medical Association Journal* 146(1): 29–33.

Fleischman, Y. 2015, November 18. *Marrying More than One Wife: The Decree of Rabbeinu Gershom—Then and Today*. Retrieved from http://dinonline. org/2015/11/18/marrying-more-than-one-wife-the-decree-of-rabbeinu -gershom-then-and-today/

Friedman, M., E. Labinsky, T. Rosenbaum, J. Schmeidler, and R. Yehuda. 2009. "Observant Married Jewish Women and Sexual Life: An Empirical Study." *Conversations: Institute for Jewish Ideas and Ideals* 5: 1–26. Retrieved from http://www.physioforwomen.com/sites/default/files/Observant_Married _Jewish_Women_0.pdf

Gillman, N. 1993. *Conservative Judaism: The New Century*. Springfield Township, NJ: Behrman House.

Glassner, B., and B. Berg. 1980. "How Jews Avoid Alcohol Problems." *American Sociological Review* 46(4): 647–664.

Goldsand, G., Z. R. S. Rosenberg, and M. Gordon. 2001. "Bioethics for Clinicians: 22. Jewish Bioethics." *Canadian Medical Association Journal* 164(2): 219–222.

Goodman, Y., and E. Witztum. 2002. "Cross-Cultural Encounters Between Care Providers: Rabbis' Referral Letters to a Psychiatric Clinic in Israel." *Social Science & Medicine* 55(8): 1309–1323.

Gorwitz, K. 1962. "Jewish Mortality in St. Louis and St. Louis County, 1955–1957." *Jewish Social Studies* (1962): 248–254.

Greenberg, D., and G. Shefler. 2002. "Obsessive Compulsive Disorder in Ultra-Orthodox Jewish Patients: A Comparison of Religious and Non-Religious Symptoms." *Psychology and Psychotherapy: Theory, Research and Practice* 75(2): 123–130.

Hanson, D. J. 1974. "Drinking Attitudes and Behaviors among College Students." *Journal of Alcohol and Drug Education* 19: 6–14.

Harrison, M. O., H. G. Koenig, J. C. Hays, A. G. Eme-Akwari, and K. I. Pargament. 2001. "The Epidemiology of Religious Coping: A Review of Recent Literature." *International Review of Psychiatry* 13(2): 86–93.

Homan, K. J., and C. J. Boyatzis. 2010. "The Protective Role of Attachment to God against Eating Disorder Risk Factors: Concurrent and Prospective Evidence." *Eating Disorders* 18(3): 239–258.

Huppert, J. D., J. Siev, and E. S. Kushner. 2007. "When Religion and Obsessive-Compulsive Disorder Collide: Treating Scrupulosity in Ultra-Orthodox Jews." *Journal of Clinical Psychology* 63(10): 925–941.

Israel and Judaism Studies. 2016. "Variants Within Judaism." Retrieved from http://www.ijs.org.au/Variants-within-Judaism/default.aspx

Kabat-Zinn, J., L. Lipworth, and R. Burney. 1985. "The Clinical Use of Mindfulness Meditation for the Self-Regulation of Chronic Pain." *Journal of Behavioral Medicine* 8(2): 163–190.

Kahn, S. M. 2000. *Reproducing Jews: A Cultural Account of Assisted Conception in Israel*. Durham, NC: Duke University Press.

Kaplan, A. 2001. "World of Love #1—Purpose of Creation." *Aish HaTorah*. Retrieved from http://www.aish.com/jl/p/wl/48929907.html

Kaplan, A., and A. Sutton. 1992. *The Handbook of Jewish Thought* (Vol. 2). Brooklyn, NY: Maznaim Publishing.

Kark, J. D., G. Shemi, Y. Friedlander, O. Martin, O. Manor, and S. H. Blondheim. 1996. "Does Religious Observance Promote Health? Mortality in Secular vs. Religious Kibbutzim in Israel." *American Journal of Public Health* 86(3): 341–346.

Kelemen, L. 1990. *Permission to Believe: Four Rational Approaches to God's Existence* (2nd ed.). Brooklyn, NY: Targum Press.

Keshet, Y., and I. Liberman. 2014. "Coping with Illness and Threat: Why Non-Religious Jews Choose to Consult Rabbis on Healthcare Issues." *Journal of Religion and Health* 53(4): 1146–1160.

Kessler, R. C., and P. D. Cleary. 1980. "Social Class and Psychological Distress." *American Sociological Review* 45(3): 463–478.

Kestenbaum, I. 1988. "The Rabbi as Caregiver: A Clinical Model." *Tradition: A Journal of Orthodox Jewish Thought* 23(3): 32–40.

Koenig, H., D. King, and V. B. Carson. 2012. *Handbook of Religion and Health*. New York: Oxford University Press USA.

Kosmin, B. A., and P. Ritterband. 1991. *Contemporary Jewish Philanthropy in America*. Lanham, MD: Rowman & Littlefield.

Krause, N., C. G. Ellison, B. A. Shaw, J. P. Marcum, and J. D. Boardman. 2001. "Church-Based Social Support and Religious Coping." *Journal for the Scientific Study of Religion* 40(4): 637–656.

Krieger, A. Y. 2010. "The Role of Judaism in Family Relationships." *Journal of Multicultural Counseling and Development* 38(3): 154–165.

Krumrei, E. J., S. Pirutinsky, and D. H. Rosmarin. 2013. "Jewish Spirituality, Depression, and Health: An Empirical Test of a Conceptual Framework." *International Journal of Behavioral Medicine* 20(3): 327–336.

Lamm, M. 1969. *The Jewish Way in Death and Mourning*. New York: Jonathan David Publishers.

Lamm, N. 1973, Fall. Review of *The Jewish Dietary Laws*, by Dayan Dr. I. Grunfeld. *Tradition: A Journal of Orthodox Jewish Thought* 14(2): 143–145.

Lazar, A., and J. P. Bjorck. 2008. "Religious Support and Psychosocial Well-Being among a Religious Jewish Population." *Mental Health, Religion and Culture* 11(4): 403–421.

Lazarus, Z., S. Pirutinsky, M. Korbman, and D. H. Rosmarin. 2015. "Dental Utilization Disparities in a Jewish Context: Reasons and Potential Solutions." *Community Dental Health* 32: 1–7.

Levav, I., R. Kohn, J. M. Golding, and M. M. Weissman. 1997. "Vulnerability of Jews to Affective Disorders." *American Journal of Psychiatry* 154(7): 941–947.

Levin, J. 2011. "Health Impact of Jewish Religious Observance in the USA: Findings from the 2000–01 National Jewish Population Survey." *Journal of Religion and Health* 50(4): 852–868.

Liebman, C. S. 1965. "Orthodoxy in American Jewish Life." *The American Jewish Year Book* (1965): 21–97.

Loewenthal, K. M. 2014. "Addiction: Alcohol and Substance Abuse in Judaism." *Religions* 5(4): 972–984.

Lyons, A. C., and T. Yilmazer. 2005. "Health and Financial Strain: Evidence from the Survey of Consumer Finances." *Southern Economic Journal* 71(4): 873–890.

Mark, N., and L. Roberts. 1993. "Ethnosensitive Techniques in the Treatment of the Hasidic Patient with Cancer." *Cancer Practice* 2(3): 202–208.

McCullough, M. E., W. T. Hoyt, D. B. Larson, H. G. Koenig, and C. Thoresen. 2000. "Religious Involvement and Mortality: a Meta-Analytic Review." *Health Psychology* 19(3): 211–222.

McCullough, M. E., and D. B. Larson. 1999. "Religion and Depression: A Review of the Literature." *Twin Research* 2(2): 126–136.

Melamed, E. 2001. "The Minor Fasts and Their Laws." *Yeshiva.co: The Torah World Gateway.* Retrieved from http://www.yeshiva.co/midrash/shiur.asp?id=2399

Merriam-Webster's Collegiate Dictionary (11th ed.). 2003. Springfield, MA: Merriam-Webster.

Meyer, M. A. 1995. *Response to Modernity: A History of the Reform Movement in Judaism.* Detroit, MI: Wayne State University Press.

Miller, M. N., and A. J. Pumariega. 2001. "Culture and Eating Disorders: A Historical and Cross-Cultural Review." *Psychiatry* 64(2): 93–110.

Mittman, I. S., J. V. Bowie, and S. Maman. 2007. "Exploring the Discourse Between Genetic Counselors and Orthodox Jewish Community Members Related to Reproductive Genetic Technology." *Patient Education and Counseling* 65(2): 230–236.

Monteiro, M. G., and M. A. Schuckit. 1989. "Alcohol, Drug, and Mental Health Problems among Jewish and Christian Men at a University." *American Journal of Drug and Alcohol Abuse* 15(4): 403–412.

Noble, A., M. Rom, M. Newsome-Wicks, K. Engelhardt, and A. Woloski-Wruble. 2009. "Jewish Laws, Customs, and Practice in Labor, Delivery, and Postpartum Care." *Journal of Transcultural Nursing* 20, no. 3 (2009): 323–333.

Nooney, J., and E. Woodrum. 2002. "Religious Coping and Church-Based Social Support as Predictors of Mental Health Outcomes: Testing a Conceptual Model." *Journal for the Scientific Study of Religion* 41(2): 359–368.

Orthodox Union. 2017. *The Kosher Primer*. Retrieved from https://oukosher.org/the
-kosher-primer/

Pargament, K. I., N. Murray-Swank, G. M. Magyar, and G. G. Ano. 2005. "Spiritual
Struggle: A Phenomenon of Interest to Psychology and Religion." In W. R.
Miller and H. D. Delane, eds., *Judeo-Christian Perspectives on Psychology:
Human Nature, Motivation, and Change*, pp. 245–268. Washington, DC:
American Psychological Association.

Pargament, K. I., B. W. Smith, H. G. Koenig, and L. Perez. 1998. "Patterns of Positive and Negative Religious Coping with Major Life Stressors." *Journal for
the Scientific Study of Religion* 37(4): 710–724.

Perkins, H. W. 1985. "Religious Traditions, Parents, and Peers as Determinants of
Alcohol and Drug Use among College Students." *Review of Religious Research*
27(1): 15–31.

Pew Research Center. 2013. "A Portrait of Jewish Americans." Retrieved from http://
www.pewforum.org/2013/10/01/jewish-american-beliefs-attitudes-culture
-survey/

Pew Research Center. 2014. "Income Distribution." Retrieved from http://www
.pewforum.org/religious-landscape-study/income-distribution/

Pew Research Center. 2015a. "Jews." Retrieved from http://www.pewforum.org
/2015/04/02/jews/

Pew Research Center. 2015b. "A Portrait of American Orthodox Jews." Retrieved
from http://www.pewforum.org/2015/08/26/a-portrait-of-american-ortho
dox-jews/

Pinhas, L., M. Heinmaa, P. Bryden, S. Bradley, and B. Toner. 2008. "Disordered Eating in Jewish Adolescent Girls." *Canadian Journal of Psychiatry* 53(9):
601–608.

Pirutinsky, S., D. D. Rosen, R. S. Safran, and D. H. Rosmarin. 2010. "Do Medical
Models of Mental Illness Relate to Increased or Decreased Stigmatization of
Mental Illness among Orthodox Jews?" *Journal of Nervous and Mental Dis-
ease* 198(7): 508–512.

Pirutinsky, S., D. H. Rosmarin, C. L. Holt, R. H. Feldman, L. S. Caplan, E. Midlarsky, and K. I. Pargament. 2011. "Does Social Support Mediate the Moder-
ating Effect of Intrinsic Religiosity on the Relationship between Physical
Health and Depressive Symptoms among Jews?" *Journal of Behavioral Medicine* 34(6): 489–496.

Pirutinsky, S., D. H. Rosmarin, K. I. Pargament, and E. Midlarsky. 2011. "Does Negative Religious Coping Accompany, Precede, or Follow Depression among
Orthodox Jews?" *Journal of Affective Disorders* 132(3): 401–405.

Pirutinsky, S., I. Schechter, A. Kor, and D. Rosmarin. 2015. "Family Size and Psychological Functioning in the Orthodox Jewish Community." *Mental Health,
Religion & Culture* 18(3): 218–230.

Regenstein, J. M. 1994. "Health Aspects of Kosher Foods." *Activities Report of the
R and D Associates (USA)* 46(1): 77–83.

Regenstein, J. M., M. M. Chaudry, and C. E. Regenstein. 2003. "The Kosher and Halal Food Laws." *Comprehensive Reviews in Food Science and Food Safety* 2(3): 111–127.

Remennick, L. 2000. "Childless in the Land of Imperative Motherhood: Stigma and Coping among Infertile Israeli Women." *Sex Roles* 43(11–12): 821–841.

Rockman, H. 1994. "Matchmaker Matchmaker Make Me a Match: The Art and Conventions of Jewish Arranged Marriages." *Sexual and Marital Therapy* 9(3): 277–284.

Rosen, D. D., D. Greenberg, J. Schmeidler, and G. Shefler. 2008. "Stigma of Mental Illness, Religious Change, and Explanatory Models of Mental Illness among Jewish Patients at a Mental-Health Clinic in North Jerusalem." *Mental Health, Religion and Culture* 11(2): 193–209.

Rosenberg, D. A., C. Swencionis, and C. J. Segal-Isaacson. 2015. "Caloric Intake on the Sabbath: A Pilot Study of Contributing Factors to Obesity in the Orthodox Jewish Community." *Journal of Religion and Health* 55(5): 1824–1831.

Rosmarin, D. H., E. J. Krumrei, and G. Andersson. 2009. "Religion as a Predictor of Psychological Distress in Two Religious Communities." *Cognitive Behaviour Therapy* 38(1): 54–64.

Rosmarin, D. H., E. J. Krumrei, and K. I. Pargament. 2010. "Do Gratitude and Spirituality Predict Psychological Distress?" *International Journal of Existential Psychology & Psychotherapy* 3(1): 1–5.

Rosmarin, D. H., K. I. Pargament, and K. J. Flannelly. 2009. "Do Spiritual Struggles Predict Poorer Physical/Mental Health among Jews?" *International Journal for the Psychology of Religion* 19(4): 244–258.

Rosmarin, D. H., K. I. Pargament, E. J. Krumrei, and K. J. Flannelly. 2009. "Religious Coping among Jews: Development and Initial Validation of the JCOPE." *Journal of Clinical Psychology* 65(7): 670–683.

Rosmarin, D. H., K. I. Pargament, and A. Mahoney. 2009. "The Role of Religiousness in Anxiety, Depression, and Happiness in a Jewish Community Sample: A Preliminary Investigation." *Mental Health, Religion and Culture* 12(2): 97–113.

Rosmarin, D. H., K. I. Pargament, S. Pirutinsky, and A. Mahoney. 2010. "A Randomized Controlled Evaluation of a Spiritually Integrated Treatment for Subclinical Anxiety in the Jewish Community, Delivered via the Internet." *Journal of Anxiety Disorders* 24(7): 799–808.

Rosmarin, D. H., S. Pirutinsky, R. P. Auerbach, T. Björgvinsson, J. Bigda-Peyton, G. Andersson, . . . E. J. Krumrei. 2011. "Incorporating Spiritual Beliefs into a Cognitive Model of Worry." *Journal of Clinical Psychology* 67(7): 691–700.

Rosmarin, D. H., S. Pirutinsky, A. B. Cohen, Y. Galler, and E. J. Krumrei. 2011. "Grateful to God or Just Plain Grateful? A Comparison of Religious and General Gratitude." *Journal of Positive Psychology* 6(5): 389–396.

Rosmarin, D. H., S. Pirutinsky, D. Greer, and M. Korbman. 2016. "Maintaining a Grateful Disposition in the Face of Distress: The Role of Religious Coping." *Psychology of Religion and Spirituality* 8(2): 134–140.

Rosmarin, D. H., S. Pirutinsky, K. I. Pargament, and E. J. Krumrei. 2009. "Are Religious Beliefs Relevant to Mental Health among Jews?" *Psychology of Religion and Spirituality* 1(3): 180–190.

Rosmarin, D. H., S. Pirutinsky, and J. Siev. 2010. "Recognition of Scrupulosity and Non-Religious OCD by Orthodox and Non-Orthodox Jews." *Journal of Social and Clinical Psychology* 29(8): 931–945.

Rumun, A. J. 2014. "Influence of Religious Beliefs on Healthcare Practice." *International Journal of Educational Resources* 2(4): 37–48.

Schechter, Y. 2012. "Creating a Resting Place for the Shechina: Ideals, Expectations and Reality in Marriage." *Klal Perspectives* 1(4): 19–27.

Schlossberger, E. S., and L. L. Hecker. 1998. "Reflections on Jewishness and Its Implications for Family Therapy." *American Journal of Family Therapy* 26(2): 129–146.

Selekman, J. 2003. "People of Jewish Heritage." In L. D. Purnell and B. J. Paulanka, eds., *Transcultural Health Care: A Culturally Competent Approach,*. pp. 234–248. Philadelphia: F. A. Davis.

Simmons, S. 2014. "Six Constant Mitzvot." *Aish HaTorah.* Retrieved from http://www.aish.com/jl/jewish-law/daily-living/2-Six-Constant-Mitzvot.html

Slochower, J. A. 1993. "Mourning and the Holding Function of Shiva." *Contemporary Psychoanalysis* 29(2): 352–367.

Smith, F. T., R. K. Hardman, P. S. Richards, and L. Fischer. 2003. "Intrinsic Religiousness and Spiritual Well-Being as Predictors of Treatment Outcome among Women with Eating Disorders." *Eating Disorders* 11(1): 15–26.

Spiro, K. 2001. "History Crash Course #39: The Talmud." *Aish HaTorah.* Retrieved from http://www.aish.com/jl/h/cc/48948646.html

Strawbridge, W. J., R. D. Cohen, S. J. Shema, and G. A. Kaplan. 1997. "Frequent Attendance at Religious Services and Mortality over 28 Years." *American Journal of Public Health* 87(6): 957–961.

Tolin, D. F., J. S. Abramowitz, B. D. Brigidi, and E. B. Foa. 2003. "Intolerance of Uncertainty in Obsessive-Compulsive Disorder." *Journal of Anxiety Disorders* 17(2): 233–242.

Wasserfall, R., ed. 2015. *Women and Water: Menstruation in Jewish Life and Law.* Waltham, MA: Brandeis University Press.

Wertheimer, J. 2010. "The High Cost of Jewish Living." *Commentary.* Retrieved from https://www.commentarymagazine.com/articles/the-high-cost-of-jewish-living/

Yeung, P. P., and S. Greenwald. 1992. "Jewish Americans and Mental Health: Results of the NIMH Epidemiologic Catchment Area Study." *Social Psychiatry and Psychiatric Epidemiology* 27(6): 292–297.

Chapter 7

Christianity—Catholic and Seventh-day Adventist Examples

Arndt Büssing and Désirée Poier

CHRISTIAN DIVERSITY

Christianity as a monotheistic religion referring to the teachings of Jesus Christ (as handed down in the New Testament of the Bible) is a theologically quite diverse religion that has separated into three larger branches and various denominations within the centuries. We can differentiate the Roman Catholic lineage (about 50% of the global Christian population; most live in Latin America), the Orthodox lineages (around 10% of all Christians; most live in Russia), and the Protestant denominations (about 40% of all Christians; most live in the United States). These latter include, for example, Calvinism, Lutheranism, Anglicanism, Methodism, Puritanism, Presbyterianism, and Adventists, among others. It is thus difficult to state the position of "Christianity" as a circumscribed and definite religious tradition. The different branches and denominations may not only differ with respect to the content of their beliefs and specific doctrines, but may also be influenced by cultural and regional characteristics. Moreover, some Catholic positions, for example, though intended to be obligatory, might be interpreted and followed differently by adherents in North Europe, South Europe, Africa, Asia, or Latin America (where more Catholics are living than in Europe). The same is true for the various Free-Church lineages with mostly independent religious authorities. Some local churches and parishes may be rather strict and others more liberal.

For purposes of this chapter, we focus on two distinct denominations within the heterogeneous group of Christianity: namely, Catholics and Seventh-day Adventists (7DAs). They both rely on the same sources of the Old and New Testament, but with different emphasis. For the 7DAs, the (prophetic) writings of Ellen G. White (1827–1915), who wrote in her publications on the benefits of a healthy lifestyle, are of outstanding importance, and have significantly influenced the health behavior of 7DAs. Other Christian groups do not acknowledge the prophetic character of her writings and thus do not following her guidance.

While the 7DA Church underlines the importance of the body (referring to 1 Corinthians 6:19[1]), others would see the development of the soul/spirit as more important (referring to Matthew 10:28,[2] Romans 8:5 and 13[3]). Therefore, ascetic lifestyles and practices that intend to "purify" the soul by ignoring the worldly realm of the body were preferred by some ancient monastic groups.

CATHOLICS

Today about 1.3 billion Catholics (1,272,281,000) live in the world (18% of world population); the largest increases have been seen in Africa and America, while in Europe the number of Catholics has decreased (Agenzia Fides 2016). The Catholic Church is mainly the Western (Latin) church and includes some of the Eastern Catholic churches, with distinct liturgy, hierarchy, and religious observances. In this church the bishop of Rome, the pope, is the main authority.

The Catholic Church and specific monastic orders run hospitals and houses for elderly and disabled persons, and they are particularly engaged in local education programs, on the one hand; and in health promotion/disease prevention programs for poor or underserved persons, on the other hand. Referring to Matthew 25:40–45, each person in need is seen as a representation of Christ, and thus helping others implies that one is helping Christ.

As stated by the 2016 *Catholic Church Statistics* report, the church runs various charity and healthcare centers around the world: More than 5,000 hospitals, most of them in the United States (29%) and Africa (24%); around 16,500 dispensaries, mainly in Africa (32%), the United States (28%) and Asia (22%); 612 care homes for people with leprosy, mainly in Asia (51%) and Africa (28%); about 15,700 homes for the elderly, the chronically ill, or people with a disability, mainly in Europe (53%) and the United States (24%); 9,500 orphanages, mainly in Asia (41); 12,600 crèches, mainly in Asia

(27%) and the United States (28%); 14,600 marriage counseling centers, mainly in the United States (39%) and Europe (39%); 3,800 social rehabilitation centers and 37,600 other kinds of institutions" (Agenzia Fides 2016).

Promoting Health: Healthy Environment and Development

Of general health relevance is Pope Francis's 2015 encyclical letter "Laudato Si," which focuses particularly on the protection of the environment, God's creation (Holy Father Francis 2015). Humankind's responsibility for pure drinking water and air as the basis of health is underlined: "One particularly serious problem is the quality of water available to the poor. Every day, unsafe water results in many deaths and the spread of water-related diseases, including those caused by microorganisms and chemical substances. Dysentery and cholera, linked to inadequate hygiene and water supplies, are a significant cause of suffering and of infant mortality" (Chapter 29). This encyclical letter underlines that social dignity, health care, and ecological responsibility are interconnected, and that a change of behavior (politically, economically, and individually) is required: "It needs educators capable of developing an ethics of ecology, and helping people, through effective pedagogy, to grow in solidarity, responsibility and compassionate care" (Chapter 210). This call for educators is also an acknowledgment of all healthcare initiatives (both governmental or nongovernmental) that run education programs focusing on responsible agriculture, healthy nutrition, health prevention, hygiene, and the like.

Promoting Health: Selected Initiatives

Hints for the role of Catholic parish communities on health promotion were given in the qualitative study by Allen et al. (2014), who conducted interviews with Catholic Latinos. The church members who were interviewed reported that prayer increases their well-being and positively impacts coping with life stresses. Prayers also seem to raise the awareness of God's role in health. Caring for people in need with material assistance such as food, clothes, and money, as well as visits to the sick, were understood as a contribution of parish communities to enhance the health of church members. Some participants reported accessing health information through their parish, for example, through flyers, announcements in parish bulletins, or announcements at the end of the Mass. However, few reported the possibility of free access to health services such as dental checkups, or screening for blood pressure or diabetes (Allen et al. 2014).

Apart from various local health initiatives, there are also several larger and global organizations.

Caritas Internationalis is a "global confederation of Catholic Church national member organizations providing humanitarian assistance, development, social services and advocacy" (Caritas Internationalis 2014). They exclusively care for the "poor, excluded or marginalized" in the world (Caritas Internationalis 2014). They explain that "food is an essential need for everyone and a lack of nutritious food not only harms health but deeply wounds people's fundamental dignity" (Caritas Internationalis 2017a). This indicates that caring for healthy food and health education programs have to go hand in hand. In line with this, Caritas Internationalis has an interesting mission statement noting that "without good health people cannot reach their full human potential"; thus, the various Caritas groups worldwide build and support local communities "to prevent the onset of illness and provide medicines and other life-saving supplies for treatment programmes" (Caritas Internationalis 2017a). Caritas Internationalis aims to "keep people in good health, especially the most poor and vulnerable." Therefore, they run hospitals, retirement homes, and also screening, prevention, and treatment programs (e.g., HIV and AIDS, tuberculosis). A further important issue is their effort to raise public and individual awareness of the interaction between poverty-related poor nutrition and living conditions and noncommunicable diseases such as diabetes, obesity, heart and lung diseases, and high blood pressure (Caritas Internationalis 2017a, 2017b).

The *Catholic Health Initiatives* are a further example of a nonprofit, faith-based health system. Its mission is to "nurture the healing ministry of the Church, supported by education and research." They underline that "fidelity to the Gospel urges us to emphasize human dignity and social justice as we create healthier communities" (Catholic Health Initiatives 2017a). Again, dignity and justice and health care are seen as an integral part of their activities motivated by their faith. As their vision, the Catholic Health Initiatives stated that their intention is to "lead the transformation of health care to achieve optimal health and well-being for the individuals and communities we serve, especially those who are poor and vulnerable." They support and sponsor various national and international healthcare initiatives run by their hospitals and participating religious congregations. Concrete examples of community benefits are free or discounted health screenings, health programs for uninsured and underserved individuals, smoking cessation programs, anti-violence programs, donations of food, meal programs, and supplies or in-kind services to help people who are poor or underserved (Catholic Health Initiatives 2017b).

The former "Pontifical Council for Health Care Workers," established in 1985, was an institution with a clear focus on the spiritual care of the sick and also spiritual support of healthcare workers' education. The council also organized international conferences on specific health care problems and published the conference proceedings in the quarterly *Dolentium Hominum*. The council's mission was to "spread, explain and defend the teachings of the Church on health issues and favors its involvement in health care practice" (The Holy See (Vatican) 2017b). Since 2017, it has been assumed by the new dicastery for "Promoting Integral Human Development" (The Holy See (Vatican) 2017a).

Health Advice: Orienting Policies and Practices

The Catechism of the Catholic Church (Libreria Editrice Vaticana 2003a) describes Catholic faith, sacraments, and doctrines and offers nonspecific instructions for health behavior, as well as ethical guidelines for behavior (referring to the Ten Commandments, virtues, sins, social justice, and so on). Christian prayer (adoration, petition, intercession, thanksgiving, praise) is explicated in a major chapter of the Catechism, and is of special relevance for mental and spiritual health.

Referring to the sacred exhortations expressed in Matthew 10:28 and Romans 8:5 and 8:13, the early church regarded self-abandonment and asceticism as signs of seriousness about following a Christian lifestyle, particularly for monks. These practices were not intended to constantly harm the body, but to actively resign from "guilty pleasures" within circumscribed periods and to focus on the sacred. The Benedictine rules (Cassian 1890), for example, advise that a monk should live his whole life as he does in the fasting period before Easter, but only a few have the necessary strength (Book V), and thus it is advised to live at least these 40 days in great sincerity. This abstinence (approved by the Benedictine abbot) is seen as an act of the monk's own will and an offering to God.

Important "sins" arise from seven negative character traits; among those relevant to health behavior are lust (debauchery, hedonism, desire) and crapulousness (immoderateness, greed, egoism). Temperance, one of the four classical cardinal virtues, is seen as helpful to deal with sensual appetites and to value the simple things in life, thereby giving order and inner balance. Fasting is not primarily a punishment of the body, but to purify the heart from desires.

The Benedictine rules, referring to the teachings of the early Christian monks living in the deserts of Egypt and Syria, advise: "For not only is drunkenness with wine wont to intoxicate the mind, but excess of all kinds of food makes it weak and uncertain, and robs it of all its power of pure and clear contemplation" (Cassian 1890, Institutes 5, 6). Book 5 is completely dedicated to discussion of the harmful "Spirit of Gluttony" (Book 5, Chapter 6). To take up food "with regard to the aim at perfect continence," the Benedictine rule recommends: "we should exercise self-restraint in the matter of the food, which we are obliged to take owing to the necessity of supporting the body" (Book 5, Chapter 8). "In order to preserve the mind and body in a perfect condition abstinence from food is not alone sufficient: unless the other virtues of the mind as well are joined to it" (Book 5, Chapter 10).

The Benedictine rules also includes advice for monks to fight the "Spirit of Fornication" (Book 6). For the Benedictine monks, it was clearly stated that if they "concentrate exclusively on the punishment of the body and do not engage the soul in abstinence from other vices, nor in holy meditation or spiritual studies," they will "never be able to attain the heights of true wholeness" (Book 6, Chapter 2). The body is clearly considered a gateway for the "evil" that seeks to misguide the religious searchers. Sexuality ("harmful passionate fever of fornication") of monks living in celibacy was seen as a hindrance to attaining "a state of full health," and thus it was advised to "add something to bodily punishment and heartfelt contrition: solitude and distance from others" (Book 6, Chapter 3). These guidelines were primarily meant for monks living in celibacy, but have influenced ethical guides for laypersons, too.

Pope Francis's encyclical letter "Laudato Si" also values acceptance of and caring for the "own body in its femininity or masculinity," so as to "respect its fullest meaning" (Chapter 155). Sexuality was thus addressed in such a way as to instruct that "we can joyfully accept the specific gifts of another man or woman, the work of God the Creator, and find mutual enrichment" (Chapter 155). This instruction is primarily meant for laypersons, not for priests, monks, and nuns who are expected to maintain celibacy (Holy Father Francis 2015).

For the Catholic Church, sexual activities are seen as an expression of love (which has its origin in God) between a married man and woman, to attain together "their human fulfilment." Sexual activities outside sacramental marriage, use of artificial contraceptives and sterilization, and interruption of pregnancy and direct abortion are a matter of strict moral concern (Pope Paul VI 1968). Not only unmarried persons but also spouses are called to self-discipline in order to "control their natural drives"; the "promotion of chastity" by educators is encouraged "so that true liberty may prevail over license and the norms of the moral law" (Pope Paul VI 1968). This vocation of chastity can be seen either as negative or as positive: according to the Catechism of the Catholic Church, it is meant as a "successful integration of sexuality within the person and thus the inner unity of man in his bodily and spiritual being" (Libreria Editrice Vaticana 2017a, #2337).

The *Theology of the Body* (Pope John Paul II 1997), a collection of catechetic teachings by Pope John Paul II (1920–2005) given between 1979 and 1984, refers to God's creation of a "man-woman duality" and the development of a self-conscious "person." These teachings can be seen as a bioethical reflection on the body concerning the moral ethics of abortion, artificial fertilization, sterilization, and assisted suicide.

The Catholic Church's prohibition of condom usage in times of HIV infection and other sexually transmitted diseases has to be seen in this light. The prohibition is based on theological and ethical considerations, not on statistical data. Despite the emotionalized debate as whether the use of condoms can significantly reduce the rate of HIV infections, particularly in underdeveloped countries, it is clear that they can prevent infections (when used regularly). Nevertheless, there is evidence that condom effectiveness is influenced not only by disease infectivity but also by the number of exposures (Mann, Stine, and Vessey 2002). Because the number of sexual partners and other health behaviors matter, abstinence is encouraged not only by the churches but also by some government programs. In a letter to the *British Medical Journal*, Amin Abboud, referring to statistical data, said that for the HIV situation in Africa, "the greater the percentage of Catholics in any country, the lower the level of HIV. If the Catholic Church is promoting a message about HIV in those countries it seems to be working" (Abboud 2005, p. 294). One may critically examine the underlying statistical data and confounding bias factors, but the main issue seems to be individuals' lifestyle and behavior. One example of a specific nonprofit organization promoting this view is the Chastity Project, which has a ministry of "Stewardship. A Mission of Faith" (Chastity Project 2017).

Fasting   Catholic tradition observes two specific periods of fasting, one during the time of penitence before Easter (Lent) and one before Christmas (Advent). In the hymnbook of the Roman Catholic Church in Germany, there is instruction to reflect on one's own lifestyle, particularly during Lent: "Do I see my life as precious; have I put it carelessly in jeopardy [e.g., by excessive physical training, nicotine, alcohol, drugs]?" (Erzbistum Köln 2014, 600/4). In contrast to this, a further reflection refers to "exaggerated worries for own health" as a negative example (Erzbistum Köln 2014, 601/1).

The 40-day fasting period before Easter (excluding the Sundays) is primarily a period of spiritual preparation. The obligation for fasting (only one meal per day) applies to persons between 18 and 60 years of age, whereas the obligation of abstinence (no meat) is intended for persons as young as age 15 and is a lifelong imperative (Bischöfliches Ordinariat Regensburg

2016). Persons who are hindered by illness or heavy work must not fast. Although strongly recommended, this fasting is nevertheless an active decision (e.g., one might choose to avoid meat, alcohol, sweets, television, dancing, etc.). Fasting during Lent is accompanied by praying, reading the scriptures, meditation, celebrating the Holy Mass, and doing acts of charity, and thus serves as an inner change to reconnect with God.

Apart from this, there is an imperative for fasting and abstinence for Catholic holidays, particularly on Ash Wednesday and Good Friday (Bischöfliches Ordinariat Regensburg 2016). Further, all Fridays in a year are days of penance during which Catholics are obligated to make a sacrifice, such as abstinence from meat and restriction of consumption (particularly foodstuffs, alcohol, and tobacco); however, they are also directed to pray, to help others, or to donate. Caring for others is an aspect of fasting mentioned in the Old Testament (Isaiah 58:6–7). The obligation for Friday penance is practiced more strictly in monasteries; it is unclear which laypersons follow these directives, either in part or not at all.

In contrast to the complex Jewish dietary laws (*Kashrut*), which must be observed all year, Catholics are not subject to such strict regulations (except abstinence from meat on Fridays, though fish is allowed). Even (moderate) alcohol consumption is allowed. So far it is unclear whether the limited fasting directive is relevant to a Catholic person's health at all. For example, Catholic priests—who are expected to live their vocation as dedicated religious persons, fast during Lent, and follow the ideals of temperance—may be obese and have problems with alcohol consumption. In fact, research has indicated that of German Catholic priests, 12% consume alcohol (apart from Communion wine) on a daily basis, compared to 8% of the general German population (Frick 2017). Also, male parish expert workers (11%) drink more than the average of the German population. Similarly, more Catholic priests and deacons than nonordained pastoral workers are overweight or even obese (Frick 2017). These effects cannot be ascribed solely to gender and age differences, because the mean Body Mass Index (BMI) remains significantly higher in priests and deacons compared to nonordained male pastoral workers. Thus, it might be that differences in the specific life situations are of greater relevance than the underlying religiosity.

Lifestyle is also implicated as an important influence on health in research involving Greek Orthodox Christian monks. Living in Mount Athos, these monks live a vegetarian or even vegan lifestyle (with rice, pasta, bread, fruits, vegetables, etc.). Their vegetarianism contributes to their favorable profiles of several health-related biomarkers (Papadaki, Vardavas, Hatzis, and Kafatos 2008). Moreover, they work and pray, have unpolluted air, and keep the rigorous fasting periods of the Orthodox Church. As a consequence, they have very low rates of coronary heart disease and cancer (Katz 2011). A study by Merakou et al. (2016) further found a quite high sense of coherence (SOC), which is an indicator of a positive global life orientation, in these Orthodox monks. The mean value on the SOC-13 scale was similar to that found in a German pastoral ministry study (Kerksieck, Büssing, Frick, Jacobs, and Baumann 2016). One may thus assume that Orthodox monks at Mount Athos have better resources to cope with stress—but they may have also lower stress *per se*, a phenomenon found also in German Catholic priests (Frick 2017).

It should be noted that the positive health effects found in Greek Orthodox monks, with their unique and regulated lifestyle, might not be easily transferable to Greek laypersons, even when they share the same denomination. Thus, the question regarding health is whether it is due to the general Greek lifestyle, with its healthy nutrition behaviors, or to the religion-related behaviors. Orthodox Christians are encouraged to keep weekly fasting days (every Wednesday and Friday, only one light meal; no meat, dairy products, olive oil, or wine); during nonfasting periods there are no generally forbidden foods. The fasting period during Lent is stricter (and the size and number of meals are smaller) and quite complicated (Orthodox Life 2017). El Chliaoutakis et al. (2002) have analyzed the health-related behavior of 250 Greek persons who have or have not adopted the Greek Orthodox Church's lifestyle (differentiated as either religious, conventional, or religiously unconcerned). Multiple regression analyses indicate that "Orthodox Religiosity" scores were positively related to feelings of relaxation and life satisfaction, good personal hygiene, and healthy nutrition. Moreover, both the highly and the moderately religious were more physically active than the unconcerned group (El Chliaoutakis et al. 2002). These effects were stable after controlling for sociodemographic data and current health status. Thus, living in accordance with the Greek Orthodox faith (including prayers and worship, scripture reading, attending church service every Sunday, fasting during Lent, practicing sacramental confession, and so on) had an influence on adherents' mental and physical health in this sample. Thus, this study suggested that it is not just the healthy Greek diet and lifestyle alone that are beneficial, but also the engagement in religious practices, given religion's positive influence on inner coherence and satisfaction in life (which may also influence psychoneuroimmunologic and neuroendocrine pathways and thus physiological activities as well).

Recommendations to Pray   The Catechism of the Catholic Church states that "the Church invites the faithful to regular prayer: daily prayers, the Liturgy of the Hours, Sunday Eucharist, the feasts of the liturgical year" (Libreria Editrice Vaticana 2017c, #2720). It explains that vocal prayer, meditation, and contemplative prayer intend "the recollection of the heart" (#2721). These forms of prayer have different qualities and intentions and were described in brief as follows:

2722 Vocal prayer, founded on the union of body and soul in human nature, associates the body with the interior prayer of the heart, following Christ's example of praying to his Father and teaching the Our Father to his disciples.

2723 Meditation is a prayerful quest engaging thought, imagination, emotion, and desire. Its goal is to make our own in faith the subject considered, by confronting it with the reality of our own life.

2724 Contemplative prayer is the simple expression of the mystery of prayer. It is a gaze of faith fixed on Jesus, an attentiveness to the Word of God, a silent love. It achieves real union with the prayer of Christ to the extent that it makes us share in his mystery.

Health-Related Effects of Praying

Several religious rituals and practices may have also psychological and physical effects. Chief among them are prayer and meditation.

Praying—which is a common religious practice of all Christian branches and denominations—can be either private or public, unstructured and spontaneous or formalized, for one's own concerns or intercessory (i.e., for others). As mentioned earlier, the practice of praying is not primarily intended to yield health benefits. Nevertheless, persons may pray for their own or other persons' health and for support in difficult times. The effects of 17 intercessory prayer studies were summarized in a meta-analysis by Hodge (2007), who found small but significant effect sizes for the use of intercessory prayer. However, most of the included studies did not show significant effects of intercessory prayer.

Apart from studies of intercessory prayer, research results on the general effects of private prayer are heterogeneous (Ladd and Spilka 2013). It should be noted that private praying may be stimulated by and done in reaction to the occurrence of significant stressors in life (e.g., illness, accidents, conflicts); thus, one may find negative associations with health indicators. However, it may also be practiced in healthier situations, such as for praise and worship; thus, one may find associations with positive psychological health and well-being. For example, in breast cancer patients from the United States, prayers were often used to cope with illness, resulting in findings of increased benefit and spiritual well-being (Levine et al. 2009). These prayers were for petitioning, comfort, or praise. In their critical review of qualitative and quantitative literature on praying, Hollywell and Walker

(2009) stated that the frequency of private prayer was mostly associated with lower levels of depression and anxiety (particularly in areas with strong religious traditions). However, most studies do not differentiate the types and motifs of prayers (e.g., ritualized, meditative, petitionary, colloquial). Hollywell and Walker (2009) found that devotional prayers were related to improved optimism, well-being and function, whereas prayers for help were related to increased distress and lower levels of functioning. Nevertheless, the associations between different types of prayer and negative affect, happiness, and life satisfaction are in most cases weak or not significant at all (Poloma and Pendleton 1989). In female cancer patients from the United States, the inverse associations between different types of prayer and depressive symptoms were marginal to weak, particularly for adoration and reception (marginal association; $r < -.20$) and thanksgiving and praying for the well-being of others (weak association; $r < -.30$) (Pérez et al. 2011). Some of these effects are indirectly mediated by rumination (e.g., thanksgiving prayer) and social support (e.g., prayer for others). Further, one cannot exclude the possibility that some effects were observed only in highly religious persons; in rather secular societies, the effects are not as strong. Indeed, in older adults from the Netherlands, no significant associations were found between the frequency of prayer (without differentiation of prayer types) and depression (Braam, Deeg, Poppelaars, Beekman, and Van Tilburg 2007).

What about Catholic priests and nonordained pastoral workers? For dedicated religious persons, praying may be an indicator of a vital spiritual life and connection with God, and thus praying might be associated with lower scores of depression and burnout, and higher scores of life satisfaction. In a sample of 7,390 Roman Catholic pastoral workers from Germany (42% priests, 13% deacons, 45% pastoral assistants and parish expert workers), frequency of praying the Liturgy of Hours (*lectio divina*) and also private praying were only marginally and inversely associated with depression, anxiety, and stress perception and marginally positively with life satisfaction (Büssing, Frick, Jacobs, and Baumann 2016a). Instead, it was the perception of transcendence that was moderately and negatively associated with depression and stress perception, and moderately positively associated with life satisfaction. In other words, in Catholic pastoral workers it is not necessarily the religious practice as a ritual which is related to better mental health indicators, but the underlying perception of the sacred—which in turn may result in more intensive religious activity such as praying to relate with God.

Contemplative Prayer/Meditation   In Christianity, there is a great variety of different meditation styles. From a theoretical point of view, one may differentiate the conventional Christian prayer, which uses words to address

God as the receiver; Centering prayer, which is more a silent, reflecting meditation that uses repetition of either a mentally articulated or quietly spoken sacred phrase (e.g., "Come, Jesus Christ"); and a Eucharistic adoration, which can be regarded as a silent meditation in front of the sacred (being present with the Holy Sacrament). "Contemplative prayer" is mentioned in the Catechism of the Catholic Church as a silent "hearing the Word of God"; it is speechless. In contrast, "meditation" is interpreted as a "quest," a longing to understand; it is a reflection of the Sacred Scriptures, holy icons, and the like. "Christian prayer tries above all to meditate on the mysteries of Christ, as in *lectio divina* or the rosary" (Libreria Editrice Vaticana 2017b, #2708).

The "Liturgy of Hours," which is mandatory for Catholic priests and deacons and practiced in monasteries, but also recommended for Catholic laypersons, involves several elements of these contemplative practices: contemplative reading of the Psalms (and other scriptures of the Old and New Testaments), silent reflection, and responding to God's words with specific ritualized prayers.

These forms of contemplative prayer and Christian meditation may calm the spirit, and can help one to focus on that which is essential in life. Nevertheless, it is not their aim to generate health and well-being—although these effects may be observed; rather, they are intended to (re)connect the person with the sacred and to deepen the relationship with God.

There are only small-sample reports on the health benefits of the Centering prayer that is in some ways similar to Eastern religious forms of silent meditation. Ferguson, Willemsen, and Castañeto (2010) investigated 15 parishioners who practiced Centering prayer for 10 weeks with 2-hour group sessions and individual practice twice a day, and 15 nonmeditating parishioners. They found that Centering prayer changed the participants' "Relationship-with-God" coping styles: namely, an increase in the collaborative style and decreases in the deferring and self-directing styles. The decrease in participants' trait-anxiety was not significant. In qualitative interviews, some of these participants reported "decreased stress and anxiety within the context of a deepened, experiential relationship with God" (Ferguson et al. 2010, p. 318). Another, rather small pilot study by Johnson et al. investigated the effects of Centering prayer in 10 women receiving outpatient chemotherapy and reported an "improvement" of emotional well-being, anxiety, depression, and faith scores (Johnson et al. 2009).

Reciting the rosary is another form of meditative prayer that begins with the Apostles Creed and Our Father prayers; moves to various repetitions of 10 Hail Marys and Glory Bes; and inserts recitation of specific Mysteries. There are only a few studies on the health-related effects of rosary recitation. In a preliminary study that enrolled 30 Catholic students (12 practiced rosary recitation and 18 control students viewed a religiously oriented video), anxiety decreased significantly in the rosary-praying group (Anastasi and Newberg 2008). With respect to autonomic cardiovascular rhythms, a study by Bernardi et al. (2001) compared the effects of rosary prayer (Hail Mary in Latin) and yoga mantras ("om mani padme om") in a group of 23 healthy adults and found an increase of existing cardiovascular rhythms and of baroreflex sensitivity in both groups when they were breathing with six breaths per minute. The underlying repetitions result in a fixed and slower respiration rate and an increase in baroreflex; the latter allows positive modulation of vascular resistance and blood pressure (Bernardi et al. 2001), which may have prognostic relevance for cardiac patients (La Rovere, Bigger, Marcus, Mortara, and Schwartz 1998). The baroreceptor reflex works to decrease a person's heart rate frequency and blood pressure when blood pressure rises (which involves an activation of the parasympathetic nervous system and inhibition of the sympathetic nervous system), and thus helps to maintain homeostasis. Meditative approaches that slow and deepen inspiration have an impact on baroreflex sensitivity, and thus may yield health benefits.

Sunday Service—The Lord's Day   For Catholics, Sunday replaces the Jewish Sabbath. The Sunday celebration of the Lord's Day and the Eucharist are obligatory for Catholics and is seen as "the heart of the Church's life" (Libreria Editrice Vaticana 2003b, #2177). On Sundays and other holy days of obligation, Catholics should avoid "work or activities that hinder the worship owed to God" and are encouraged instead to perform "works of mercy" and also engage in "appropriate relaxation of mind and body" (#2185). Keeping the Lord's Day on Sunday means having time for devotion and family. Sunday is seen as the necessary "time for reflection, silence, cultivation of the mind, and meditation which furthers the growth of the Christian interior life" (Libreria Editrice Vaticana 2003c, #2186). This Sunday obligation may also yield health benefits, as it helps to avoid or reduce stress and to focus on the essential aspects in life.

However, the Sunday service is only rarely practiced, particularly in Northern Europe. The number of participating Catholics in Germany, for example, decreased from 50% in 1950 to 10% in 2015 (Deutsche Bischofskonferenz 2015). This is in sharp contrast to nonordained laypersons who are employed as Catholic pastoral workers; among them, 75% participated in the Eucharist regularly on the weekends, 20% several times per week, and 5% daily (Büssing, Frick, Jacobs, and Baumann 2016b). Thus, what is recommended or even obligatory in theory is often not practiced in reality by laypersons, who may be identified as Catholics only by denomination, not by practice and heart.

Faith as Resource to Influence Healthful Eating Behavior

The ancient Benedictine abbess Hildegard von Bingen (1098–1179 CE) had several visions of God which inspired her writings about medicine and health. According to her teachings, important rules for a healthy lifestyle are the strengthening of the soul (through meditation, prayer, and fortifying one's own virtues to fight weakness), and detoxification of the body according to the ancient theory of the Four Temperaments from Greco-Roman medicine (humor[al]ism), which also includes fasting and lifestyle regulation (balance between work and leisure time; proper amounts of sleep, etc.). She strongly encouraged healthful and balanced nutrition (later termed the "Hildegard Diet") and is one of the ancestors of modern phytotherapy. Part 2 of her book *Liber Divinorum Operum* (about God's acting in the world and in humans) is "Causae et Curae" (about the origins and treatments of diseases) and sets out her insights about medicine and health (von Bingen 2011). Several of her lifestyle recommendations are still pertinent to and beneficial from today's point of view, although her discussion of underlying causes based on the humoralist system of medicine are mostly outdated.

Interestingly, qualitative interviews, done to evaluate a Christian, church-based, healthy, intuitive eating and weight management program for individuals belonging mainly to the Christian faith, indicated that although faith plays a central role in daily living, eating behavior and diet are not necessarily seen in relation to God. Reasons offered for not using their faith as a resource to change eating behavior and reduce weight included that the issues they experienced "were too trivial for God to be interested in" and that weight management was "something they had to deal with by themselves" (Patel, Lycett, Coufopoulos, and Turner 2017, p. 5). Health-promoting programs based on Christian principles may, however, help these individuals to see faith as a resource to support the change to a healthier lifestyle, by getting God's help and strength for behavior changes through prayer, by changing motivation to adapt eating behavior, and by promoting self-love in the way God loves them (Patel et al. 2017).

Currently, there is no general Catholic recommendation for healthy nutritional habits, although tacit suggestions of beneficial diets are found in several local and superregional initiatives. The American national weekly newspaper *Our Sunday Visitor* (printed by a U.S. Roman Catholic publishing company) published an article by Emily Stimpson Chapman (2015) about "The Catholic Diet." This article presents a number of questions to be used as a "repentance reflection" and alludes to the practice of healthy nutritional behaviors (e.g., "Do I practice prudence by eating foods that nourish my body—fruits, vegetables, meat and whole grains—and avoiding foods that harm my body—heavily processed food, junk food and too many sweets?"; "Do I avoid drinking too much, never drinking to the point of drunkenness?"), fasting practices (e.g., "Do I fast when the Church fasts— abstaining from meat on Fridays in Lent, eating only one meal on Ash Wednesday and Good Friday and making some sacrifice on Fridays through-out the year?"), and gratitude (e.g., "Do I pray before every meal, even when in a restaurant, giving thanks to God for the food he's provided?"; "Do I thank those who have prepared a meal for me or served me in their home?"). All these questions are intended as a "fitness regimen for your soul" (Stimpson Chapman 2015).

Survival Benefit of Christian Monks

The German-Austrian cloister studies investigate the determinants of health and longevity in monastic persons, particularly with respect to gender and longevity. Marc Luy (2002) compared the mortality of more than 11,000 Catholic nuns and monks with data of the general German population (from 1890 to 1995). A key finding was that the mortality differences between women and men in the general population increased after World War II, whereas they were more or less stable in the monastic persons, indicating that not only biological factors were active (Luy 2002). Interestingly, the monks were living longer than men in the general population, whereas nuns had a life expectancy similar to that of women in the general population. The sur-vival benefit of monks seems to be attributable to their regulated and less stressful lifestyle (Luy and Wegner 2011). However, it should be noted that closer examination of the nuns revealed differential effects, in that the sur-vival benefit of younger nuns was similar to that of monks, but lower for the older nuns; this difference in survival benefit for young and old nuns is prob-ably due to stress and selection effects (tuberculosis of young nuns) in the second half of the 19th century and at the beginning of the 20th century.

SEVENTH-DAY ADVENTISTS

The Seventh-day Adventist Church is a Protestant denomination refer-ring to the scriptures of the Old and the New Testament of the Bible. Its roots go back to 1863, with its beginnings in the eastern parts of the United States (Fraser 2003; General Conference of Seventh-day Adventists 2016). The 7DA church statistics for 2014 and 2015, published in 2016, report that 19.1 million (19,126,438) 7DAs live in the world (3% of the world popula-tion), most in Inter-America (19%), East-Central Africa (17%), Southern Africa-Pacific (18%), and South America (13%) (Seventh-day Adventist Church Office of Archives, Statistics, and Research 2016).

Contrary to other Christians, members of the 7DA Church regard the Saturday as the weekly Sabbath (from Friday sunset to Saturday sunset) instead of Sunday as memorial of creation. The Saturday is seen as a day of worship and rest (General Conference of Seventh-day Adventists 2016).

Health Guides: Orienting Policies and Practices

The 7DA Church's understanding of the Holy Scriptures is formulated in 28 fundamental beliefs (General Conference of Seventh-day Adventists 2016). These beliefs also give instructions for parishioners' health behavior based on the idea of the body as the temple of the Holy Spirit (1 Corinthians 6:19). In all aspects of life, individuals are encouraged to enhance their health and to avoid behavior that is harmful to their bodies (General Conference of Seventh-day Adventists 2016).

The "Official Statements" of the 7DA Church about sexual behavior identify adultery, premarital sex, and obsessive sexual behavior as "sexual practices which are contrary to God's expressed will." Further, they regard "sexual abuse of spouses, sexual abuse of children, incest, homosexual practices (gay and lesbian), and bestiality . . . [as] among the obvious perversions of God's original plan" (Seventh-day Adventist Church 1987). To prevent HIV infection and AIDS, 7DAs see it as their mission to educate particularly younger people who are "growing up in an era of moral laxity" and "need to be taught biblical principles regarding sexuality and God's design that sexual intimacy be experienced within the protection of the marriage covenant" (Seventh-day Adventist Church 2000). They clearly uphold the ideal of abstinence from premarital sex and fidelity in marriage.

With respect to abortion, it is taught that "prenatal life must not be thoughtlessly destroyed" and that "abortion should be performed only for the most serious reasons" (Seventh-day Adventist Church 1992). 7DAs aim to "offer gracious support to those who personally face the decision concerning an abortion," hoping to help Christians who are in a personal crisis to consider their alternatives—without inappropriate "attitudes of condemnation" (Seventh-day Adventist Church 1992). An important issue is the intention "to assist in alleviating the unfortunate social, economic, and psychological factors that add to abortion and to care redemptively for those suffering the consequences of individual decisions on this issue" (Seventh-day Adventist Church 1992).

A significant contribution to the emergence of a consciousness for health in the Black 7DA Church was made by their co-founder, Ellen G. White (1827–1915 CE), who wrote in her publications on the benefits of a healthy lifestyle that included adequate rest, water, regular exercise, sunlight, and air (White 2006). Encouraged lifestyle practices include a vegetarian diet, and the avoidance of alcohol, tobacco, drugs, and other stimulants such as narcotics, coffee, and tea (General Conference of Seventh-day Adventists 2016; White 2006). Some 7DAs also abstain from highly refined food, sweets, and hot spices (Jarvis and Northcott 1987; Phillips et al. 1980). The diet should include fruits, nuts, grains, and vegetables: this is, as stated by White (2006, p. 297), "the diet chosen for us by our creator." Seasonal food should be selected and be prepared in as natural a way as possible (White 2006). These recommendations result in a diet similar to that of the Greek Ortho-dox monks living at Mount Athos, as discussed earlier.

As part of its great efforts for health and well-being, the 7DA Church has also issued guidelines on immunization. 7DAs are encouraged to be vac-cinated to prevent disease, although this is not a requirement or dogma of the 7DA Church. It is an individual's choice to be immunized or not (Seventh-day Adventist Church 2015).

Before entering the 7DA Church as members through baptism, candi-dates are instructed about the fundamental beliefs and practices of the 7DA Church in a baptismal class or individually. They accept the fundamental beliefs and commit by saying, "I believe that my body is the temple of the Holy Spirit; and I will honor God by caring for it, avoiding the use of that which is harmful, and abstaining from all unclean foods; from the use, man-ufacture, or sale of alcoholic beverages; from the use, manufacture, or sale of tobacco in any of its forms for human consumption; and from the mis-use of or trafficking in narcotics or other drugs" (General Conference of Seventh-day Adventists 2016, p. 48). Nevertheless, the extent to which Adventists follow the church's encouraged lifestyle vary from person to per-son; possibly wide variances in this factor should be taken into account when interpreting study results (Butler et al. 2008; Montgomery et al. 2007; Phillips 1975). This becomes particularly obvious when considering the characteristics of study participants in the cohort of 90,156 7DAs enrolled in the Adventists Health Study-2. The majority of church members are non-smokers (99%) and nondrinkers (93%), but a vegetarian diet is followed only by approximately 50% of 7DAs (Butler et al. 2008).

Promoting Health

The mission of the 7DA Church involves Christ-like living, meaning "[i]llustrating the lordship of Jesus in our lives by moral, ethical, and social behaviors that are consistent with the teachings and example of Jesus" (Seventh-day Adventist Church 2009). As stated by the General Conference of Seventh-day Adventists Executive Committee, church members intend to "make healthful living and the healing of the sick a priority" and are devoted "to humble service, ministering to individuals and populations most affected by poverty, tragedy, hopelessness, and disease" (Seventh-day Adventist Church 2009).

As is true of many other faiths, there are significant efforts in the 7DA Church to enhance public health, supported by many activities to promote healthy lifestyle patterns in church members. As stated in the *Seventh-day Adventist Church Manual*, a document published by the General Conference that coordinates the global ministry, "the church believes its responsibility to make Christ known to the world includes a moral obligation to preserve human dignity by promoting optimal levels of physical, mental, and spiritual health" (General Conference of Seventh-day Adventists 2016, p. 93). Besides caring for sick people, the 7DA Church regards the prevention of disease as part of its responsibility; it accomplishes this through promoting optimal health and effective health education. To give this task an institutional base, health ministries in 7DA churches are considered part of the church structure to fulfill their mission to promote health. Establishing a Health Ministries Leaders or a Health Ministries council are two of several ways to implement the field of healthful living in 7DA churches (General Conference of Seventh-day Adventists 2016). The Adventist health ministries' task as part of the General Conference of the 7DA Church is "to serve the Health Ministries needs of the world church." It offers news, information on special events, and articles related to various health issues. It also publishes the free quarterly *Health Connection Newsletter* which reports on the worldwide developments in 7DA Health Ministries (Adventist Health Ministries 2017).

Promoting Health: Selected Initiatives

The Adventist Development and Relief Agency (ADRA) is a global humanitarian organization of the 7DA Church whose mission is to deliver "relief and development assistance to individuals in more than 130 countries—regardless of their ethnicity, political affiliation, or religious association" (ADRA 2017). The international commitment is fulfilled by health-related projects in partnership with communities; for example, by working with "healthy communities" to improve and sustain health by shifting health behavior; and adopting "a community-level approach to address unique needs of populations, including capacity building of health professionals, increasing access to health information and health facilities, and improving the quality of health resources" (ADRA 2017). According to its own statements, ADRA is also involved in projects "ensuring access to safe water, hygienic sanitation facilities, and educating families and communities on hygiene practices that are vital to good health." A further integral part of this work is the promotion of nutrition awareness, by "focusing on farmers' increase of food supply, income and savings for food purchasing" or by promoting healthy nutrition behavior (ADRA 2017).

The 7DA Church also uses other ways to promote its beliefs regarding healthy life and to serve its mission by educating scientists, healthcare professionals, and scholars. One example is the Loma Linda Adventist Health Sciences Center, which aims to "continue Christ's healing and teaching ministry" and to serve the Seventh-day Adventist Church in its mission "to make man whole" physically, intellectually, emotionally, and spiritually (Loma Linda University 2017).

Adventist Health International is a management-organization part of Loma Linda University; its purpose is to "utilize the health care understanding, strength, and commitment of the Seventh-day Adventist church to mobilize expertise, personnel, and other resources to promote quality health for all" (Adventist Health International 2017). The organization supports 7DA mission hospitals in Asia, Africa and America (Adventist Health International 2017).

The great commitment of the 7DA Church to promotion of public health is also shown in the delivery of health care. The 7DA Church currently runs 385 clinics and dispensaries, 175 hospitals and sanitariums, 169 nursing/retirement or orphanages/children's homes, 15 medical centers, and 22 food companies (Seventh-day Adventist Church Office of Archives, Statistics, and Research 2016).

Health Behavior (Empirical Data)

The focus on the body and the characteristically healthy lifestyle promoted in the 7DA Church is thought to be responsible for better health status and higher life expectancies in church members compared to non-Adventists (Fraser and Shavlik 2001; Le and Sabaté 2014). A number of studies investigated the positive impact of the unique lifestyle of 7DA members on health-related outcomes over the years in different countries. Three major health studies were conducted: the Adventist Mortality Study (1958–1966), the Adventist Health Study-1 (1974 and 1988), and the Adventist Health Study-2 (2002–2006/07).

Life Expectancies and Mortality   The results of the Adventist Health Study-2, for which 96,000 study participants from the United States and Canada were recruited, showed an association between vegetarian diets and lower all-cause mortality, with a mortality rate of 6.05 (95% confidence interval [CI], 5.82–6.29) deaths per 1,000 person-years; more robust results were found for men. When comparing all forms of vegetarianism documented in 7DA study participants, a significantly reduced risk for all-cause mortality compared to non-vegetarians in the study cohort was found (0.88; 95% CI, 0.80–0.97; adjusted for age, smoking, race, sex, education, exercise, alcohol, marital status, menopause, geographic region, and hormone therapy) (Orlich et al. 2013; Orlich and Fraser 2014). Further, it was noted that "[t]he adjusted HR for all-cause mortality in vegans was 0.85 (95% CI, 0.73–1.01); in lacto-ovo–vegetarians, 0.91 (95% CI, 0.82–1.00); in pesco-vegetarians, 0.81 (95% CI, 0.69–0.94); and in semi-vegetarians, 0.92 (95% CI, 0.75–1.13) compared with non-vegetarians" (Orlich et al. 2013, p. 1230).

Previous research had indicated higher life expectancies and lower mortality in 7DAs compared to the general population/non-Adventists (e.g., Berkel and De Waard 1983; Fønnebø 1992a; Fraser and Shavlik 2001; Lemon, Walden, and Woods 1964). Fraser and Shavlik, for example, reported higher life expectancies for 30-year old California Adventists (study period 1976–1988) compared to other white Californians: 7.28 years in men and 4.42 years in women (Fraser and Shavlik 2001). Fønnebø et al. found a substantially significant lower mortality in Norwegian 7DA Church members entering the church before the age of 19 compared to the general population (41% lower in females and 31% lower in males) (Fønnebø 1992a; Fønnebø 1994). Berkel and de Waard (1983) confirmed the beneficial effect of the 7DA healthy lifestyle patterns by comparing 7DAs from the Netherlands with the total Dutch population (study period 1968–1977). The authors reported highly significant differences in total mortality, with more favorable results for 7DA members (Berkel and De Waard 1983). There is also evidence that the length of time one is a member of the 7DA Church is important for mortality. Fønnebø found that individuals converting to the 7DA Church after the age of 35 seemed to have smaller benefits in mortality than individuals who entered the church before age 19 (Fønnebø 1992a).

Cancer   One of the major health studies focusing on a cohort of 7DAs, the Adventist Health Study-2 (study period 2002–2007), compared all vegetarians (vegans, pesco-vegetarians, lacto-ovo-vegetarians, and semi-vegetarians) with non-vegetarians and found a significantly reduced risk for all cancers in 7DA vegetarians (HR: 0.92; 95% CI: 0.85; 0.99). The protective association between vegetarianism and all types of cancer combined for both sexes was statistically significant only in the cohort with a vegan diet. A significantly reduced risk for cancer of the gastrointestinal tract was reported for lacto-vegetarians (HR=0.75; 95% CI: 0.60; 0.93), who ate poultry, fish, and red meat less than once a month and dairy and eggs once or more per month (Tantamango-Bartley, Jaceldo-Siegl, Fan, and Fraser 2013).

Further, comparisons between 7DA members and non-Adventists/ general population indicate beneficial effects of the 7DA lifestyle with regard to cancer incidences. Thygesen et al. (2012) followed Danish Adventists between 1943 and 2008 and reported on lower cancer incidences for men and women in comparison to the general Danish population (standardized incidence ratio for male: 91; 95% CI (81; 103) and female: 97; CI (89; 106)). This was found especially for lifestyle-related cancers such as oral cavity, lung, stomach, liver, cervix, and esophagus cancer (Thygesen et al. 2012). The beneficial effects of the 7DA lifestyle on cancer incidence and lower risk of death by cancer compared to non-7DAs was also reported in previous publications on other cohorts: for example, California Adventists (Mills, Beeson, Phillips, and Fraser 1994; Wynder, Lemon, and Bross 1959; Phillips et al. 1980) and male Danish Adventists (study period 1939–1963) (Jensen 1983). Contrary to that, Fønnebø and Helseth (1991) found no significant difference between the standardized incidence ratio for cancer in Norwegian Adventists and that of the general population.

Metabolic Risk Factors and Metabolic Syndrome   The vegetarian diet encouraged for 7DA Church members may play an important role in influencing their health status. There is evidence, after adjusting for demographic and other lifestyle factors, that vegetarian dietary patterns beneficially lower levels in metabolic risk factors such as glucose, triglycerides, blood pressure, waist circumference, and Body Mass Index (BMI) compared to nonvegetarian eating patterns in a cohort of 7DA Church members (Rizzo et al. 2011). There is in fact evidence that Adventists following the recommended vegetarian diet have a lower risk for metabolic syndrome (OR 0.44, 95% CI 0.30; 0.64) compared to 7DAs with nonvegetarian dietary pattern (Rizzo, Sabaté, Jaceldo-Siegl, and Fraser 2011). However, in a Norwegian study (study period: 1973–1987) comparing Adventists and non-Adventists (sex-, age-, and residence-matched controls), no significant differences in BMI were found (Fønnebø 1992b). Within the cohort of 7DA Church members in the Adventist Health Study-2, the prevalence of Type 2 diabetes was 3.2% among lacto-ovo-vegetarians, 2.9% among vegans, 6.1% among semi-vegetarians, 4.8% among pesco-vegetarians, and 7.6% among non-vegetarians (Tonstad, Butler, Yan, and Fraser 2009). Generally, studies found a reduced risk for Type 2 diabetes among all types of vegetarianism compared to the nonvegetarian dietary pattern (Tonstad et al. 2009; Tonstad et al. 2013).

Bible Study, Prayer and Sabbath Keeping

For 7DAs, devotional Bible study and being with God in prayer are of utmost importance. Praying means to listen to God instead to the flood of distracting voices of the mass media. The advice to keep the Sabbath should be seen in this respect. During Sabbath, a time of worship and praying, all unnecessary work should be avoided, so that neither daily labor nor secular media will distract the believer from God (General Conference of Seventh-day Adventists 2016, 144–45). Nevertheless, the Sabbath is also the time to "visit the sick and work for the salvation of souls" (General Conference of Seventh-day Adventists 2016, p. 145). Thus, "man is to leave the occupations of his daily life, and devote those sacred hours to healthful rest, to worship, and to holy deeds" (General Conference of Seventh-day Adventists 2016, 145). Such strictures regarding praying and Scripture reading and avoidance of "unnecessary" work also promote slowing down life and avoiding stress, thereby helping one to focus on the sacred in life.

Is It the Lifestyle or Religion?

All these data indicate that the healthy lifestyle of 7DAs is of outstanding relevance—and this lifestyle is shaped by their underlying religious belief. Morton, Lee, and Martin (2016) attempted to clarify which component of the 7DA lifestyle was most responsible for the lower all-cause mortality: vegetarian diet and physical activity (exercises), personality factors (depression, neuroticism), or religious issues such as positive religious support, religious engagement, or engagement in the church. The findings were rather complex, as "Religious Engagement and Church Activity operate through the mediators of health behavior, emotion, and social support to decrease mortality risk" (p. 106). The relationships between religious engagement and mortality were "indirect through positive Religious Support, Emotionality, and lifestyle mediators" (Morton et al. 2016, p. 106)). Further, Morton et al. reported that "Church Activity has a direct positive effect on mortality as well as indirect effects through Religious Support, Emotionality, and lifestyle mediators (diet and exercise)" (Morton, Lee, and Martin 2016, p. 106). Religious engagement (i.e., religious self-perception, intrinsic religiosity, religious coping) and church activity (i.e., worship attendance, Sabbath responsibilities) were thus recognized as important variables with health relevance, as they influence the health behavior of 7DAs.

CONCLUSIONS

Christianity is a diverse religion with at least three major branches and many denominations and churches; all share several core principles, but may be different in specific interpretations of the Scriptures and also in their doctrines. They all rely on similar, basic religious practices such as praying, meditation/contemplation, Scripture reading, keeping the Sabbath/Sunday, and certain fasting periods; however, specific lifestyle and health behavior recommendations may differ greatly among Christian churches and denominations. While 7DAs and Greek Orthodox monks may live as (strict or part-time) vegetarians, Catholics do not (other than abstaining from eating meat on Fridays and during Lent). While 7DAs avoid alcohol, Orthodox Christians and Catholics may drink alcohol moderately. None of them intend religious fasting to help reduce weight; instead, it is a spiritual activity of preparation.

The 7DA Church and the Greek Orthodox Church in particular promote a healthy lifestyle and good care for the body which is the "temple of the Holy Spirit" (1 Corinthians 6:19); for Catholics there are no such clear-cut recommendations. Explanations for these differences in lifestyle practices and approaches to healthy living are difficult to elucidate. One possible reason might be differing interpretations of sacred scriptures such as Romans 14:17–18: "For the kingdom of God is not a matter of eating and drinking, but of righteousness, peace and joy in the Holy Spirit, because anyone who serves Christ in this way is pleasing to God and receives human approval."

Similar beneficial effects of religious beliefs on health behaviors are also noted in Christian denominations other than 7DA. For example, Mormons who follow strict religious doctrines are more likely to engage in beneficial health behavior, particularly with respect to use of intoxicants, food, and social support (de Diego Cordero and Romero 2017). In contrast, conflicts with the norms of the religious group (e.g., sexual identities, gender-related role models) were related to lower mental and physical health (de Diego Cordero and Romero 2017). This phenomenon can be found in any community that relies on strict rules and prohibitions, instead of encouraging personal insight and understanding of how lifestyle choices may affect one's health and well-being.

Christians do know and value the public health behavior and nutrition recommendations, but not all observe them; nor do all follow the often strict ethical and religious laws and recommendations of their respective church or denomination. In most cases one has to differentiate between health-related effects due to the general lifestyle (according to the respective religious views and recommendations), and specific religious practices (e.g., praying, meditation, fasting) that may have an influence on mental and physical health and well-being. Of course, spirituality should not be reduced to a useful tool to generate health and well-being; this would thwart its primary aim.

Several of these lifestyle issues are not unique and can also be found in nonreligious persons. The short-term effects of Christian meditation/

contemplation are probably similar to those garnered from mindfulness meditation (deriving from the Buddhist tradition). More important are the long-term effects of religion: a change of attitudes and behavior in the case of a conversion, to become a more compassionate and caring person who sees and hears the needs of the world; and to "discover the action of God in the soul, but also to discover God in all things" (Holy Father Francis 2015, Chapter 233).

ACKNOWLEDGMENT

Many thanks to Christoph Jacobs and Klaus van Treeck for their helpful suggestions and comments as this chapter was being developed.

NOTES

1. "Do you not know that your bodies are temples of the Holy Spirit, who is in you, whom you have received from God? You are not your own." (1 Corinthians 6:19); all Holy Bible verses are from the *New International Version.*

2. "Do not be afraid of those who kill the body but cannot kill the soul. Rather, be afraid of the One who can destroy both soul and body in hell" (Matthew 10:28).

3. "Those who live according to the flesh have their minds set on what the flesh desires; but those who live in accordance with the Spirit have their minds set on what the Spirit desires." (Romans 8: 5)

"For if you live according to the flesh, you will die; but if by the Spirit you put to death the misdeeds of the body, you will live." (Romans 8: 13)

REFERENCES

Abboud, A. 2005. "Searching for Papal Scapegoats Is Pointless." *BMJ (Clinical Research Ed.)* 331 (7511): 294. doi:10.1136/bmj.331.7511.294

Adventist Development and Relief Agency (ADRA). 2017. "About ADRA." Retrieved from https://adra.org/about-adra/

Adventist Health International. 2017. "What Is Adventist Health International." Retrieved from http://www.ahiglobal.org/main/main/

Adventist Health Ministries. 2017. "Adventist Health Ministries." Retrieved from http://healthministries.com/

Agenzia Fides. 2016, October 21. "Vatican—World Mission Day—Catholic Church Statistics 2016." Retrieved from http://www.fides.org/en/news/61026-VATI CAN_WORLD_MISSION_DAY_CATHOLIC_CHURCH_STATIS-TICS_2016#.WH4ZCH0vvS0

Allen, J. D., B. Leyva, M. I. Torres, H. Ospino, L. Tom, S. Rustan, and A. Bartholomew. 2014. "Religious Beliefs and Cancer Screening Behaviors among Catholic

Latinos: Implications for Faith-Based Interventions." *Journal of Health Care for the Poor and Underserved* 25(2): 503–526. doi:10.1353/hpu.2014.0080

Anastasi, M. W., and A. B. Newberg. 2008. "A Preliminary Study of the Acute Effects of Religious Ritual on Anxiety." *Journal of Alternative and Complementary Medicine* 14(2): 163–165. doi:10.1089/acm.2007.0675

Berkel, J., and F. De Waard. 1983. "Mortality Pattern and Life Expectancy of Seventh-day Adventists in the Netherlands." *International Journal of Epidemiology* 12(4): 455–459.

Bernardi, L., P. Sleight, G. Bandinelli, S. Cencetti, L. Fattorini, J. Wdowczyc-Szulc, and A. Lagi. 2001. "Effect of Rosary Prayer and Yoga Mantras on Autonomic Cardiovascular Rhythms: Comparative Study." *BMJ: British Medical Journal* 323(7327): 1446–1449.

Bischöfliches Ordinariat Regensburg. 2016. "Amtsblatt Für Die Diözese Regensburg." Retrieved from http://www.bistum-regensburg.de/typo3conf/ext/mediathek_main/uploads/3/02-2016.pdf

Braam, A. W., D. J. H. Deeg, J. L. Poppelaars, A. T. F. Beekman, and W. Van Tilburg. 2007. "Prayer and Depressive Symptoms in a Period of Secularization : Patterns among Older Adults in the Netherlands." *American Journal of Geriatric Psychiatry* 15(4): 273–281.

Büssing, A., E. Frick, C. Jacobs, and K. Baumann. 2016a. "Health and Life Satisfaction of Roman Catholic Pastoral Workers: Private Prayer Has a Greater Impact than Public Prayer." *Pastoral Psychology* 65(1): 89–102. doi:10.1007/s11089-015-0672-2

Büssing, A., E. Frick, C. Jacobs, and K. Baumann. 2016b. "Self-Attributed Importance of Spiritual Practices in Catholic Pastoral Workers and Their Association with Life Satisfaction." *Pastoral Psychology*, December, 1–16. doi:10.1007/s11089-016-0746-9

Butler, T. L., G. E. Fraser, W. L. Beeson, S. F. Knutsen, R. P. Herring, J. Chan, . . . K. Jaceldo-Siegl. 2008. "Cohort Profile: The Adventist Health Study-2 (AHS-2)." *International Journal of Epidemiology* 37(2): 260–265. doi:10.1093/ije/dym165

Caritas Internationalis. 2014. "Code of Ethics & Code of Conduct for Staff." Retrieved from https://www.caritas.org/includes/pdf/CodesEthicsConduct.pdf

Caritas Internationalis. 2017a. "Food." Retrieved from http://www.caritas.org/what-we-do/food/

Caritas Internationalis. 2017b. "Health and HIV." Retrieved from http://www.caritas.org/what-we-do/health/

Cassian, J. 1890. "The Twelve Books on the Institutes of the Coenobia and the Remedies for the Eight Principal Faults." Retrieved from http://www.osb.org/lectio/cassian/inst/index.html

Catholic Health Initiatives. 2017a. "Catholic Health Initiatives." Retrieved from http://www.catholichealthinitiatives.org/

Catholic Health Initiatives. 2017b. "Community Benefit—Catholic Health Initia-
    tives." Retrieved from http://www.catholichealthinitiatives.org/community
    -benefit

Chastity Project. 2017. "Chastity Project." Retrieved from http://chastityproject
    .com/

de Diego Cordero, R., and B. B. Romero. 2017. "Health Impacts of Religious Prac-
    tices and Beliefs Associated with The Church of Jesus Christ of Latter-
    Day Saints." *Journal of Religion and Health*, January, 1–10. doi:10.1007/
    s10943-016-0348-y

Deutsche Bischofskonferenz. 2015. "Kirchliche Statistik-Tabelle: Katholiken und
    Gottesdienstteilnehmer 1950–2015." Retrieved from http://www.dbk.de
    /zahlen-fakten/kirchliche-statistik/?tx_igmedienkatalog_pi1%5Bcatsearch
    %5D=113&tx_igmedienkatalog_pi1%5Bshow%5D=1&cHash=57f6cf7b6f
    24fd14183105c8219559c7

El Chliaoutakis, J., I. Drakou, C. Gnardellis, S. Galariotou, H. Carra, and M. Chl-
    iaoutaki. 2002. "Greek Christian Orthodox Ecclesiastical Lifestyle: Could It
    Become a Pattern of Health-Related Behavior?" *Preventive Medicine* 34(4):
    428–435. doi:10.1006/pmed.2001.1001

Erzbistum Köln. 2014. *Gotteslob: Katholisches Gebet- und Gesangbuch* (2nd ed.).
    Stuttgart, Germany: Katholisches Bibelwerk.

Ferguson, J. K., E. W. Willemsen, and M. V. Castañeto. 2010. "Centering Prayer
    as a Healing Response to Everyday Stress: A Psychological and Spiritual
    Process." *Pastoral Psychology* 59(3): 305–329. doi:10.1007/s11089-009
    -0225-7

Fønnebø, V. 1992a. "Mortality in Norwegian Seventh-day Adventists 1962–1986."
    Journal of Clinical Epidemiology 45(2): 157–167. doi:10.1016/0895-4356
    (92)90008-B

Fønnebø, V. 1992b. "Coronary Risk Factors in Norwegian Seventh-day Adventists:
    A Study of 247 Seventh-day Adventists and Matched Controls—The Car-
    diovascular Disease Studies in Norway." *American Journal of Epidemiology*
    135(5): 504–508.

Fønnebø, V. 1994. "The Healthy Seventh-day Adventist Lifestyle: What Is the
    Norwegian Experience?" *American Journal of Clinical Nutrition* 59(5):
    1124S–1129S.

Fønnebø, V., and A. Helseth. 1991. "Cancer Incidence in Norwegian Seventh-day
    Adventists 1961 to 1986: Is the Cancer-Life-Style Association Overesti-
    mated?" *Cancer* 68(3): 666–671. doi:10.1002/1097-0142(19910801)68:3<666::
    AID-CNCR2820680338>3.0.CO;2-L

Fraser, G. E. 2003. *Diet, Life Expectancy, and Chronic Disease: Studies of Seventh-
    day Adventists and Other Vegetarians.* Oxford, UK: Oxford University Press.

Fraser, G. E., and D. J. Shavlik. 2001. "Ten Years of Life: Is It a Matter of Choice?"
    Archives of Internal Medicine 161(13): 1645–1652. doi:10.1001/archinte
    .161.13.1645

Frick, E. 2017. "Psychosomatische Gesundheit?" In K. Baumann, A. Büssing, E. Frick, C. Jacobs, and W. Weig, eds., *Zwischen Spirit und Stress. Die Seelsorgenden in den deutschen Diözesen*, pp. 71–138. Würzburg, Germany: Echter.

General Conference of Seventh-day Adventists. 2016. *Seventh-day Adventist Church Manual.* Hagerstown, MD: Secretariat, General Conference of Seventh-day Adventists.

Hodge, D. R. 2007. "A Systematic Review of the Empirical Literature on Intercessory Prayer." *Research on Social Work Practice* 17(2): 174–187. doi:10.1177/1049731506296170

Hollywell, C., and J. Walker. 2009. "Private Prayer as a Suitable Intervention for Hospitalised Patients: A Critical Review of the Literature." *Journal of Clinical Nursing* 18(5): 637–651. doi:10.1111/j.1365-2702.2008.02510.x

Holy Bible. 2008. *The New International Version.* Grand Rapids, MI: Zondervan.

Holy Father Francis. 2015. "Encyclical Letter LAUDATO SI' of the Holy Father Francis on 'Care for the Common Home.'" Retrieved from http://w2.vatican.va/content/francesco/en/encyclicals/documents/papa-francesco_20150524_enciclica-laudato-si.html

The Holy See (Vatican). 2017a. "Apostolic Letter Issued 'Motu Proprio' by the Supreme Pontiff Francis Instituting the Dicastery for Promoting Integral Human Development." Retrieved from http://w2.vatican.va/content/francesco/en/motu_proprio/documents/papa-francesco-motu-proprio_20160817_humanam-progressionem.html

The Holy See (Vatican). 2017b. "Pontifical Council for Health Pastoral Care." Retrieved from http://www.vatican.va/roman_curia/pontifical_councils/hlthwork/documents/rc_pc_hlthwork_pro_20051996_en.html

Jarvis, G. K., and H. C. Northcott. 1987. "Religion and Differences in Morbidity and Mortality." *Social Science & Medicine* 25(7): 813–824. doi:10.1016/0277-9536(87)90039-6

Jensen, O. M. 1983. "Cancer Risk among Danish Male Seventh-day Adventists and Other Temperance Society Members." *Journal of the National Cancer Institute* 70(6): 1011–1014.

Johnson, M. E., A. M. Dose, T. B. Pipe, W. O. Petersen, M. Huschka, M. M. Gallenberg, . . . M. H. Frost. 2009. "Centering Prayer for Women Receiving Chemotherapy for Recurrent Ovarian Cancer." *Oncology Nursing Forum* 36(4): 421–428. doi:10.1188/09.ONF.421-428

Katz, N. 2011. "How Do Mount Athos Monks Stay So Healthy?" Retrieved from http://www.cbsnews.com/news/how-do-mount-athos-monks-stay-so-healthy/

Kerksieck, P., A. Büssing, E. Frick, C. Jacobs, and K. Baumann. 2016. "Reduced Sense of Coherence Due to Neuroticism: Are Transcendent Beliefs Protective Among Catholic Pastoral Workers?" *Journal of Religion and Health*, October, 1–15. doi:10.1007/s10943-016-0322-8

Ladd, K. L., and B. Spilka. 2013. "Prayer: A Review of the Empirical Literature." In K. I. Pargament, J. J. Exline, and J. W. Jones, eds., *APA Handbook of Psychology, Religion, and Spirituality (Vol. 1): Context, Theory, and Research,* pp. 293–310. Washington, DC: American Psychological Association.

La Rovere, M. T., J. T. Bigger, F. I. Marcus, A. Mortara, and P. J. Schwartz. 1998. "Baroreflex Sensitivity and Heart-Rate Variability in Prediction of Total Cardiac Mortality after Myocardial Infarction." *Lancet* 351(9101): 478–484.

Le, L., and J. Sabaté. 2014. "Beyond Meatless, the Health Effects of Vegan Diets: Findings from the Adventist Cohorts." *Nutrients* 6(6): 2131–2147. doi:10.3390/nu6062131

Lemon, F. R., R. T. Walden, and R. W. Woods. 1964. "Cancer of the Lung and Mouth in Seventh-day Adventists: Preliminary Report on a Population Study." *Cancer* 17(4): 486–497. doi:10.1002/1097-0142(196404)17:4<486::AID-CNCR2820170410>3.0.CO;2-Z

Levine, E. G., C. Aviv, G. Yoo, C. Ewing, and A. Au. 2009. "The Benefits of Prayer on Mood and Well-Being of Breast Cancer Survivors." *Supportive Care in Cancer* 17(3): 295. doi:10.1007/s00520-008-0482-5

Libreria Editrice Vaticana. 2003a. "Catechism of the Catholic Church." Retrieved from http://www.vatican.va/archive/ENG0015/_INDEX.HTM

Libreria Editrice Vaticana. 2003b. "Catechism of the Catholic Church—You Shall Love the Lord Your God with All Your Heart, and with All Your Soul, and With All Your Mind, Article 3: The Third Commandment; II. The Lord's Day, 2177." Retrieved from http://www.vatican.va/archive/ENG0015/_P7O.HTM

Libreria Editrice Vaticana. 2003c. "Catechism of the Catholic Church—You Shall Love the Lord Your God with All Your Heart, and with All Your Soul, and With All Your Mind, Article 3: The Third Commandment; II. The Lord's Day, 2186." Retrieved from http://www.vatican.va/archive/ENG0015/_P7O.HTM

Libreria Editrice Vaticana. 2017a. "Catechism of the Catholic Church—The 6 Commandment: II. The Vocation to Chastity, 2337." Retrieved from http://www.vatican.va/archive/ENG0015/_P9N.HTM

Libreria Editrice Vaticana. 2017b. "Catechism of the Catholic Church—The Life of Prayer, Article 1: Expressions of Prayer, II: Meditation, 2708." Retrieved from http://www.vatican.va/archive/ENG0015/_P9L.HTM

Libreria Editrice Vaticana. 2017c. "Catechism of the Catholic Church—The Life of Prayer: Article 1: Expressions of Prayer, In Brief, 2720." Retrieved from http://www.vatican.va/archive/ENG0015/_P9N.HTM

Loma Linda University. 2017. "About Loma Linda University Health." Retrieved from http://home.llu.edu/about-us/about-loma-linda-university-health

Luy, M. 2002. "Warum Frauen Länger Leben: Erkenntnisse Aus Einem Vergleich von Kloster-Und Allgemeinbevölkerung." Retrieved from http://www.ssoar.info/ssoar/handle/document/33398

Luy, M., and C. Wegner. 2011. "Lebe Langsam-Stirb Alt. Eine Geschlechterspezifische Studie über Klosterleben und Lebenserwartung." *Ärzte Woche* 24(46): 16.

Mann, J. R., C. C. Stine, and J. Vessey. 2002. "The Role of Disease-Specific Infectivity and Number of Disease Exposures on Long-Term Effectiveness of the Latex Condom." *Sexually Transmitted Diseases* 29(6): 344–349.

Merakou, K., S. Taki, A. Barbouni, E. Antoniadou, D. Theodoridis, G. Karageorgos, and J. Kourea-Kremastinou. 2016. "Sense of Coherence (SOC) in Christian Orthodox Monks and Nuns in Greece." *Journal of Religion and Health* (First publication online May 5, 2016). doi:10.1007/s10943-016-0244-5

Mills, P. K., W. L. Beeson, R. L. Phillips, and G. E. Fraser. 1994. "Cancer Incidence among California Seventh-day Adventists, 1976–1982." *American Journal of Clinical Nutrition* 59(5): 1136S–1142S.

Montgomery, S., P. Herring, A. Yancey, L. Beeson, T. Butler, S. Knutsen, . . . G. Fraser. 2007. "Comparing Self-Reported Disease Outcomes, Diet, and Lifestyles in a National Cohort of Black and White Seventh-day Adventists." *Prevention of Chronic Disease* 4(3): A62.

Morton, K. R., J. W. Lee, and L. R. Martin. 2016. "Pathways from Religion to Health: Mediation by Psychosocial and Lifestyle Mechanisms." *Psychology of Religion and Spirituality* 9(1): 106–117. doi:10.1037/rel0000091

Orlich, M. J., and G. E. Fraser. 2014. "Vegetarian Diets in the Adventist Health Study 2: A Review of Initial Published Findings." *American Journal of Clinical Nutrition* 100 (Suppl. 1): 353S–358S. doi:10.3945/ajcn.113.071233

Orlich, M. J., P. N. Singh, J. Sabaté, K. Jaceldo-Siegl, J. Fan, S. Knutsen, . . . G. E. Fraser. 2013. "Vegetarian Dietary Patterns and Mortality in Adventist Health Study 2." *JAMA Internal Medicine* 173(13): 1230–1238. doi:10.1001/jamainternmed.2013.6473

Orthodox Life. 2017. "The Fasting Rule of the Orthodox Church." Retrieved from http://www.abbamoses.com/fasting.html

Papadaki, A., C. Vardavas, C. Hatzis, and A. Kafatos. 2008. "Calcium, Nutrient and Food Intake of Greek Orthodox Christian Monks During a Fasting and Non-Fasting Week." *Public Health Nutrition* 11(10): 1022–1029. doi:10.1017/S1368980007001498

Patel, R., D. Lycett, A. Coufopoulos, and A. Turner. 2017. "Moving Forward in Their Journey: Participants' Experience of Taste & See, a Church-Based Programme to Develop a Healthy Relationship with Food." *Religions* 8(1): 14. doi:10.3390/rel8010014

Pérez, J. E., A. R. Smith, R. L. Norris, K. M. Canenguez, E. F. Tracey, and S. B. DeCristofaro. 2011. "Types of Prayer and Depressive Symptoms among Cancer Patients: The Mediating Role of Rumination and Social Support." *Journal of Behavioral Medicine* 34(6): 519–530. doi:10.1007/s10865-011-9333-9

Phillips, R. L. 1975. "Role of Life-Style and Dietary Habits in Risk of Cancer among Seventh-day Adventists." *Cancer Research* 35(11 Pt. 2): 3513–3522.

Phillips, R., L. Garfinkel, J. W. Kuzma, W. L. Beeson, T. Lotz, and B. Brin. 1980. "Mortality among California Seventh-day Adventists for Selected Cancer Sites." *Journal of the National Cancer Institute* 65(5): 1097–1107.

Poloma, M. M., and B. F. Pendleton. 1989. "Exploring Types of Prayer and Quality of Life: A Research Note." *Review of Religious Research* 31(1): 46–53. doi:10.2307/3511023

Pope John Paul II. 1997. *The Theology of the Body Human Love in the Divine Plan.* Boston: Pauline Books & Media.

Pope Paul VI. 1968. "Encyclical Letter Humanae Vitae of the Supreme Pontiff Paul VI on the Regulation of Birth." Retrieved from http://w2.vatican.va/content/paul-vi/en/encyclicals/documents/hf_p-vi_enc_25071968_humanae-vitae.html

Rizzo, N. S., J. Sabaté, K. Jaceldo-Siegl, and G. E. Fraser. 2011. "Vegetarian Dietary Patterns Are Associated with a Lower Risk of Metabolic Syndrome." *Diabetes Care* 34(5): 1225–1227. doi:10.2337/dc10-1221

Seventh-day Adventist Church. 1987. "Official Statements—Sexual Behavior." Retrieved from https://www.adventist.org/en/information/official-statements/statements/article/go/-/sexual-behavior/

Seventh-day Adventist Church. 1992. "Official Statements—Abortion." Retrieved from https://www.adventist.org/en/information/official-statements/guidelines/article/go/-/abortion/

Seventh-day Adventist Church. 2000. "Official Statements Guidelines—AIDS Epidemic." Retrieved from https://www.adventist.org/en/information/official-statements/guidelines/article/go/-/aids-epidemic/

Seventh-day Adventist Church. 2009. "Mission Statement of the Seventh-day Adventist Church." Retrieved from https://www.adventist.org/en/information/official-statements/statements/article/go/-/mission-statement-of-the-seventh-day-adventist-church/

Seventh-day Adventist Church. 2015. "Official Statements—Immunization." Retrieved from https://www.adventist.org/en/information/official-statements/guidelines/article/go/-/immunization/

Seventh-day Adventist Church Office of Archives, Statistics, and Research. 2016. "2016 Annual Statistical Report." Retrieved from http://documents.adventistarchives.org/Statistics/ASR/ASR2016.pdf

Stimpson Chapman, E. 2015. "The Catholic Diet." Retrieved from https://www.osv.com/Article/TabId/493/ArtMID/13569/ArticleID/17819/The-Catholic-Diet.aspx

Tantamango-Bartley, Y., K. Jaceldo-Siegl, J. Fan, and G. Fraser. 2013. "Vegetarian Diets and the Incidence of Cancer in a Low-Risk Population." *Cancer Epidemiology and Prevention Biomarkers* 22(2): 286–294. doi:10.1158/1055-9965.EPI-12-1060

Thygesen, L. C., N. C. Hvidt, H. P. Hansen, A. Hoff, L. Ross, and C. Johansen. 2012. "Cancer Incidence among Danish Seventh-day Adventists and Baptists." *Cancer Epidemiology* 36(6): 513–518. doi:10.1016/j.canep.2012.08.001

Tonstad, S., T. Butler, R. Yan, and G. E. Fraser. 2009. "Type of Vegetarian Diet, Body Weight, and Prevalence of Type 2 Diabetes." *Diabetes Care* 32(5): 791–96. doi:10.2337/dc08-1886

Tonstad, S., K. Stewart, K. Oda, M. Batech, R. P. Herring, and G. E. Fraser. 2013. "Vegetarian Diets and Incidence of Diabetes in the Adventist Health Study-2." *Nutrition, Metabolism and Cardiovascular Diseases* 23(4): 292–299. doi:10.1016/j.numecd.2011.07.004

von Bingen, H. 2011. *Ursprung und Behandlung der Krankheiten: Causae et Curae (Hildegard von Bingen-Werke Band II)*. Beuron, Germany: Beuroner Kunstverl.

White, E. G. 2006. *The Ministry of Healing*. Telico Plains, TN: Digital Inspiration.

Wynder, E. L., F. R. Lemon, and I. J. Bross. 1959. "Cancer and Coronary Artery Disease among Seventh-day Adventists." *Cancer* 12(5): 1016–1028. doi:10 .1002/1097-0142(195909/10)12:5<1016::AID-CNCR2820120523>3.0 .CO;2-2

Chapter 8

Islam and Health

Mona M. Amer

When people think of "religion," what often comes to mind is a belief system that is associated with specific traditions and rituals. Islam distinguishes itself from other faiths by incorporating a comprehensive way of life with guidelines for all aspects of daily activity and even for death. There are special supplications for virtually every action a person can take during the day, whether entering a home, using the bathroom, donning a new piece of clothing, studying for an exam, eating a meal, taking transportation, hearing thunder, or preparing for sleep. For Muslims who make an effort to recite such supplications, the entire day is a form of remembrance of God. Islam is, moreover, not only a personal way of life: it also incorporates standards for family, social, economic, political, legal, and environmental systems.

Given the all-encompassing experience of Islam, it is natural that beliefs and practices that relate to health and well-being are also incorporated. This chapter first orients the reader to the sources of jurisprudence and main beliefs and rituals endorsed by the Islamic faith. Next, concepts related to health and healing are discussed. These concepts underlie many of the daily lifestyle practices that are discussed in the fourth section. Finally, research is presented on the health consequences of the main rituals in Islam: the daily prayers, fasting during Ramadan, and the hajj pilgrimage to Mecca and other holy sites.

THE ISLAMIC WAY OF LIFE

The Islamic knowledge base on how to conduct worldly affairs is vast and complex. There are two main sources of information regarding the Islamic way of life. The first and foremost is the Qur'an, which contains verses from God that were revealed to Prophet Muhammad (PBUH[1]) through the angel Gabriel over a period spanning a little more than two decades. Prophet Muhammad (PBUH) was not literate, and thus the verses were recited, memorized, and transferred to others who memorized and wrote them down. After his death, the 114 chapters or *surahs* of the Qur'an were compiled, each comprising a series of verses (Esposito 2011). To this day there is only one version of the Qur'an. Viewed as the word of God, the Qur'an is believed by Muslims to be infallible and unquestionable.

The second source of knowledge about Islamic beliefs and practices is the *Sunnah*, which refers to the traditions and example of Prophet Muhammad (PBUH). After his death, religious scholars preserved and codified his behavior by collecting thousands of *hadiths*, or sayings, that were attributed to him or observed about him. Most of the hadiths were based on the experiences of the direct companions of the Prophet (PBUH), who verbally described to others what they had heard and seen. Scholars such as Ibn Malik, Al Bukhari, and Muslim applied intensive research to verify the authenticity and validity of each hadith, focusing particularly on the integrity of the chain of transmitters of the hadith. The Sunnah is essential to following Islam, because while the Qur'an presents a general framework, the sayings and actions of Prophet Muhammad (PBUH) provide greater details and distinctions on how to understand and implement the framework (McCloud, Hibbard, and Saud 2013).

When questions are raised regarding the Islamic view, or judgments must be made on new situations or issues that arise as a function of the evolution of modern society, *ijtihad* is used. This term refers to the use of deductive logic among Islamic scholars to draw a conclusion, or *fatwa*, based on consensus and analogy. To come to these conclusions, scholars draw from the Qur'an and the Sunnah. This process allows Islam to flexibly adapt to modern times while staying constant to its principles (Al-Qaradawy n.d.).

Of course, not all Muslims adopt or even are familiar with the vast array of concepts and edicts found in Islam, and there is diversity among Muslims in terms of thought and practice. Although the Qur'an admonishes people who pick and choose parts of religion to follow based on what suits them, in reality this may happen; some people may adopt some parts of the Islamic way of life while ignoring or rejecting others. Muslims may differ in specific beliefs and rituals as a result of adhering to different branches of Sunni and Shi`a Islam. Additionally, Islam is the second largest religion in the world after Christianity; about one-fifth of the world's population is Muslim, distributed across every region and nation. As a consequence, local cultural mores often contradict or obfuscate Islamic dictates, producing a tremendous variety of traditions and behavioral practices among Muslims. Notwithstanding all these forms of diversity, there are some core threads that tie together and define the worldwide community of Muslims: These include the basic articles of faith as well as the five pillars of Islam.

Shared among Muslims worldwide are six articles of faith: the beliefs in God, angels, Day of Judgment, predestination, prophets, and the holy books. God, translated as *Allah* in Arabic, is believed to be one transcendent omnipotent power who created and controls the universe. He has no son or partner or companion, and has absolute perfection and infallibility (Al-Qaradawy n.d.). As directed in the Qur'an: "Say: He is Allah, the One and Only; Allah, the Eternal, Absolute; He begetteth not, nor is He begotten; And there is none like unto Him (112:1–4)."[2] God is merciful and forgiving; all-knowing and all-seeing; pre-eternal and perpetual (Tarsin 2015). It is the human duty to worship and follow God. In fact, the word *Islam* comes from the Arabic root *sa-la-ma,* which is the root for the words "peace" and "submission." This signifies that the overall purpose of Islam is to submit oneself to God, and indeed God states in the Qur'an that He created humankind only to worship Him (51:56).

Muslims also believe in angels, unseen creatures made from light who serve as messengers for God. Angels carry peoples' prayers up to God and keep record of peoples' daily actions. These actions will be reviewed on the Day of Judgment, which is believed to be the time of resurrection during which all humans will be assembled and each will receive word of their final destination in the Afterlife, whether Heaven or Hell. Belief in the Afterlife motivates Muslims to conduct themselves piously on earth with the best of deeds (Tarsin 2015). A related core belief in Islam is that of pre-destination, or God's divine decree over what will happen. However, there is a constant tension in the religious scholarship between pre-destination and limited free will. This theological debate is perhaps beyond the scope of human understanding, but Islam emphasizes the importance of each person's responsibility for his or her own actions (Denny 2011).

To help people meet this responsibility and support them in learning the best ways of worship, God sent prophets and messengers who gave guidance on how to implement God's intentions on earth. The prophets established justice, and led their peoples by example (Al-Qaradawy n.d.). Muslims believe in the line of previous prophets starting from Adam and ending with Muhammad. The Qur'an makes reference to 25 prophets, including Abraham, Noah, David, Solomon, Joseph, Moses, and Jesus (peace be upon them). Muslims believe that Prophet Muhammad (PBUH) is the last and final prophet who came with the final set of comprehensive guidelines for people to follow. Many prophets received scriptures from God that documented guidelines; for example, Moses had the Torah, David had the Psalms, and Jesus had the Gospel. As described earlier, the Qur'an is believed to be the final and purest text because, unlike previous scriptures, it has not been corrupted or modified by humans since the time of its revelation (Denny 2011).

The Qur'an lays out the five pillars, or foundations, of Islam. These are the minimal acts of worship that define a person as Muslim. The first is the *shahada*, or the testimony that "there is no God but God and Prophet Muhammad is His messenger." This proclamation is sufficient for someone to enter the folds of Islam and forms the basis of all Muslim belief and behavior (Denny 2011). The *shahada* is repeated numerous times throughout the day, such as during prayer.

Second is the *salat*, or obligatory prayers, which break the day with scheduled opportunities for the worshiper to meet God in prayer. The timings of the prayers, which are based on the position of the sun, include dawn, around noon, mid-afternoon, sunset, and in the evening. The daily prayers follow a structured sequence of physical movements that are aligned with recitations from the Qur'an and supplications. Muslims must perform the prayers while in a state of purity, and thus ablution (*wudu'*) is made before prayers during which the hands, mouth, nose, face, arms, head, ears, and feet are washed with a particular order and set of movements (Tarsin 2015).

The third foundation of Islam is fasting from dawn to dusk during the holy month of Ramadan, which is described in more detail later in this chapter. The fourth pillar is the *zakat*, which is the required almsgiving. Muslims should pay a percentage of their saved wealth annually to people who are in need, including those who are poor and destitute, and wayfarers. The zakat is a form of worship that purifies one's money, reminds one that all wealth is a temporary loan from God, and ensures financial support for those who are less fortunate (Denny 2011). Finally, any Muslim who is physically and financially able to should perform the *hajj* once in the lifetime. This fifth pillar of Islam is a pilgrimage to holy sites located in Saudi Arabia. The hajj entails participating in rituals that represent the paths that Prophet Abraham (PBUH) and Prophet Muhammad (PBUH) took centuries before. This annual visitation of about 3 million people is a mass migration and human gathering that is unparalleled in scope and historical continuity (Shujaa and Alhamid 2015).

As can be seen by the description of the five pillars, there is a rhythmic flow to the Islamic way of life. The main foundations are based on the cycles of the day and night (shahada and daily prayers), year (Ramadan fasting and zakat), and lifetime (hajj). These rituals are the minimum requirements.

Muslims are encouraged to pray, fast, and give charity more often than what is prescribed, and to take the lesser pilgrimage, or *umrah*, to the holy sites in Mecca. Also implicit in the five pillars is encouragement for Muslims to engage in constant worship and appreciation for God's blessings. These are the core values that underlie Muslims' views on all aspects of daily living, including concepts of health and illness.

ISLAMIC VIEWS ON HEALTH AND HEALING

When considering the views on health in Islam, it is important to recognize that the concepts of mind, body, and spirit are interwoven. A human being has a body and soul, with the soul continuing for eternity even after the body has died (Saniotis 2015). Muslims are instructed to care for the physical body and nurture the soul. The psyche (*nafs*), heart (*qalb*), and mind (`*aql*) are viewed as complementary and together constitute healthy well-being. These terms do not carry the rigid body-mind distinction found in modern medicine; instead, their definitions are often fluid, holistic, and overlapping. For example, the *nafs* refer to the self, and there are different types or levels of the nafs mentioned in the Qur'an. Yet the nafs may also sometimes connote the soul or the ego (Saniotis 2015, Deuraseh and Abu Talib 2005).

The *qalb* represents not only the physical organ of the heart but also the source of reason, wisdom, compassion, emotion, and spiritual closeness (Saniotis 2015, Haque 2004). Prophet Muhammad (PBUH) said, "Beware, in the body there is a piece of flesh; if it is sound, the whole body is sound and if it is corrupt the whole body is corrupt, and hearken it is the heart" (Al-Bukhari 2:49, Muslim 10:3882).[3] At a physiological level, this saying illustrates the systemic interconnections of the body systems; metaphorically, it also warns against sins, or diseases of the heart such as hatred, envy, miserliness, arrogance, anger, and others. As for the `*aql*, it is defined as the highest level of intellect and reasoning (Haque 2004). Yet through contemplating the signs of God's existence, this intellect may be the pathway for enhancing spirituality.

It is an obligation to care for all these interconnected aspects of well-being. Muslims believe that health is a blessing that one should thank God for and not take for granted. Because one's body is seen as a gift from God, the body has rights over the person. Muslims expect to be judged by God for how they cared for their bodies in times of health and illness (Zaman 1997; Yosef 2008). The suffering experienced during illness is viewed as a pathway to earning rewards from God for being patient, or as expiation of sins (al-Shahri and al-Khenaizan 2005). Prophet Muhammad (PBUH) said: "No fatigue, no disease, nor sorrow, nor sadness, nor hurt, nor distress befalls a Muslim, even if it were the prick he receives from a thorn, but Allah expiates some of his sins for that" (Al-Bukhari 70:545). As such, despite any pain, illness is conceived as conferring benefits on the person. The faith accords high importance to visiting those who are sick and praying for them. Conversely, the person who is ill is believed to be closer to God, so people often ask the ailing person to pray for them (Koenig and Al Shohaib 2014).

When Muslims fall ill with any ailment, they are encouraged in Islam to pursue avenues for healing. This could include modern medicine, traditional healing practices, spiritual healing such as prayer and reading the Qur'an, or any other type of healthcare behavior that does not contradict any tenets or guidelines of the faith. This is because Muslims believe that healing is always possible and it is a duty to care for the body that God blessed one with (al-Shahri and al-Khenaizan 2005). Prophet Muhammad (PBUH) said: "There is no disease that Allah has created, except that He also has created its treatment" (Al-Bukhari 71:582) and, "There is a remedy for every malady, and when the remedy is applied to the disease it is cured with the permission of Allah, the Exalted and Glorious" (Muslim 26:5466). These statements foster optimism that a cure is possible even if it is not yet known to humankind. With regard to fatalistic views that illness is delivered by God and only He can deliver health, the majority consensus among scholars is that people with illnesses should actively seek treatment and then leave the outcome to God's will (Koenig and Al Shohaib 2014). As the Qur'an states, "[It is God] Who created me, and it is He Who guides me; Who gives me food and drink, and when I am ill, it is He Who cures me; Who will cause me to die, and then to life (again)" (26:78–81).

In Islam, death is defined as the moment when the angel of death visits the dying person and releases his or her soul to God. Therefore, someone who is brain-dead but has other parts of the body functioning would not be considered dead. For those who are experiencing terminal illness, even if painful, it is not permissible to end one's life because life is owned by God. Muslims with terminal illness may prefer to remain at home for their final period on earth and to die there. At home they can more easily participate in religious practices such as prayers and modest dress. After death the person is buried quickly. Postmortem examination, such as autopsy for educational purposes, is generally not conducted because the body belongs to God and should be treated in a dignified manner. Death signifies the juncture between the life on earth and the events that happen after death, which end with the permanent Afterlife. Muslims believe that after a transitional phase they will each be independently judged by God on their worldly actions and accordingly face eternal Afterlife in either Heaven or Hell (Sarhill, LeGrand, Islambouli, Davis, and Walsh 2001; Sheikh 1998).

LIFESTYLE PRACTICES AND HEALTH

To earn the positive judgment of God, devout Muslims invest time and energy in avoiding sins and adopting practices that are in accordance with the faith. As mentioned earlier, Islam encompasses guidelines for all aspects of daily life from waking to sleep. This includes bathroom hygiene, modest dress, manners and good etiquette, and others. These injunctions match the natural state of humans, have reasonable explanations behind them, and emphasize moderation (Al-Qaradawy n.d.). Many of the lifestyle practices that were encouraged in the Qur'an and were modeled by Prophet Muhammad (PBUH) have important salutary outcomes for and influences on health and well-being. These include guidelines for eating, teeth cleaning, avoidance of drugs and tobacco, physical activity, social relationships, and sleep.

Eating and Nutrition

With regard to meals, the Islamic way of life encourages moderation. This is mentioned in the Qur'an: "O Children of Adam! wear your beautiful apparel at every time and place of prayer: eat and drink: But waste not by excess, for Allah loveth not the wasters" (7:31). Prophet Muhammad (PBUH) instructed people to avoid sleeping immediately after eating meals or it will harden the heart. He also advised to fill the stomach with one-third food and one-third drink, and to leave one-third empty for easy breathing (Tahir-ul-Qadri 2005). These are all useful instructions against overeating.

The diet and food preferences of Muslims show much diversity around the world, as they are influenced by regional, cultural, and socioeconomic factors. The variety of foods and encouragement of a nutritionally balanced diet is illustrated by the more than 30 different types of foods that are mentioned in the Qur'an, including meats, grains, vegetables, and fruits (Tarighat-Esfanjani and Namazi 2016). The Qur'an says: "O ye who believe! Eat of the good things that We have provided for you, and be grateful to Allah, if it is Him ye worship" (2:172). Yet there are types of things that are forbidden to eat in Islam, including pork, blood, and carrion. Although there may be multiple reasons for the prohibition of pork, many have surmised that one of the reasons may be the propensity of pigs to carry parasites and infectious diseases, especially in hot climates. Hygienic reasons may also be the basis for the prohibition of carrion such as meat from animals who died from disease, accidents, or being killed by other animals (Toda and Morimoto 2001). For terrestrial animals that are lawful to eat, such as cattle, sheep, and chicken, the animal should be slaughtered by cutting the throat while reciting a prayer; this is similar to the Jewish Kosher regulations.

There are other aspects of Islamic practice that also influence food intake. The cycle of eating and sleeping is aligned with Islamic rituals that improve health status. For example, longer prayers take place after the larger lunch and dinner meals, whereas the shortest prayer is at dawn when the stomach is empty. During the month of Ramadan, additional prayers are recommended at night, which is not long after the *iftar* or breaking of the fast with large meals. This kind of light exercise found in the prayer cycles can help maintain weight and is hypothesized to positively affect cholesterol levels (Tahir-ul-Qadri 2005).

Miswak Tooth Stick

The *miswak* is a chewing stick, most commonly from the *Salvadora persica* plant, that is used to clean and polish the teeth. Prophet Muhammad (PBUH) encouraged people to use the miswak often, at least prior to each of the five daily prayers. The miswak continues to be used around the Muslim world, particularly in Saudi Arabia and other Gulf countries. The miswak contains fluoride and other substances, and is effective in reducing plaque, gingivitis, and tooth decay. In fact, in many studies it was found to be superior to contemporary tooth-brushing for those benefits. It also has beneficial antimicrobial effects that are not found with the toothbrush, thereby reducing one's risk for periodontal disease (al-Otaibi 2004; Halawany 2012). Regardless of whether a person uses miswak or a toothbrush, in general there is an awareness of dental hygiene in Islam.

Alcohol and Drugs

Decades of medical and psychological literature have shown that psychoactive drugs, including illicit drugs and alcohol, have the potential to cause significant damage to health, mental health, and social relationships, not to mention their negative repercussions on society. All intoxicants are prohibited in Islam because they both cause harm to the body and also precipitate behaviors that are harmful to the self or others (Yosef 2008). Three verses in the Qur'an demonstrate the incremental prohibition of intoxicants. First, people were instructed to eschew intoxicants when praying, because it would interfere with concentration on the prayer. The second verse encourages people to abstain by noting that despite any benefits, the sins and harms are worse than the benefits. The third verse prohibits intoxicants altogether as the work of Satan (Koenig and Al Shohaib 2014).

The Qur'an refers to intoxicants with the word *khamr*, which in essence comes from the Arabic root for the concept of veiling; essentially, it indicates that the substance veils the mind. Therefore, the prohibition is believed by most scholars to refer to any substance that has psychoactive properties and thus has the potential to affect perception, cognition, and the like. In recent decades the Arabic word *khamr* has been more commonly used to connote wine, so there are Muslims around the world who believe that only alcohol is prohibited and that other substances are permissible. However, Prophet Muhammad (PBUH) had already clarified that "Every intoxicant is khamr and every intoxicant is forbidden" (Muslim 23:4966). He also said: "If a large amount of anything causes intoxication, a small amount of it is prohibited" (Abudawud 26:3673), and he warned that God curses anyone who produces, drinks, serves, carries, sells, buys, or otherwise benefits from the production and sales of khamr. These very strict guidelines regarding intoxicants represent a primary prevention strategy that significantly lowers the chance of a Muslim using or abusing drugs.

Tobacco

Because intoxicants are prohibited, a question of debate among Islamic scholars has been the status of tobacco products, which have addictive properties without salient psychoactive effects. There are no direct texts in the Qur'an and Sunnah that forbid the consumption or use of tobacco, so historically it was considered an acceptable behavior. The prevalence of smoking and chewing tobacco is disproportionately high across Muslim-majority countries compared to other nations, especially among men (Toda and Morimoto 2001; Ghouri, Atcha, and Sheikh 2006). However, in recent decades greater awareness has arisen regarding the serious negative physical consequences of tobacco and smoking, bolstering the view that it is not aligned with Islamic teachings.

Nowadays the majority of Islamic scholars classify tobacco use and smoking as at least discouraged, if not outright forbidden, due to negative impacts on the body and wasting of money (Ghouri, Atcha, and Sheikh 2006). Knowledge of these fatwas about smoking may not significantly alter smoking behavior (Radwan et al. 2003). Nevertheless, intrinsic religiosity and religious commitment are associated with reduced rates of smoking and increased attempts at cessation among smokers, indicating that Muslims who are more connected with their faith may avoid tobacco use. Therefore, religion can be a potential vehicle for anti-smoking programming, especially for those who are more religious (Toda and Morimoto 2001; Alzyoud, Kheirallah, Ward, Al-Shdayfat, and Alzyoud 2015).

Physical Activity

The positive benefits of physical exercise in promoting health and preventing illness are undisputable. Physical exercise is encouraged in Islam for both men and women. Prophet Muhammad (PBUH) modeled a physically active lifestyle such as walking fast and working with his hands in the fields (Yosef 2008). There are many references to sports, such as wrestling, fencing, hunting, horseback riding, running, and swimming, in the Qur'an and the Sunnah, and some specifically pertain to the value of maintaining a fit body in order to be prepared in case of war (Kahan 2003).

In general, Muslims believe that participating in exercise and sport is important for both health and recreation. Among more religious Muslims, such activities may even be seen as intricately linked with religious faith, as obligatory behaviors in order to care for one's body. Yet despite positive values associated with physical activity, there may be religious, cultural, and logistical barriers to participating in exercise, particularly for women. For example, women may prefer to exercise in private, same-sex spaces or at home where they can avoid being observed by men and can remove the veil and clothing items that may be cumbersome in sport. Additionally, some women may turn to their fathers or husbands for permission to be involved in sport. As a result, opportunities for women to participate in physical activity can be limited, especially in competitive sports. It is therefore not surprising that the rates of participation in sport are lower among women compared to men in Muslim-majority countries (Walseth and Fasting 2003; Wray 2002).

For Muslims living as minorities in regions such as in North America and Europe, challenges to engaging in physical activity can be further exacerbated by cultural and social pressures. For example, Muslim girls living in Western countries generally have positive experiences in physical education classes and value the health benefits of exercise. However, for older adolescents, religious accommodations are important, such as offering private changing rooms and shower spaces, allowing youths to cover their hair and body according to religious principles, not requiring swimming when fasting, and avoiding close contact with the opposite sex. When the school or college environment is rigid and not sensitive to these needs, Muslim girls may become frustrated and resentful. Such overall insensitivity and lack of accommodation may dampen their motivation to engage in physical activity or lead to withdrawal from physical education classes (Dagkas and Benn 2006; Kahan 2003). Involvement in extracurricular activities and sports clubs may be reduced among adult women for similar reasons (Strandbu 2005; Zaman 1997).

Social Relationships

Maintaining respectful and strong bonds with family, friends, and neighbors is an important virtue among Muslims that is encouraged in the Qur'an and the Sunnah. These behaviors are described in the famous compilation of morals and manners called *Riyadh Us-Saliheen* (Gardens of the Righteous), recorded by Imam Al-Nawawi in the 13th century. Family members, especially parents and mothers, are to be treated with respect and kindness. Extended family relationships should be nurtured. Marriage in Islam carries high distinction and honor, so Muslims are encouraged to marry and extramarital relationships are prohibited. Friendship is valued, and true friendship is seen to be a form of love for the sake of Allah. With respect to all acquaintances, Islamic etiquette promotes tolerance and kindness while denouncing backbiting, lying, or any other behaviors that sow discord and ill feelings among people.

The encouragement to foster healthy relationships extends beyond people in one's inner circle of connections, also including the wider society. Muslims experience an attachment with and responsibility toward the worldwide community of Muslims, called the *ummah*. Moreover, prejudice, racism, and intergroup conflict are discouraged. It is stated in the Qur'an: "And among His Signs is the creation of the heavens and the earth, and the variations in your languages and your colours: verily in that are Signs for those who know" (30:23) and "O mankind! We created you from a single (pair) of a male and a female, and made you into nations and tribes, that ye may know each other (not that ye may despise each other). Verily the most honoured of you in the sight of Allah is (he who is) the most righteous of you. And Allah has full knowledge and is well acquainted (with all things)" (49:13).

These directives for social interactions carry positive effects for health and well-being. For example, a large volume of health and social research has shown that social support is a preventive factor for physical and psychological conditions and is a key resource for coping and resilience. Social relationships, including marriage, are associated with positive psychological well-being and longevity of life (Koenig and Al Shohaib 2014). Additionally, discrimination and intergroup conflict can increase physiological stress, mental health concerns, and negative health outcomes for members of the targeted group (Pascoe and Richman 2009; Paradies 2006). Therefore, when tolerance and intergroup harmony are emphasized, these risk factors may be reduced.

Sleep

Sleep is another aspect of daily activity that has been given attention in the Islamic way of life. The Qur'an uses different Arabic words to describe different types of sleep; these align with modern-day understanding of the stages of the sleep cycle (BaHammam 2011). The importance of sleep was highlighted by Prophet Muhammad (PBUH), who instructed worshipers to prioritize sleep over continuing to pray when feeling drowsy. He said, "... offer prayers and also sleep at night, as your body has a right on you" (Bukhari 31:196).

The etiquette of sleep in Islam contains specific recommendations that are associated with positive health. Based on the Sunnah, Muslims are encouraged to maintain early bedtime by sleeping after the *esha* prayer and to wake up early at dawn for the *fajr* prayer. It is advised to perform the ablution prior to sleep, which (as discussed later in this chapter) prevents risk of disease and enhances relaxation. Muslims were instructed by Prophet Muhammad (PBUH) to lie on the right side of the body while sleeping. Recent studies have shown that this position has benefits for the heart and autonomic nervous system. Also encouraged is modification of the environment so that it is dark and peaceful, and so that the material that one is sleeping on is clean. Moreover, taking a mid-day nap is integrated in the Islamic lifestyle, and recent research has shown that such naps are associated with improved cognition, memory, and alertness (BaHammam 2011).

RELIGIOUS RITUALS AND HEALTH

As is shown by the preceding discussion, positive health outcomes are associated with the daily activities of the Islamic lifestyle, from waking time to sleep. Beneficial health outcomes related to important rituals such as prayer, fasting, and the hajj have also been documented in decades of medical research.

Daily Prayers and Ablution

The five daily prayers have physical, mental, emotional, spiritual, and social benefits, some of which are similar to the documented benefits of yoga and meditation. It is a form of exercise because the prayer includes shifting body positions among standing, bowing, resting on the shins, and prostrating. As such, the prayer stretches different muscle groups in the body (Zaman 1997) and improves posture, coordination, and balance (Bhat, Murtaza, Sharique, and Jabin 2014). The position of prostration in particular relies on several joints and muscles, and over time can strengthen the body. For example, the neck muscles are strengthened, which can reduce muscle strain and prevent pain caused by the wearing down of discs and vertebrae in the neck (Sayeed and Prakash 2013). Orthopedic benefits also come from the movement of the joints, which increases blood flow into the joint areas (Bhat et al. 2014). Even more than that, the functioning of many body systems—including respiratory, cardiovascular, digestive, and endocrine—is improved as a consequence of the pressuring, squeezing, relaxing, and shifting of different muscles and the enhancement of blood flow created by prayer movements (Bhat et al. 2014).

Prayer, especially the bowing and prostration positions, as well as the ablution wash that is conducted before praying, help activate the brain cooling system, thereby reducing risk for overheating (Irmak 2014). During prayer, many parts of the body touch the floor, including feet, hands, knees, and head. This causes a healthy grounding or "earthing" effect whereby mobile electrons in the earth flow into the body (Irmak 2014). There are also suggestions that electromagnetic energy is released during prayer, which increases relaxation (Sayeed and Prakash 2013).

Relaxation, or emotional calmness, may occur for the person who is praying, and there are many potential explanations for that. The rituals that take place prior to the prayer (washing ablution, and reminding oneself of the intention and purpose of prayer) serve as cues to focus on the prayer and avoid thinking of worldly matters (Sayeed and Prakash 2013). Electro-encephalographic (EEG) records of brain activity while people are praying show increased amplitude of alpha waves in the parietal and occipital regions during prostration. This signifies a parasympathetic or relaxation response, potentially due to the eyes focusing on one point on the floor when the head is on the floor (Doufesh, Faisal, Lim, and Ibrahim 2012). Praying also serves as a buffer against anxiety and depression (Al-Krenawi and Graham 2000).

The physical aspects of prayer can positively influence cognitive functioning. During the prostration the head is touching the floor, so the head is lower than the heart. Therefore, increased blood supply travels to the brain, which can have positive impacts on cognitive acuity, concentration, and memory (Sayeed and Prakash 2013). Enhancement of greater attention and concentration during the prayer can even be demonstrated with EEG, revealed by increased gamma activity in the brain (Doufesh, Ibrahim, and Safari 2016). Memory can also be improved through the constant recitation of verses from the Qur'an during the prayer (Bhat et al. 2014). In older adults, those who pray regularly show better cognitive functioning than those who do not pray regularly, similar to the positive effects on cognition that result from exercise (Bai, Ye, Zhu, Zhao, and Zhang 2012).

The prayer is also an opportunity to put aside life's demands and concentrate on one's relationship with God, thereby enhancing spirituality and God consciousness (Zaman 1997). People who are concentrating in prayer experience higher levels of connectedness with God and surrendering to Him, states that are associated with changes in brain activity as measured by single photon emission computed tomography (Newberg et al. 2015). This kind of transcendental connection with God exposes the person to the omniscient and omnipotent powers of God (Al-Krenawi and Graham 2000).

The prayer is not merely an individual endeavor; prayers can be performed in congregate settings at home or at the mosque. Joining the Friday sermon and prayer at the mosque is an important religious ritual that is obligatory for men and optional for women. Congregate praying provides additional benefits to the worshiper, including strengthening social networks and receiving emotional and social support. People who pray with a group may also experience greater social warmth, selflessness, familiarity, and group cohesion, as well as reduced prejudice toward persons from different cultural backgrounds who are sharing the same prayer. All of these benefits can positively impact psychological well-being (Al-Krenawi and Graham 2000).

In addition to the health advantages of the formal prayers, the ablution or *wudu'* that is conducted prior to praying brings further benefits. Ablution includes hand washing, which helps remove germs and potential sources of infection. Gargling removes food particles in the mouth, thereby improving oral health and reducing risk for common colds. Similarly, washing the nostrils removes germs, dust, and allergens, and washing the feet and toes can prevent fungal infection. The circular or massaging motions using when washing the face and neck (for those who include the neck in the ablution) can invigorate and relax the person (Bhat et al. 2014). Overall, people feel refreshed and relaxed after the ablution.

Fasting

During the Islamic month of Ramadan, Muslims fast from dawn to dusk. *Fasting* refers to abstaining from food, drink, and sexual relations. Also emphatically discouraged during the time of the fast are behaviors that are not accepted in Islam, such as backbiting, lying, shouting at others, and so on. This is because Ramadan is meant to be a holy month, with increased observance and performance of prayers and good deeds to bring oneself closer to God. By abstaining from food and drink, Muslims are reminded of the daily blessings they have which people who are poor do not. They develop humility, patience, and self-discipline. As such, Ramadan is a month of spiritual elevation (Denny 2011; A. S. Ahmed 2002).

The effects of fasting on different aspects of body functions has been a longstanding area of inquiry for medical researchers; more than a thousand publications address this topic. It is important to note that fasting is discouraged in Islam if it may compromise a person's health. For example, people who are ill, travelers, women who are menstruating, and prepubertal children are exempted from fasting. However, the determination of illness versus health is often made by patients themselves, with some Muslims preferring to share the collective spirit of Ramadan by fasting even if this constitutes a hardship on their bodies. Systematic reviews have documented that fasting can be safe for patients with a wide range of medical conditions. Even though it is usually acceptable, individualized consultation with a medical professional is still recommended for patients with hypertension (Alinezhad-Namaghi and Salehi 2016), diabetes (Rouhani and Azadbakht 2014), renal/kidney diseases (Bragazzi 2014; Emami-Naini, Roomizadeh, Baradaran, Abedini, and Abtahi 2013), and pregnant women (Rouhani and Azadbakht 2014; Mirsane and Shafagh 2016). Fasting is generally not recommended for persons with active ulcers (Bragazzi et al. 2015) or high-risk or Type I diabetes (Bragazzi et al. 2015).

With regard to healthy adults who do not have any significant illness, a review of more than a hundred investigations published over five decades concluded that glucose levels remain stable during Ramadan. Similarly, systematic reviews and meta-analyses have shown no significant changes in kidney function (Rouhani and Azadbakht 2014), endocrine functions (Azizi 2010), risk for cardiovascular events (Turin et al. 2016; Salim, Al Suaidi, Ghadban, Alkilani, and Salam 2013), and neuropsychiatric status (Azizi 2010). Serum lipid levels, however, may change depending on any shifts in body weight and the amount and quality of meals consumed during the month (Azizi 2010). Changes in lipid levels also depend on gender, with many studies showing reduced levels of cholesterol and triglyceride among men and increased high-density lipoprotein among women (Rouhani and Azadbakht 2014). Regarding weight loss, meta-analyses of studies in different parts of the world conclude that although weight loss during the month could be significant, especially for males (Kul, Savas, Ozturk, and Karadag 2014), the weight is typically regained soon after Ramadan ends (Sadeghirad, Motaghipisheh, Koladooz, and Haghdoost 2012; Rouhani and Azadbakht 2014). So, in summary, there does not seem to be evidence of any long-term negative repercussions of fasting on physical well-being. With respect to mental health, subjective well-being such as happiness and life satisfaction increases with Ramadan fasting (Campante and Yanagizawa-Drott 2015).

Many Muslims may try to take advantage of Ramadan to make enduring changes to their health-related behaviors. For instance, Islamic fasting has been recommended as a safe way to prevent and control obesity, particularly because it entails both reduction in caloric intake and behavioral modification (Khan and Khattak 2002). Another example is the reduction of tobacco consumption. Because most Muslims believe that tobacco consumption is also prohibited during the time of the fast, Ramadan provides a natural opportunity for smoking reduction and cessation. Some authors have argued for the strategic benefits of aligning smoking reduction and cessation programming with Ramadan (Aveyard, Begh, Sheikh, and Amos 2011; Suriani, Zulkefli, Chung, and Zainal 2015). At the same time, it should be acknowledged that Ramadan may be a challenging time for Muslim smokers, who may report less religious interest and commitment, and may have more negative Ramadan experiences compared to nonsmokers (Khan, Watson, and Chen 2013). Therefore, the effectiveness of tobacco interventions related to Ramadan is likely to be moderated by level of religiosity.

Hajj

The hajj is a journey of spiritual cleansing that includes opportunities to draw closer to God and ask for sins to be forgiven while facing physically arduous rituals. The hajj includes a great deal of travel among and within the holy sites, such as the *tawaf* or circumambulation around the Kaaba in Mecca. Much of this movement is performed on foot. As such, it is physically exhausting even for youths. Because it may take decades before one has the financial means to make the pilgrimage, hajj travelers are often older and may already be suffering from medical conditions. Moreover, tens of thousands of travelers come from lower-income nations where preventive health care is minimal. The most common causes of death during the hajj are cardiac arrest and heat stroke. Means to prevent this include water sprinklers, drinking fountains, and umbrellas. Other causes of injury or death have been accidents and stampedes. These have decreased over the years—with an absence of serious incident over the past decade—as a result of new transportation systems and more effective crowd management (Q. Ahmed, Arabi, and Memish 2006; Shujaa and Alhamid 2015).

In addition to the personal strain and risk of injury during the hajj, the crowding of millions of people in small geographical locations, sometimes in high temperatures, raises the risk for the spread of infectious disease and poses a significant annual public health challenge. The primary concerns in the past have been meningococcal disease, as well as respiratory tract infections such as pneumonia, tuberculosis, pertussis, and influenza. Because of previous outbreaks, the Saudi government requires pilgrims to have taken the meningitis vaccine before they can receive the vise to perform hajj. The government recommends the influenza vaccine for everyone, and pneumococcal vaccine for those above age 65. Also recommended are face masks. The government immediately takes action if pilgrims are coming from regions where there is an epidemic of disease, such as during previous outbreaks of Ebola, SARS, avian flu, and MERS coronavirus. Actions may include banning, delaying entry to, or screening the pilgrims (Q. Ahmed, Arabi, and Memish 2006; Shujaa and Alhamid 2015).

There are many additional health risks at the hajj. The prospect of having to prepare and properly store food for millions of people can be challenging. Gastrointestinal problems such as traveler's diarrhea and food poisoning are among the primary sources of burden on the hundreds of free healthcare clinics distributed throughout the cities hosting the hajj rituals. Efforts to contain these problems have included barring pilgrims from carrying perishable foodstuffs, monitoring food services provided by the hajj organizing companies and hotels, and encouraging vaccination against hepatitis. Further risks of the hajj are skin infections and exacerbation of skin conditions, as well as bloodborne diseases spread by nonsterile blades that are used in the ritual of shaving hair (Q. Ahmed, Arabi, and Memish 2006; Memish 2007).

Aside from the risk of physical illness, there is a risk for mental health problems. The hajj experience can be stressful, especially for those traveling for the first time to a foreign location with language barriers and crowded conditions. For a minority of pilgrims, this may exacerbate existing psychiatric concerns such as depression, anxiety, and panic. Pilgrims with these conditions can and do seek help at any of the available psychiatric care clinics found along the hajj route (Özen 2010). One study found that female pilgrims reported less emotional well-being a few months after the hajj, possibly a consequence of the physical or financial stress of the journey (Clingingsmith, Khwaja, and Kremer 2009). However, for the vast majority of pilgrims the hajj may contribute to positive psychological well-being. There are many moments of emotional catharsis during the hajj, including the ritual of stoning the devil Satan, which symbolizes the release from guilt and sin. This kind of psychological cleansing and the conviction that previous sins are erased leaves the hajj traveler feeling rejuvenated and optimistic, with a sense of resolution and readiness to begin a new phase in life (Al-Krenawi and Graham 2000).

As much as there are individual impacts on the person performing the hajj, it is also a communal experience. Prior to the hajj, people mend any interpersonal conflicts so that they can meet God without any unfinished business (Al-Krenawi and Graham 2000). During hajj, groups of pilgrims support one another, and it is not permissible to engage in any kind of argumentation or speaking ill of another person (Koenig and Al Shohaib 2014). After completing the hajj and returning home, the person may occupy a higher social status and will be expected to demonstrate a high level of moral etiquette, such as showing ongoing kindness, virtues, and adherence to the faith (Al-Krenawi and Graham 2000). These characteristics of the hajj support the strengthening of social relationships and community health. Pilgrims who return from hajj show greater desire for peace and harmony, tolerance for intergroup diversity, and support for gender equity (Clingingsmith, Khwaja, and Kremer 2009).

CONCLUSION

From the daily routine of brushing one's teeth to the lifetime event of performing the hajj, the Islamic way of life is a comprehensive framework that for the most part enhances physical, mental, emotional, social, and spiritual well-being. Devout Muslims believe in the importance of nurturing and protecting the blessing of their bodies. Yet there is a difference between the faith and the people, with not all Muslims applying the daily lifestyle modeled by Prophet Muhammad (PBUH) and not all Muslims performing the required rituals. Nevertheless, given how extensively positive health is associated with Islam, it would be reasonable to integrate Islam into disease prevention and health promotion programs, especially for individuals and communities that are more devout.

NOTES

1. PBUH is the abbreviation for "peace be upon him," which is a form of respect accorded to the prophets.

2. Quotations from the Qur'an are taken from the translation of Abdullah Yusuf Ali. Citations include the number of the chapter followed by the number of the verse.

3. Citations for hadiths in this chapter refer to the name of the compilation of hadith, followed by the chapter and hadith number.

REFERENCES

Ahmed, A. S. 2002. *Islam Today: A Short Introduction to the Muslim World*. London: I.B. Tauris Publishers.

Ahmed, Q. A., Y. M. Arabi, and Z. A. Memish. 2006. "Health Risks at the Hajj." *Lancet* 367 (9515): 1008–1015. doi:10.1016/S0140-6736(06)68429-8

Alinezhad-Namaghi, M., and M. Salehi. 2016. "Effects of Ramadan Fasting on Blood Pressure in Hypertensive Patients: A Systematic Review." *Journal of Fasting and Health* 4(1): 17–21.

Al-Krenawi, A., and J. R. Graham. 2000. "Islamic Theology and Prayer: Relevance for Social Work Practice." *International Social Work* 43(3): 289–304. doi:10.1177/002087280004300303

al-Otaibi, M. 2004. "The Miswak (Chewing Stick) and Oral Health: Studies on Oral Hygiene Practices of Urban Saudi Arabians." *Swedish Dental Journal Supplement* 167: 2–75.

Al-Qaradawy, Y. n.d. *Introduction to Islam*. n.p.: Islamic Inc. Publishing and Distribution. Retrieved from http://www.muslim-library.com/dl/books/English_Introduction_to_Islam.pdf

al-Shahri, M. Z., and A. al-Khenaizan. 2005. "Palliative Care for Muslim Patients." *Journal of Supportive Oncology* 3(6): 432–436.

Alzyoud, S., K. A. Kheirallah, K. D. Ward, N. M. Al-Shdayfat, and A. A. Alzyoud. 2015. "Association of Religious Commitment and Tobacco Use among Muslim Adolescents." *Journal of Religion and Health* 54(6): 2111–2121. doi:10.1007/s10943-014-9921-4

Aveyard, P., R. Begh, A. Sheikh, and A. Amos. 2011. "Promoting Smoking Cessation Through Smoking Reduction during Ramadan." *Addiction* 106: 1379–1380. doi:10.1111/j.1360-0443.2011.03432.x

Azizi, F. 2010. "Islamic Fasting and Health." *Annals of Nutrition and Metabolism* 56(4): 273–282. doi:10.1159/000295848

BaHammam, A. S. 2011. "Sleep from an Islamic Perspective." *Annals of Thoracic Medicine* 6: 187–192. doi:10.4103/1817-1737.84771

Bai, R., P. Ye, C. Zhu, W. Zhao, and J. Zhang. 2012. "Effect of Salat Prayer and Exercise on Cognitive Functioning of Hui Muslims Aged Sixty and Over." *Social Behavior & Personality* 40(10): 1739–1748. doi:10.2224/sbp.2012.40.10.1739

Bhat, R. A., S. T. Murtaza, M. Sharique, and F. Jabin. 2014. "Unity of Health through Yoga and Islamic Prayer 'Salah.'" *Academic Sports Scholar* 3(10): 1–6.

Bragazzi, N. L. 2014. "Ramadan Fasting and Chronic Kidney Disease: A Systematic Review." *Journal of Research in Medical Sciences* 19(7): 665–676.

Bragazzi, N. L., W. Briki, H. Khabbache, I. Rammouz, S. Mnadla, T. Demaj, and M. Zouhir. 2015. "Ramadan Fasting and Infectious Diseases: A Systematic Review." *Journal of Infection in Developing Countries* 9(11): 1186–1194. doi:10.3855/jidc.5815

Campante, F., and D. Yanagizawa-Drott. 2015. "Does Religion Affect Economic Growth and Happiness? Evidence from Ramadan." *Quarterly Journal of Economics* 130(2): 615–658. doi:10.1093/qje/qjv002

Clingingsmith, D., A. I. Khwaja, and M. R. Kremer. 2009. "Estimating the Impact of the Hajj: Religion and Tolerance in Islam's Global Gathering." *Quarterly Journal of Economics* 124(3): 1133–1170. doi:10.1162/qjec.2009.124.3.1133

Dagkas, S., and T. Benn. 2006. "Young Muslim Women's Experiences of Islam and Physical Education in Greece and Britain: A Comparative Study." *Sport, Education and Society* 11(1): 21–38. doi:10.1080/13573320500255056

Denny, F. M. 2011. *An Introduction to Islam.* New York: Pearson Education.

Deuraseh, N., and M. Abu Talib. 2005. "Mental Health in Islamic Medical Tradition." *International Medical Journal* 4(2): 76–79.

Doufesh, H., T. Faisal, K.-S. Lim, and F. Ibrahim. 2012. "EEG Spectral Analysis on Muslim Prayers." *Applied Psychophysiology and Biofeedback* 37(1): 11–18. doi:10.1007/s10484-011-9170-1

Doufesh, H., F. Ibrahim, and M. Safari. 2016. "Effects of Muslims Praying (Salat) on EEG Gamma Activity." *Complementary Therapies in Clinical Practice* 24: 6–10. doi:10.1016/j.ctcp.2016.04.004

Emami-Naini, A., P. Roomizadeh, A. Baradaran, A. Abedini, and M. Abtahi. 2013. "Ramadan Fasting and Patients with Renal Diseases: A Mini Review of the Literature." *Journal of Research in Medical Sciences* 18(8): 711–716.

Esposito, J. L. 2011. *What Everyone Needs to Know about Islam: Answers to Frequently Asked Questions, from One of America's Leading Experts.* Oxford, UK: Oxford University Press.

Ghouri, N., M. Atcha, and A. Sheikh. 2006. "Influence of Islam on Smoking among Muslims." *British Medical Journal* 332(7536): 291–294. doi:10.1136/bmj.332.7536.291

Halawany, H. S. 2012. "A Review on Miswak (Salvadora persica) and Its Effect on Various Aspects of Oral Health." *Saudi Dental Journal* 24(2): 63–69. doi:10.1016/j.sdentj.2011.12.004

Haque, A. 2004. "Religion and Mental Health: The Case of American Muslims." *Journal of Religion and Health* 43(1): 45–58. doi:10.1023/B:JORH.000 0009755.25256.71

Irmak, M. K. 2014. "Medical Aspects of Ablution and Prayer." *Journal of Experimental & Integrative Medicine* 4(2): 147–149. doi:10.5455/jeim.291213.hp.010

Kahan, D. 2003. "Islam and Physical Activity: Implications for American Sport and Physical Educators." *Journal of Physical Education, Recreation & Dance* 74(3): 48–54. doi:10.1080/07303084.2003.10608470

Khan, A., and M. M. A. K. Khattak. 2002. "Islamic Fasting: An Effective Strategy for Prevention and Control of Obesity." *Pakistan Journal of Nutrition* 1(4): 185–187.

Khan, Z. H., P. J. Watson, and Z. Chen. 2013. "Smoking, Muslim Religious Commitments, and the Experience and Behaviour of Ramadan in Pakistani Men." *Mental Health, Religion & Culture* 16(7): 663–670. doi:10.1080/13674676.2 012.712956

Koenig, H. G., and S. Al Shohaib. 2014. *Health and Well-Being in Islamic Societies: Background, Research, and Applications.* Geneva: Springer International. doi:10.1007/978-3-319-05873-3

Kul, S., E. Savas, Z. A. Ozturk, and G. Karadag. 2014. "Does Ramadan Fasting Alter Body Weight and Blood Lipids and Fasting Blood Glucose in a Healthy Population? A Meta-analysis." *Journal of Religion and Health* 53: 929–942. doi:10.1007/s10943-013-9687-0

McCloud, A. B., S. W. Hibbard, and L. Saud. 2013. *An Introduction to Islam in the 21st Century.* West Sussex, UK: Wiley-Blackwell.

Memish, Z. A. 2007. "Muslim Pilgrimage." In A. Wilder-Smith, E. Schwartz, and M. Shaw, eds., *Travel Medicine: Tales behind the Science*, pp. 253–262. Amsterdam: Elsevier.

Mirsane, S. A., and S. Shafagh. 2016. "A Narrative Review on Fasting of Pregnant Women in the Holy Month of Ramadan." *Journal of Fasting and Health* 4(2): 53–56.

Newberg, A. B, N. A. Wintering, D. B. Yaden, M. R. Waldman, J. Reddin, and A. Alavi. 2015. "A Case Series Study of the Neurophysiological Effects of Altered States of Mind during Intense Islamic Prayer." *Journal of Physiology-Paris* 109(4–6): 214–220. doi:10.1016/j.jphysparis.2015.08.001

Özen, Ş. 2010. "Sociodemographic Characteristics and Frequency of Psychiatric Disorders in Turkish Pilgrims during Hajj." *Dicle Tip Dergisi* 37(1): 8–15.

Paradies, Y. 2006. "A Systematic Review of Empirical Research on Self-Reported Racism and Health." *International Journal of Epidemiology* 35(4): 888–901. doi:10.1093/ije/dyl056

Pascoe, E. A., and L. S. Richman. 2009. "Perceived Discrimination and Health: A Meta-analytic Review." *Psychological Bulletin* 135(4): 531–554. doi:10.1037/a0016059.supp

Radwan, G. N., E. Israel, M. El-Setouhy, F. Abdel-Aziz, N. Mikhail, and M. K. Mohamed. 2003. "Impacts of Religious Rulings (Fatwa) on Smoking." *Journal of the Egyptian Society of Parasitology* 33(3): 1087–1101.

Rouhani, M. H., and L. Azadbakht. 2014. "Is Ramadan Fasting Related to Health Outcomes? A Review on the Related Evidence." *Journal of Research in Medical Sciences* 19(10): 987–992.

Sadeghirad, B., S. Motaghipisheh, M. J. Z. Kolahdooz, and A. A. Haghdoost. 2012. "Islamic Fasting and Weight Loss: A Systematic Review and Meta-analysis." *Public Health Nutrition* 17(2): 396–406. doi:10.1017/S1368980012005046

Salim, I., J. Al Suwaidi, W. Ghadban, H. Alkilani, and A. M. Salam. 2013. "Impact of Religious Ramadan Fasting on Cardiovascular Disease: A Systematic Review of the Literature." *Current Medical Research & Opinion* 29(4): 343–354. doi:10.1185/03007995.2013.774270

Saniotis, A. 2015. "Understanding Mind/Body Medicine from Muslim Religious Practices of Salat and Dhikr." *Journal of Religion and Health* Online First: 1–9. doi:10.1007/s10943-014-9992-2

Sarhill, N, S. LeGrand, R. Islambouli, M. P. Davis, and D. Walsh. 2001. "The Terminally Ill Muslim: Death and Dying from the Muslim Perspective." *American Journal of Hospice & Palliative Care* 18(4): 251–255. doi:10.1177/104990910101800409

Sayeed, S. A., and A. Prakash. 2013. "The Islamic Prayer (Salah/Namaaz) and Yoga Togetherness in Mental Health." *Indian Journal of Psychiatry* 55: 224–230. doi:10.4103/0019-5545.105537

Sheikh, A. 1998. "Death and Dying—A Muslim Perspective." *Journal of the Royal Society of Medicine* 91(3): 138–140.

Shujaa, A., and S. Alhamid. 2015. "Health Response to Hajj Mass Gathering from Emergency Perspective: Narrative Review." *Turkish Journal of Emergency Medicine* 15(4): 172–176. doi:10.1016/j.tjem.2015.02.001

Strandbu, A. 2005. "Identity, Embodied Culture and Physical Exercise: Stories from Muslim Girls in Oslo with Immigrant Backgrounds." *Young: Nordic Journal of Youth Research* 13(1): 27–45. doi:10.1177/1103308805048751

Suriani, I., N. A. M. Zulkefli, C. S. Chung, and M. S. Zainal. 2015. "Factors Influencing Smoking Behaviour Changes during Ramadan among Malay Male Students." *Journal of Fasting and Health* 3(3): 97–102.

Tahir-ul-Qadri, M. 2005. *Islam on Prevention of Heart Diseases.* Lancashire, UK: Minhaj Welfare Foundation.

Tarighat-Esfanjani, A., and N. Namazi. 2016. "Nutritional Concepts and Frequency of Foodstuffs Mentioned in the Holy Quran." *Journal of Religion and Health* 55(3): 812–819. doi:10.1007/s10943-014-9855-x

Tarsin, A. 2015. *Being Muslim: A Practical Guide.* Davie, FL: Sandala Inc.

Toda, M., and K. Morimoto. 2001. "Health Practice in Islam: The Cultural Dependence of the Lifestyle Formation." *Environmental Health and Preventive Medicine* 5: 131–133. doi:10.1007/BF02918287

Turin, T. C., S. Ahmed, N. S. Shommu, A. R. Afzal, M. Al Mamun, M. Qasqas, . . . N. Berka. 2016. "Ramadan Fasting Is Not Usually Associated with the Risk of Cardiovascular Events: A Systematic Review and Meta-analysis." *Journal of Family and Community Medicine* 23(2): 73–81. doi:10.4103/2230-8229.181006

Walseth, K., and K. Fasting. 2003. "Islam's View on Physical Activity and Sport: Egyptian Women Interpreting Islam." *International Review for the Sociology of Sport* 38(1): 45–60. doi:10.1177/10126902030381003

Wray, S. 2002. "Connecting Ethnicity, Gender, and Physicality: Muslim Pakistani Women, Physical Activity and Health." In S. Scraton and A. Flintoff, eds., *Gender and Sport: A reader*, pp. 127–140. London: Routledge.

Yosef, A. R. O. 2008. "Health Beliefs, Practice, and Priorities for Health Care of Arab Muslims in the United States." *Journal of Transcultural Nursing* 19(3): 284–291. doi:10.1177/1043659608317450

Zaman, H. 1997. "Islam, Well-Being and Physical Activity: Perceptions of Muslim Young Women." In G. Clarke and B. Humberstone, eds., *Researching Women and Sport*, pp. 50–67. Houndmills, UK: Palgrave Macmillan. doi:10.1007/978-1-349-25317-3_4

Chapter 9

Sufism and Optimal Health

*Saloumeh Bozorgzadeh, Nasim Bahadorani,
and Mohammad Sadoghi*

INTRODUCTION

Sufism is known as the mystical dimension of Islam.[1] As described by His Holiness Salaheddin Ali Nader Angha, Sufism is "the reality of religion" (2011, p. 91). This means "experiencing God in one's inner self, submitting to Him, and loving Him with one's mind, heart, and soul, until no other but the Beloved remains" (Angha 2000b, p. 3). Thus, Sufism is a "way of love, a way of devotion, and a way of knowledge" (Angha 2003, p. 35). Its teachings promote physical, cognitive, emotional, and spiritual health, which enables one to attain a state of balance: oneness with the Divine Beloved. There are different orders in Islamic Sufism, and their practices vary. This chapter focuses on the health-oriented teachings of the Maktab Tarighat Oveyssi (MTO) Shahmaghsoudi®, School of Islamic Sufism®. His Holiness Salaheddin Ali Nader Angha, or Professor Angha[2] as he is referred to by his students, is the current Sufi Master of the school.

ISLAMIC SUFISM AND HEALTH

Health is more than a physical state. Knowing this, for more than 1,400 years Islamic Sufism has taught its students how to reach a state of optimal health by developing the spiritual dimension and expanding the innate capacities and talents that lie within each individual. Moreover, within this tradition it is held that through self-knowledge one's ultimate potential is discovered, and balance is restored to the individual's life. Thus, as taught by Professor Angha, well-being is achieved when the physical, cognitive, emotional, and spiritual aspects of an individual's life are balanced and in harmony (Angha 2002b).

It is important to point out that there is a plethora of information on the physical, cognitive, and emotional aspects of health. However, the spiritual dimension is often neglected by science due to its seemingly intangible or unobservable qualities, despite recent research that has demonstrated significant positive correlations between spirituality and health outcomes (Koenig 2003; Hooker, Masters, and Carey 2014; Koenig 2012). To illuminate the importance of developing one's spirituality for good health, it is taught that human beings have two dimensions, physical and spiritual (Angha 2002b). The physical dimension includes the physical body, the senses, the emotions, the mind, and their interactions with the outside world. It follows the laws of nature, and is externally focused on the physical, mental, and social aspects of the individual. It constantly makes comparisons and wants more; therefore, it has insatiable needs and desires. In contrast, it is held that the spiritual dimension is eternal and is found within each individual (Angha 2002b). This dimension is connected to Existence, to God; thus, it is all-knowing. It is taught that both of these dimensions need to be fully developed and constantly nurtured to experience the harmony and balance necessary to achieve optimal health. The two dimensions are not separate from each other, but are connected through a point of union in the heart. The goal of Islamic Sufism is discovery of this point of union, called the capital "I" or "Source of Life," which is the true self, as it contains both dimensions of one's being. This Source of Life is not bounded by race, ethnicity, culture, or gender and is "the true value of each individual" (Angha 2002b, p. 125). It is constant and remains steady throughout time, physical changes, and external conditions. As the cells of the body multiply and die, the essence of the individual remains. This is due to the inner, true self—the "I." Because it is connected with Existence, which is constant and eternal, when discovered, it provides an individual with a greater span of knowledge that is not based on sensory input.

Thus, a central focus of Islamic Sufism is on self-knowledge, as it is "a method, a way, a discipline that teaches each person the science of exploring his or her being" (Angha 2011, p. 73). This holistic method teaches individuals to observe, understand, and develop both dimensions of themselves to their full potential. The knowledge of one's true identity helps clarify each individual's purpose and provides a framework for all that one does. This includes an understanding of what one needs in order to achieve optimal health and balance. With an understanding that one's identity is more than just the physical dimension, issues related to this physical world have less of a stressful effect on one's well-being. Of course, the physiological systems of the human body continue to do their part as they react to events and send pain signals, regulate autonomic functions, and so forth. However, biological reactions such as pain are understood as being part of the physical system as opposed to having a greater meaning to the person or defining him or her. This adds an element of psychological resilience when dealing with worldly stressors.

BALANCE AND HARMONY

A central tenet of belief is that balance and harmony are essential for health and well-being; when something is out of balance, dis-order or dis-ease ensues. Islamic Sufism teaches how to re-establish balance between the physical and spiritual dimensions of the human being. The student, or seeker, actively applies the teachings to himself or herself, watching to not overdo or underdo in any aspects of life. The physical body is maintained, and eating, sleeping, exercise, and activities are monitored to ensure that they are not out of equilibrium. Emotions and reactions to the environment are examined by the individual in the same way. Using a metaphorical example of the growth of an apple seed, in order for it to prosper and develop a trunk, branches, and leaves, the earth in which the seed is planted must be balanced. It cannot be too dry, wet, acidic, and so on. The tree must be in a stable and healthy environment in order for it to ultimately present its true identity, that of an apple tree. The same is true for human beings.

Thus, it is held that one must actively endeavor to maintain homeostasis in the physical dimension (physiologically, cognitively, emotionally, socially, etc.) in order to provide a healthy and harmonious environment for the spiritual dimension to thrive. Focusing only on the external/physical factors results in an undeveloped and neglected spiritual dimension. Conversely, strictly fixating on spirituality will come at the cost of neglecting one's physical, emotional, cognitive, and social aspects. If only one dimension of the individual is developing, disharmony will occur. This disharmony can cause distress, depression, anxiety, negative emotions, and low energy (Angha 2002b). Seekers are taught to evaluate and dispel that which does not serve them. The beliefs, values, and judgments that are based upon familial, societal, and cultural practices, but which have no true basis or utility for the individual, are dismissed, and truth is sought from the point of union in the heart, the Source of Life. This point determines what is needed for balance and, as it is connected with Existence, it is independent of the needs, ego, selfishness, and desires of the physical realm. It is governed by a higher standard, that of a vast and infinite existence. As a result, resilience, strength, and creativity spring from this point. This affects not only an individual's health and presence, but also his or her interactions with and contributions to society.

ELECTROMAGNETIC CENTERS AND HEART

It is taught that the human body is equipped with 13 electromagnetic centers, and the spiritual dimension is developed through the activation and balance of these electromagnetic centers (Angha 2002b). These centers are often ignored by science due to the lack of instrumentation to properly measure them. However, they connect the physical to the spiritual dimension and allow individuals to discover their spiritual dimension. The main center, the Source of Life, located in the crista terminalis of the heart (S. M. S. Angha 1999; Angha 2002b), is the point where extraordinary traits emerge. These traits and qualities, often associated with saints, such as creativity, love, peace, wisdom, and compassion, are not products of the environment but are innate to the human being. Just as balancing the physical dimension supports spiritual development, these inherent spiritual traits support the physical realm.

This paradigm, which focuses on the heart, stands in stark contrast to how Western traditions view the human being. The American Psychological Association defines *psychology* as "the scientific study of the behavior of individuals and their mental processes" (Gerrig and Zimbardo 2002). As individuals go through life, they interact with the world around them using their senses. They accumulate memories, and create notions and varying schemas in order to make sense of their surroundings and themselves. Their family, school, work, religious institution, society, and culture all play an important role in the development of their personality, morals, worldview, and health. As they encounter new information, they adapt it to their established worldview. The brain and its processes are central to this paradigm, as the brain is presumed to control the body and heart. However, it is held that the brain and senses are part of the physical realm and as such are limited in their abilities to discover truth (Angha 2002b). Thus, the senses have a restricted range within which they operate (for example, only a small portion of the light spectrum can be observed by the eyes), and the brain, like a computer, continues to operate with whatever information it was programmed. The Sufi paradigm seeks to depend on something less variable than the brain and senses. From the Sufi perspective, the heart controls all. Because the Source of Life in the heart is connected to Existence, which is vast and infinite, it is the heart with its connection to infinite knowledge that commands the brain, which in turn commands the body (Angha 2002b). The heart is the first organ to develop in a fetus. At approximately 21 days after conception, it is a mass of cells with a pulse beat that forms into the heart (Angha 2011). From the knowledge in the heart, nerve cells branch out to form the brain and the rest of the organs. Throughout life, the brain and all other organs are dependent upon the heart (Angha 2011). Evidence of support for this type of influence by the heart is reported in research suggesting that heart transplant recipients, post-transplant, take on personality characteristics that paralleled those of the donor's personality, memories, and preferences (Pearsall, Schwartz, and Russek 2000). It suggests that the transplanted hearts may still continue to hold cellular and possibly systemic memory that influences the perceptions, memories, and lifestyle preferences of the transplant recipient. Transplanted hearts function effectively and independently without any neural connections to the brain (Vanderbilt Health n.d.). Thus, to achieve balance within this paradigm, as His Holiness Shah Maghsoud Sadegh Angha advises, "enlighten the channel that extends from your heart to your brain and do not allow the heart and the brain to live apart, like two unfriendly neighbors unaware of each other" (S. M. S. Angha 1986, p. 62). The practices of Islamic Sufism promote the union of heart and brain.

THE PRACTICES OF ISLAMIC SUFISM

The practices of Islamic Sufism nurture both the physical and spiritual dimensions of the human being and lead to a state of optimal health. From the spiritual dimension, they allow the seeker to discover his or her true identity and anchor the individual within his or her stable being. From the physical dimension, they bring balance to the physical, emotional, cognitive, and social aspects of the individual. The individual is encouraged to study, and examine every action in light of his or her purpose, questioning whether or not the act is beneficial to both the physical and spiritual dimensions. Considering the physical body to be a vehicle that carries the human being through this spiritual quest, each individual must safeguard this precious gift from harm in order to attain the final goal, which in Islamic Sufism is self-knowledge.

It is taught that there are three levels of practices that lead to self-cognition. The first level of practice is referred to as *shariat*. It involves the basic practices in religion such as fasting and prayers that at the surface level provide discipline to the self, and are necessary for purification of the physical body, which subsequently benefits the inner being. Many people stop at the level of shariat, and do not progress further into deeper levels (Angha 2002a). The second level is called *tarighat* and is the way of the Sufi. It involves concentration of the mind and energies, purification of the individual from worldly attachments and desires that bind the soul, and unification of the inner being with God. This level requires laser-focused concentration on gathering thoughts and energy on the stable center within the heart—the Source of Life. An example is the practice of *salat* (daily prayers). The physical act of doing them is *shariat*. Ensuring an understanding of the words, and postures, while concentrating all your thoughts and energies on one purpose and actively remaining present with the postures and intention is *tarighat*. Finally, the third level is arriving at the state of oneness or unity where both dimensions are presenting the exact same thing, called *haghighat*. All of the practices revolve around remembrance of one goal, which can be called unity with Existence, self-knowledge, or optimal health. To promote this state of holistic health, students of Islamic Sufism follow practices including *salat* (daily prayers), fasting, *zikr* (remembrance), Tamarkoz® (discussed later), weekly classes, spiritual readings, *khidmat* (service), *khums* (alms), retreats, and dietary restrictions.

SALAT (DAILY PRAYERS)

"Remember Me; I will remember you."

—Holy Qur'an 2:152

Remembrance of one's beloved throughout the day is natural for many people. In Islamic Sufism, the Beloved is God, and devotional prayers (*salat*) five times a day are in remembrance of Him. True worship is performed with adoration, humility, awe, and gratitude. It does not stem from fear, desires for acquisition of worldly materials, or out of habit or obligation. To worship with full adoration, one should be in the present moment, and the body, mind, and soul should all say the same thing. Professor Angha defines a human being as "a unique masterpiece" (Angha 2002a, p. 37), capable of direct union with God. To worship is to come to know Him. During prayer, concentration and focus on one's goal, which is union with God, is important, and the precise methodology is provided in Islamic Sufism. As the seeker performs the prayers on a daily basis at dawn, noon, mid-afternoon, sunset, and nightfall, a healthy structure is brought into one's day-to-day life. The exact explanation for the purpose and meaning of the postures of salat are provided in the book *Al-Salat* (1998) by His Holiness Shah Maghsoud Sadegh Angha.

There have been several studies on the physiological and psychological benefits of daily practice of salat. Sayeed and Prakash (2013) note that most joints and muscles in the body are exercised during salat. They emphasize the importance of prostration, which is performed 34 times per day.

During prostration, the body is inverted, so the head is positioned lower than the heart, leading to an increased blood supply, which is shown to improve cognitive abilities. Prostration causes a grounding effect of the electromagnetic field of the body that is hypothesized to have a calming effect on the individual due to the observed amplification of alpha waves in the brain (Doufesh, Faisal, Lim, and Ibrahim 2012). Henry (2015) suggests that Islamic prayers produce spiritual energy, reduce stress, improve subjective well-being, and encourage self-forgiveness as a process of personal healing. Bai et al. (Bai, Ye, Zhu, Zhao, and Zhang 2012) describe salat as a type of mind concentration with tranquilizing effects, different from conventional meditation, with physical health benefits. Patients with age-related disabilities had improved blood flow and increased musculoskeletal fitness (Reza, Urakami, and Mano 2001). Studies using electroencephalograms demonstrated that during salat, high amplitudes of alpha waves were generated, which are associated with a relaxation state and focus (Doufesh et al. 2012; Doufesh, Ibrahim, Ismail, and Ahmad 2014). Furthermore, Doufesh et al.'s (2014) study suggests that salat increases parasympathetic activity and decreases sympathetic activity; regular practice of salat promotes relaxation, reduces anxiety, and decreases the risk of cardiovascular disease.

FASTING

For 30 days during the month of Ramadan, Islam requires healthy adults to fast from the consumption of food and beverages from before dawn to after sunset. In addition, one fasts from gossip, negative thoughts, idle behavior, attachments, sex, and habits while gathering and concentrating all energies toward one's ultimate goal of self-knowledge, of cognizing one's true self. Specific Ramadan prayers are recited in the morning before the fast and in the evening before breaking the fast. In addition to Ramadan, students are encouraged to fast for three days each month. Fasting is considered a method of purification in which the individual (i.e., the seeker) abstains from all earthly urges and desires while gathering and concentrating all energies toward his or her ultimate purpose. This requires concentration. The precise meaning of concentration is discussed in a later section of this chapter.

There is steadily mounting evidence that fasting produces a wide range of very positive physical health benefits. Ramadan fasting has been shown to significantly reduce low-density lipoprotein (LDL) cholesterol concentration and elevate high-density lipoprotein (HDL) cholesterol concentration (Adlouni, Ghalim, Benslimane, Lecerf, and Saïle 1997; Qujeq, Bijani, Kalavi, Mohiti, and Aliakbarpour 2001; Ara, Jahan, Sultana, Choudhury, and Yeasmin 2016); to be effective in reducing the systolic and diastolic blood pressure (Salahuddin, Ashfak, Syed, and Badaam 2014); and to significantly reduce body fat (Saedeghi, Omar-Fauzee, Jahromi, Abdullah, and Rosli 2012; Salahuddin et al. 2014). Brandhorst et al. developed a fasting mimicking diet (FMD) program (two to five days per month) through which they found that fasters improved metabolism, immune, and cognitive functions; decreased inflammation, bone loss, and cancer; and extended longevity in mice. In humans, they found a reduction in multiple risk factors for diabetes, cardiovascular diseases, cancer, and aging (Brandhorst et al. 2015). Klempel, Kroeger, and Varady (2013) showed that an alternate day fasting (ADF) program results in a reduction of LDL cholesterol and triacylglycerol concentrations. Mattson, Longo, and Harvie (2016) observed that intermittent fasting improved age-related disorders (e.g., diabetes, cancer, and cardiovascular diseases) and neurological disorders (e.g., stroke and Alzheimer's and Parkinson's disease) in laboratory rats. They further note the similarity in how cell responses to exercise and to intermittent fasting both promote improved cognitive functions and brain-healthy lifestyles. Their findings are further explained from an evolutionary standpoint: Humans evolved in an environment where food was often scarce. Therefore, to obtain food, the brain was forced to function at its best when the individual was physically active and hungry.

ZIKR (REMEMBRANCE)

One of the defining practices of Islamic Sufism is *zikr*. The word *zikr* literally translates as "remembrance," specifically remembrance of the Divine Beloved, known as Existence or God. It is a Sufi chant, a song of love, to reunite each individual with his or her true self. It is a practice of harmony and unification. There are many different types of zikr, including *Sama*[3] (sacred movement). The most common zikr, practiced in weekly sessions, involves students sitting cross-legged on the ground with a straight back. They close their eyes, clear their minds from thoughts and desires, and focus on their heart. They melodically chant or sing a specific phrase or word, typically from a Sufi love poem or the name of the Beloved. As they sing, they move their bodies from left to right in the shape of an infinity sign (∞). This movement matches the pattern of the electromagnetic energy in the heart. Each person lightly taps his or her knees with the palms of the hands. This light tapping is like a metronome that keeps the pace, and activates the electromagnetic centers in the knees and palms. As everyone chants together, they sing and move in unison, with one voice, one movement. This creates one wave-like movement and creates harmony with the electromagnetic fields.

Zikr meditation has been shown to significantly lower subjective indices of anxiety and pain severity, and has been suggested for use in clinical practice as an intervention before and after abdominal surgery (Soliman and Mohamed 2013). The Istanbul Memorial Hospital's intensive care unit utilizes Sufi music and Sufi songs on cardiac patients prior to surgery (Barnell 2012). Although music is not a substitute for conventional treatment, the doctors (Erol Can and Bingür Sönmez) note that the approach lowers heart rate, as well as systolic and diastolic blood pressure, and improves oxygen delivery and oxygen saturation of the blood (Barnell 2012). Similar music therapies have been implemented by Janigro of the Cleveland Clinic (2010) for soothing neurosurgical patients during surgery. These findings suggest that music therapy may reduce patient anxiety, lowering blood pressure, and reducing the need for medication intake; these factors often result in quicker patient recovery and shorter hospital stays. A related study on choir groups has shown that during slow chanting, their respiration aligns, and then their heartbeats synchronize (Vickhoff et al. 2013). Grünhagen (2014) reported that during chanting, an increased occurrence of slow alpha brain waves was measured; these waves are linked to meditative and relaxed states. They further note that chanting also results in deeper breathing, increased oxygen intake, and increased levels of serotonin and endorphins, which create a joyful feeling. Chanting activates the parasympathetic nervous system; there is a reduction of stress hormones, strengthening of the immune system, lowering of blood pressure, and slowing of the heart rate. Grünhagen (2014) also reported that individuals who regularly sing are more resilient both emotionally and mentally.

Music therapy studies of rhythmic entrainment, which closely resembles rhythmic chanting, have shown it to have profound health benefits, such as improved cognitive, speech, and language rehabilitation; studies have also linked rhythmic music to brain rehabilitation (Thaut, McIntosh, and Hoemberg 2015; Schneider, Schönle, Altenmüller, and Münte 2007; Altenmüller, Marco-Pallares, Münte, and Schneider 2009; Grau-Sánchez et al. 2013). It has also been shown to reduce pain intensity and anxiety levels in intensive-care patients (Uyar and Korhan 2011) and decrease depression levels and systolic blood pressure in the elderly (Gök Ugur et al. 2016). Furthermore, in a study with pretest, posttest, and follow-up testing, music therapy reduced anger and psychological symptoms in an intervention group compared to a control (Sezer 2012). Rhythmic auditory stimulation has been shown to be effective to enhance gait training in patients who suffer from hemiparetic stroke (Thaut et al. 2007) and Parkinson's disease (Spaulding et al. 2013). Music therapy is also shown to be beneficial for motor-skills rehabilitation in children with cerebral palsy disease (Wang et al. 2013). Other potential benefits of music therapy are improvement of motor functioning in individuals with autism (Hardy and LaGasse 2013) and enhancement of cognitive functions in children (Miendlarzewska and Trost 2014).

TAMARKOZ®

Tamarkoz® is an experiential practice unique to the MTO Shahmagh-soudi® School of Islamic Sufism. The word *tamarkoz* in Farsi literally means concentration, but in Sufism more precisely means "concentration of abilities and energies." The precise methods of this practice include deep breathing, mind and body relaxation, Movazeneh® (meditative movements unique to this school of Sufism), visualization, energy activation, concentration, and heart meditation. These breathing and movement practices enable the individual to quiet the mind; let go of all attachments, labels, and boundaries imposed by society or one's self; and reach a state of deep concentration. This results in a healthier and a more balanced body, benefiting both physical and spiritual dimensions, and ultimately allowing the individual to tap into the power of the heart and discover his or her true identity. What differentiates this relaxation technique from other meditative traditions is the emphasis on heart concentration.[4]

Professor Angha (2000a, pp. 316–323) uses an analogy to illustrate these concepts. He teaches that the brain is a receiver similar to a radio. To facilitate thinking, the brain is tuned to receive and transmit certain wave frequencies (p. 316). The process of attuning the brain to new waves is mental concentration (p. 318). To concentrate on a subject, one needs to gather, to collect, to converge, to consolidate all relevant constituents of the subject as closely as possible (p. 323). In the context of the brain, he defines concentration as "dismissal of unrelated waves and subsequent immersion in those relevant to the subject" (p. 324). Examples of this can be found throughout history in sciences and arts. Creativity and theories seem to spring from nowhere when the recipient is focused. Just as Isaac Newton understood gravity from seeing an apple falling, the knowledge is present and all that is needed is a healthy receptor. Professor Angha (2011) further points out that the brain's limited receptivity can only be overcome through heart concentration, which is the true meaning of meditation (p. 335). Thus, it is recognized that "[t]he heart is the seat of knowledge in the teachings of Sufism. This is why meditation in the heart is so crucial and important" (Angha 2011, p. 121).

As to the deep breathing component, Professor Angha (2000a) stresses the importance of supplying the necessary amount of oxygen to the body. He explains that oxygen strengthens the immune system; it plays an essential role in disease control and improves the treatment of cancer and AIDS patients. He notes that normal breathing results in intake of only 0.5 liter of air—far below the 5-liter lung capacity of an average person; therefore, through deep breathing, an individual can substantially increase oxygen intake (pp. 137–139).

Health benefits of some forms of meditation are well-established in scientific research, including meditation to improve health, including deep breathing (Allen and Friedman 2012; Evers, Starr, and Starr 2007; Paul, Elam, and Verhulst 2007; Seaward 2009), guided visualization (Margolin, Pierce, and Wiley 2011; Newberg and Waldman 2010), movement balancing or movement meditation (Caldwell, Harrison, Adams, Quin, and Greeson 2010; Carmody and Baer 2008; Wolf et al. 1996; Yeh et al. 2004), and spirituality (Alexander, Robinson, Orme-Johnson, and Schneider 1994; Koenig 2012; McKinney and McKinney 1999; Wachholtz and Pargament 2005). In preliminary studies at the University of California, Berkeley (Bahadorani 2015, 2016a, 2016b, 2016c), Tamarkoz® (the Sufi experiential technique of deep breathing, and mind and body relaxation) was shown to significantly decrease perceived stress and heart rate, and significantly increase positive emotions and daily spiritual experiences in participants. The quasi-experimental 18-week design, with pretest, posttest, and follow-up, compared the deep breathing and relaxation group to a stress management resources group and a waitlist control group. Half of the participants in the deep breathing and relaxation group were atheists or agnostics, but had significant increases in daily spiritual experiences; thus, the technique is not limited to those who self-designate as religious or who declare a religious affiliation. This technique also seems to show some advantages over the usual stress management resources offered by a campus health center, as it provides a mechanism by which spirituality and positive emotions are increased even among individuals with no religious ideology (Bahadorani 2016a, 2016b, 2016c). A pilot study on the effects of Tamarkoz® involving heart patients at Kaiser Permanente Hospital (Crumpler 2005) demonstrated statistically significant decline in depression among participants. Additionally, reports from the cardiology department suggested reduced utilization of nursing services by participants in the study (Crumpler 2005). Another pilot study (in breast cancer patients) focused on effects of Tamarkoz®, including visualization, Movazaneh®, and breath awareness on the emotional state and DNA repair (Crumpler 2002). Increase in levels of emotional distress is noted to decrease the efficiency of DNA repair, which may influence the recurrence of a disease such as breast cancer. Results from this study (Crumpler 2002) indicated that greater involvement in these Sufi practices were correlated with lower levels of emotional distress and higher levels of emotional well-being. Participants who practiced longer periods of these relaxation techniques were also found to maintain highly functional DNA repair systems.

WEEKLY CLASSES/READINGS

Students of Islamic Sufism attend weekly classes at authorized centers, which are located throughout the world. The current Sufi Master lectures at these classes and the students experience zikr and prayer. Centers often offer other classes that complement the teachings. The sessions are broadcast to more than 500,000 students worldwide. Students are given homework and come prepared to actively engage in the sessions. In addition, students spend time reading the Holy Books (such as the Qur'an, Bible, and Torah) as well as books about Sufism, Islam, and the sciences. There have been many studies demonstrating the positive effects of Qur'anic readings. Mottaghi, Esmaili, and Rohani (2011) found that such reading decreases anxiety in athletes before competition. In addition, Rana and North (2007) found that rhythmic Qur'anic recitation significantly decreased depression levels in hospitalized patients.

The centers are operated by the local students under the supervision of the Sufi Master. Just as the teachings promote spiritual growth, the activities at the centers promote growth of the physical dimension as well. Students are encouraged to step out of their comfort zones in order to learn. For example, someone who may not know how to cook is put in charge of the kitchen. This causes individuals to push past their limitations and learn in order to complete the task. In addition, students work together on many tasks. Professor Angha has often described the act of working together as being like rocks along the shore. With each wave they rub against one another and smooth away the rough edges. This sense of cooperation and collaboration carries over into each student's personal life and is reflected in interactions with their environment and society.

KHIDMAT (SERVICE)

Charity work, volunteer work, and community service are considered important. The service not only helps the community, but also encourages humility within oneself, reduces the ego, and develops a sense of responsibility to help others. This altruism is not for the purpose of doing good deeds to be rewarded by God, or even to expect thanks in return. It is for the purpose of benefiting humanity, improving camaraderie, and bringing some measure of ease to the lives of people, as well as allowing each individual to grow and learn from the experience.

KHUMS (ALMS)

The act of giving of one's own wealth to help those in need or for good causes serves as part of a purification process to get rid of one's attachments to material things and to money. Of course, one should live the best life possible within one's means, but not become consumed with, addicted to, or attached to one's worldly possessions. Therefore, the practice of regularly giving of one's wealth to those who are in need is an important purification process to help one detach from the love of worldly possessions.

RETREATS

Every year, retreats are offered. Retreats are usually two to three days long. Retreats offer a joyful, friendly, and relaxing atmosphere, so one can simply let go of all everyday habits, worries, and constant distraction by the digital world. This opportunity allows one to nurture and revitalize both physical and spiritual dimensions and often results in a profound personal experience. To achieve these goals, retreats employ a wide array of activities, including theme-driven workshops, various relaxation techniques, zikr, creative projects, and outdoor activities, which are all focused to tap into the individual's inner being.

DIETARY RESTRICTIONS

The dietary restrictions in Islamic Sufism are abstaining from alcohol and pork, and are intended solely for the health of the individual, so he or she can function in balance and health. It is well known that during pregnancy, it is crucial for women to abstain from alcohol; otherwise the health of the fetus is put at risk (Virji 1991; Abel 1982; Hanson, Streissguth, and Smith 1978). It is also very well known that drinking can, and often does, harm one's health, including liver damage (Bellentani et al. 1997), DNA damage (Brooks 1997), weakened immune system (Cook 1998), and brain damage and dysfunction (Harper and Matsumoto 2005), to name a few. The negative effects of alcoholism also threaten the whole fabric of society and result in substantial economic burden (World Health Organization 2007). "Excessive alcohol use led to approximately 88,000 deaths and 2.5 million years of potential life lost (YPLL) each year in the United States from 2006–2010, shortening the lives of those who died by an average of 30 years" (Centers for Disease Control and Prevention 2016).

St. Augustine of Hippo (2011) stated: "By eating and drinking we restore the daily losses of the body . . . health is the reason for our eating and drinking . . . What is sufficient for health is not enough for pleasure" (pp. 214–215). Therefore, eating and drinking are a method for restoring the necessary nutrients to the body in order to maintain a healthy state that will assist the individual in reaching his or her goal. Muslims share the injunction against eating pork with Jews. The Bible (Leviticus

11:7–8, Isaiah 66:17, Deuteronomy 14:8) and the Qur'an (2:173, 5:3, 6:145, 16:115) make it very clear that pork should not be eaten. In Islam, a dietary restriction is designed to guide the individual to reach his or her optimal health state in order to fulfill his or her purpose. There is no compulsion; healthiness cannot be forced or enforced on anyone. The desire must arise from within. A true inner desire to achieve a goal reinforces the necessary lifestyle behavior, including dietary restrictions, to achieve it. As it is stated in the Holy Qur'an, "Let there be no compulsion in religion. Truth stands out clear from error" (2:256).

OTHER HEALTH BENEFITS AND POTENTIAL RISKS

Islamic religious moral beliefs have shown positive impacts on mental stability in adolescents (Pajević, Hasanović, and Delić 2007) and war veterans who experienced several war traumas (Hasanović and Pajević 2015) in Bosnia. Hasanović and Pajević (2010) also report that Islamic moral belief negatively correlates with the severity of tobacco and alcohol abuse.

As Islamic Sufism concentrates on the internal, not the external, world, Sufi spiritual practices may be less effective and perhaps stressful to those who are strongly extrinsically motivated. Being a student of Sufism is also risky for those who live in countries governed by Islamic radicals and fundamentalists. Both historically and today, Sufis have been the target of persecution due to their desire for an intimate, personal, and direct relationship with God. Some locations have banned the practice of zikr. Sufis have been tortured, jailed, and killed, and Islamic militants have destroyed Sufi shrines, mausoleums, and places of worship. The authors note that there are no known negative health outcomes associated with the practice of this worldview and heeding of its basic principles. However, problems may occur when people ignore the principles, the major one being the necessity of a teacher.

THE SUFI MASTER AND KNOWLEDGE

"Whoever travels without a guide needs two hundred years for a two days' journey."

—Rumi (Schimmel 2011, p. 103)

Islamic Sufism recognizes that a Sufi Master is needed to aid one in the perils of the spiritual journey, and is introduced through the heart. Islamic Sufism is learned through one's own guided experience, so having a legitimate teacher is essential. The Sufi Master has made the complete journey, so he can enlighten and guide others to find the way to the source of knowledge within. The Sufi Master guides the individual on the path to self-knowledge, and teaches that cognition can be obtained through self-discipline, purification, concentration, meditation, and prayer.

The succession of Masters within Sufism dates back to the time of the Holy Prophet of Islam (peace be upon him) and Oveys Gharani, who is the founding father of Islamic Sufism. Each Sufi Master appoints the next. As a result, the teachings of Islamic Sufism have never been left unattended or left to people's imaginations and interpretations.

Professor Angha uses the following example to illustrate the need for a teacher. He explains that a seed has all the knowledge that it needs to grow roots, branches, leaves, and bear fruit. There is nothing that the seed must do. However, for that seed to manifest its full potential, it must be planted in the proper soil, raised under suitable conditions, and tended by the hand of a caring and knowledgeable gardener. It is the gardener who knows the full potential of the seed and has the knowledge and ability to care for the seed until it becomes a tree and reaches its full growth. Thus, it is recognized that the Sufi Master brings joy, hope, stability, peace, and love to the lives of the students, which results in expansive creativity that has influenced literature, poetry, music, art, architecture, philosophy, medicine, and science. The Sufi Master teaches how to live a healthy, balanced life through self-knowledge and experiencing tranquility. Without a teacher, one can easily neglect the spiritual dimension and focus primarily on the physical, as that is the dimension individuals are most familiar with. As previously mentioned, this can lead to instability, disorder, and disease.

COMMONALITIES WITH OTHER FAITHS

"If the prophets—Buddha, Moses, Jesus, and Mohammad (peace be upon them)—were in one room, would they fight? The answer is obvious, of course not."

—Angha 2002a, pp. 13–14

Sufism is called "The Way of Love." All the major religious groups teach the importance of love, and from love flow the qualities of goodness, kindness, compassion, and other positive characteristics that religions teach, each in their own way. When one loves, warmth and tenderness permeate every cell. One's being is suffused with the radiance of a delicate energy. Boundaries, restrictions, barriers melt away like butter melting in the warm sun. Ego and egotism vanish. Anxieties and fears evaporate like fog burned away by sunshine, and one is filled with a quiet joy. Memories of the past fade away and expectations of the future dissolve. Everywhere one looks, beauty is seen, a reflection of what is within. Being right becomes irrelevant; being perfect becomes irrelevant; all else in existence becomes irrelevant. The chattering brain is quiet and still, and the heart opens like a blossoming flower. There is only the moment, only the Beloved . . . It is a state all wish to attain and to sustain. Call it bliss, call it ecstasy, call it whatever: all have tasted it, glimpsed it, hoped for it, yearned for it, and experienced it, however briefly.

All faiths have in common a desire to unite the finite human to the infinite. The faith practices, created in differing times and circumstances, were prescribed for that purpose. Now, centuries later, on the surface, these faiths may look very different, even though the purpose and goal is the same: to know God, Existence, "I," Brahman, Universe, Nirvana, or whatever term a particular religion uses for this end. Indeed, all faith practices encourage this union, and their views toward humanity—love and compassion for one's fellow humans—are also common ideologies. As Professor Angha has taught, "human beings have an innate need to know," and religion fills that need. Thus, at the core, religions may all be seen to be the same; they are different rivers attempting to reach the same sea.

Further, religions often engage in similar types of practices, such as prayers, fasting, attending religious classes, readings, service, alms, dietary restrictions, and so on, even though the specifics of these practices vary. For example, during Ramadan Muslims fast from food, drink, sex, and all extraneous thoughts and desires. For Yom Kippur, Jews fast from work, food, drink, sex, bathing/washing, anointing, and wearing leather shoes. Though Christian denominations fast differently during Lent, typically during Lent Christians fast from meat and/or individuals pick something that is habitual or important to them to give up. In Buddhism, again there are varying practices, but monks abstain from solid foods after noon. Thus, as can be seen from these examples of fasting, we may recognize that there is a central commonality among various faith groups even though the specific details of each practice may vary.

Islamic Sufism focuses on the internal processes (*tarighat*) of its faith practices to achieve unity with Existence (*haghighat*). For that reason, the students of Islamic Sufism are of varying faiths. In an instructional session, you can have a Muslim, Jew, and Christian all sitting next to each other. The practice of Islamic Sufism allows each seeker to practice their faith, wholly, and not just in the physical dimension, where it seems so varied. As Professor Angha teaches, Sufism is the reality of religion, and religion is the reality of each individual. As he further elaborates, "Sufism is the essence of the Prophets' teaching" (2011, p 19). It is a teaching to guide the never-ending quest, which begins and ends in the individual, to fulfill the seeker's inner desire, to know, to reunite the seeker with the beloved, to cognize and annihilate in the infinite tapestry of existence. Bayazid Bastami, the great ninth century Sufi, described the history of Sufism as follows: "Its seeds were set at the time of Adam, they sprouted under Noah and flowered under Abraham. Grapes formed at the time of Moses, and they ripened at the time of Jesus. In the time of Mohammad, they were made into pure wine" (Angha 2011, p. 20).

CONCLUSION

The practices of Islamic Sufism are designed to allow each individual to attain balance and equilibrium within his or her stable center. The purpose of all Sufi practices is concisely contained in the statement: "The divine message is heard on the horizons of equilibrium" (S. M. S. Angha 1986, p. 3). Any underdoing or overdoing in the broadest sense will inevitably result in imbalance and instability, which disturbs and hinders spiritual growth, and can cause physical illness if it exceeds the body's internal threshold. Professor Angha reminds his students that with everything they do, they must ask themselves: Am I developing my weakness or my health? Today's scientific inquiry most frequently examines only the benefits that religious practices bring to the physical body, while the role of faith practices in developing a stable and balanced human being is seen as secondary at best. Moreover, faith practices are often viewed either as a limited way to enhance existing medical treatments, or as a way to make medical procedures sensitive to the spiritual belief of patients (Koenig 1998, p. xxxi). Given the all-encompassing role of Sufi practices, scientific curiosity suggests that we should fundamentally rethink the role of religious principles in medicine.

When the person is spiritually and physically balanced and in harmony with all of existence, optimal health is experienced. From an Islamic Sufism perspective, this is the human being presenting as a comprehensive whole. The person has shed the embellishments that have been gathered from the world, the deficiencies that stem from desires and temporary wants, and the veil of self-image. Only then is the true identity of each person known, which is the rightful dignity of each human being. Thus, as Professor Angha teaches, "[a] prosperous human society is attained through the outward and inward harmony of each of its members, and their harmonious existence in a unified system" (1987, p. 59).

NOTES

1. Though Sufism is not separate from Islam, "conservative" Muslims have not always been accepting of the practices of Islamic Sufism.

2. Hereafter in this chapter, we use the title "Professor Angha" when referring to His Holiness Salaheddin Ali Nader Angha.

3. More information about *Sama* can be found at http://www.zendehdelan.org/.

4. To gain a deeper understanding of brain, mind, and concentration, one can study the detailed and comprehensive scientific framework developed by Professor Angha (2000a) in his book, *Expansion and Contraction Within Being (Dahm)*.

REFERENCES

Abel, E. L. 1982. "Consumption of Alcohol during Pregnancy: A Review of Effects on Growth and Development of Offspring." *Human Biology* 54(3): 421–453.

Adlouni, A., N. Ghalim, A. Benslimane, J. M. Lecerf, and R. Saïle. 1997. "Fasting during Ramadan Induces a Marked Increase in High-Density Lipoprotein Cholesterol and Decrease in Low-Density Lipoprotein Cholesterol." *Annals of Nutrition and Metabolism* 41(4): 242–249.

Alexander, C. N., P. Robinson, D. W. Orme-Johnson, and R. H. Schneider. 1994. "The Effects of Transcendental Meditation Compared to Other Methods of Relaxation and Meditation in Reducing Risk Factors, Morbidity, and Mortality." *Homeostasis in Health and Disease* 35: 243–263.

Allen, B., and B. H. Friedman. 2012. "Positive Emotion Reduces Dyspnea during Slow Paced Breathing." *Psychophysiology* 49(5): 690–696.

Altenmüller, E., J. Marco-Pallares, T. F. Münte, and S. Schneider. 2009. "Neural Reorganization Underlies Improvement in Stroke-Induced Motor Dysfunction by Music-Supported Therapy." *Annals of the New York Academy of Sciences* 1169(1): 395–405.

Angha, S. A. N. 1987. *Peace*. Verdugo City, CA: M.T.O. Shahmaghsoudi® Publications.

Angha, S. A. N. 2000a. *Expansion and Contraction Within Being (Dahm)*. Riverside, CA: M.T.O. Shahmaghsoudi® Printing and Publication Center.

Angha, S. A. N. 2000b. *Sufism: The Reality of Religion*. Riverside, CA: M.T.O. Shahmaghsoudi® Publications.

Angha, S. A. N. 2002a. *Sufism: A Bridge Between Religions*. Riverside, CA: M.T.O. Shahmaghsoudi® Publications.

Angha, S. A. N. 2002b. *Theory "I": The Unlimited Vision . . . of Leadership*. Riverside, CA: M.T.O. Shahmaghsoudi® Printing & Publication Center.

Angha, S. A. N. 2003. *Sufism and Faith*. Martinez, CA: M.T.O. Shahmaghsoudi® Publications.

Angha, S. A. N. 2011. *Sufism Lecture Series*. Great Britain: M.T.O. Publications®.

Angha, S. M. S. 1986. *The Mystery of Humanity*. Lanham, MD: University Press of America.

Angha, S. M. S. 1998. *Al-Salat: The Reality of Prayer in Islam*. Riverside, CA: M.T.O. Shahmaghsoudi® Publications.

Angha, S. M. S. 1999. *Dawn*. Riverside, CA: M.T.O. Shahmaghsoudi® Publications.

Ara, T., N. Jahan, N. Sultana, R. Choudhury, and T. Yeasmin. 2016. "Effect of Ramadan Fasting on Total Cholesterol (TC) Low Density Lipoprotein

Cholesterol (LDL-C) and High Density Lipoprotein Cholesterol (HDL-C) in Healthy Adult Males." *Journal of Bangladesh Society of Physiologists* 10(2): 46–50.

Augustine of Hippo. 2011. *Confessions.* Peabody, MA: Hendrickson Publishers.

Bahadorani, N. 2015. "Implications of a Sufi Meditation on Reducing Stress, Increasing Positive Emotions and Increasing Spirituality for University Students." Presentation at the143rd Annual American Public Health Association Meeting and Convention, Chicago, IL, October 31-November 4.

Bahadorani, N. 2016a. "Implications of Tamarkoz® on Reducing Stress, Increasing Positive Emotions and Increasing Spirituality for University Students." Presentation at the American Psychology Association Division 36 Mid-Year Conference, Brooklyn, NY, March 11–12.

Bahadorani, N. 2016b. "Implications of Tamarkoz® on Reducing Stress, Increasing Positive Emotions and Increasing Spirituality for University Students." Poster presentation at the Division 36 Hospitality Suites at the American Psychology Association Convention in Denver, CO, August 4.

Bahadorani, N. 2016c. "Implications of Tamarkoz® on Reducing Stress for University Students." Presentation at the International Congress of Behavioral Medicine, Melbourne, Australia, December 7–11.

Bai, R., P. Ye, C. Zhu, W. Zhao, and J. Zhang. 2012. "Effect of *Salat* Prayer and Exercise on Cognitive Functioning of Hui Muslims Aged Sixty and Over." *Social Behavior and Personality: An International Journal* 40(10): 1739–1747.

Barnell, R. 2012. *Neonatal Nightingales: Live Parental and Neonatal Nurse Infant-Directed Singing as a Beneficial Intervention for the Health and Development of Infants in Neonatal Care.* (Unpublished master's thesis). University of Wolverhampton, UK.

Bellentani, S., G. Saccoccio, G. Costa, C. Tiribelli, F. Manenti, M. Sodde, . . . G. Brandi. 1997. "Drinking Habits as Cofactors of Risk for Alcohol Induced Liver Damage." *Gut* 41(6): 845–850.

Brandhorst, S., I. Y. Choi, M. Wei, C. W. Cheng, S. Sedrakyan, G. Navarrete, . . . S. Di Biase. 2015. "A Periodic Diet that Mimics Fasting Promotes Multi-System Regeneration, Enhanced Cognitive Performance, and Healthspan." *Cell Metabolism* 22(1): 86–99.

Brooks, P. J. 1997. "DNA Damage, DNA Repair, and Alcohol Toxicity: A Review." *Alcoholism: Clinical and Experimental Research* 21(6): 1073–1082.

Caldwell, K., M. Harrison, M. Adams, R. H. Quin, and J. Greeson. 2010. "Developing Mindfulness in College Students through Movement-Based Courses: Effects on Self-Regulatory Self-Efficacy, Mood, Stress, and Sleep Quality." *Journal of American College Health* 58(5): 433–442.

Carmody, J., and R. A. Baer. 2008. "Relationships between Mindfulness Practice and Levels of Mindfulness, Medical and Psychological Symptoms and Well-Being in a Mindfulness-Based Stress Reduction Program." *Journal of Behavioral Medicine* 31(1): 23–33.

Centers for Disease Control and Prevention. 2016, July. "Fact Sheets: Alcohol Use and Your Health." Retrieved from https://www.cdc.gov/alcohol/fact-sheets /alcohol-use.htm

Cleveland Clinic. 2010. "Cleveland Clinic Neurological Institute Annual Report 2010." Retrieved from https://my.clevelandclinic.org/ccf/media/files/Neuro logical_Institute/Neurological-Institute-2010-Year-In-Review.pdf

Cook, R. T. 1998. "Alcohol Abuse, Alcoholism, and Damage to the Immune System: A Review." *Alcoholism: Clinical and Experimental Research* 22(9): 1927–1942.

Crumpler, C. 2002. "Sufi Practices, Emotional State, and DNA Repair: Implications for Breast Cancer." *Science of the Soul* 4(1), 25–37.

Crumpler, C. 2005. "Tamarkoz (Sufi Meditation) for Heart Patients: A Pilot Study." *Sufi Psychology Journal: Science of the Soul* 7(1): 9–10.

Doufesh, H., T. Faisal, K.-S. Lim, and F. Ibrahim. 2012. "EEG Spectral Analysis on Muslim Prayers." *Applied Psychophysiology and Biofeedback* 37(1): 11–18.

Doufesh, H., F. Ibrahim, N. A. Ismail, and W. A. W. Ahmad. 2014. "Effect of Muslim Prayer (*Salat*) on α Electroencephalography and Its Relationship with Autonomic Nervous System Activity." *Journal of Alternative and Complementary Medicine* 20(7): 558–562.

Evers, C., C. Starr, and L. Starr. 2007. *Biology Today and Tomorrow with Physiology* (2nd ed.). Belmont, CA: Thomson Brooks/Cole.

Gerrig, R. J., and P. G. Zimbardo. 2002. "Glossary of Psychological Terms." In *Psychology and Life* (16th ed.). Boston: Allyn & Bacon. Retrieved from http:// www.apa.org/research/action/glossary.aspx

Gök Ugur, H., Y. Y. Aktaş, O. S. Orak, O. Saglambilen, and İ. A. Avci. 2016, September 3. "The Effect of Music Therapy on Depression and Physiological Parameters in Elderly People Living in a Turkish Nursing Home: A Randomized-Controlled Trial." *Aging & Mental Health*: 1–7. http://dx.doi.org /10.1080/13607863.2016.1222348

Grau-Sánchez, J., J. L. Amengual, N. Rojo, M. V. de las Heras, J. Montero, F. Rubio, . . . A. Rodríguez-Fornells. 2013. "Plasticity in the Sensorimotor Cortex Induced by Music-Supported Therapy in Stroke Patients: A TMS Study." *Frontiers in Human Neuroscience* 7: 494.

Grünhagen, C. 2014. "Healing Chants and Singing Hospitals: Towards an Analysis of the Implementation of Spiritual Practices as Therapeutic Means." *Scripta Instituti Donneriani Aboensis* 24: 76–88.

Hanson, J. W., A. P. Streissguth, and D. W. Smith. 1987. "The Effects of Moderate Alcohol Consumption during Pregnancy on Fetal Growth and Morphogenesis." *Journal of Pediatrics* 92(3): 457–460.

Hardy, M. W., and A. B. LaGasse. 2013. "Rhythm, Movement, and Autism: Using Rhythmic Rehabilitation Research as a Model for Autism." *Frontiers in Integrative Neuroscience* 7: 19. doi.org/10.3389/fnint.2013.00019

Harper, C., and I. Matsumoto. 2005. "Ethanol and Brain Damage." *Current Opinion in Pharmacology* 5(1): 73–78.

Hasanović, M., and I. Pajević. 2010. "Religious Moral Beliefs as Mental Health Protective Factor of War Veterans Suffering from PTSD, Depressiveness, Anxiety, Tobacco and Alcohol Abuse in Comorbidity." *Psychiatria Danubina* 22 (2): 203–210.

Hasanović, M., and I. Pajević. 2015. "Religious Moral Beliefs Inversely Related to Trauma Experiences Severity and Presented Posttraumatic Stress Disorder among Bosnia and Herzegovina War Veterans." *Journal of Religion and Health* 54(4): 1403–1415.

Henry, H. M. 2015. "Spiritual Energy of Islamic Prayers as a Catalyst for Psychotherapy." *Journal of Religion and Health* 54(2): 387–398.

Hooker, S. A., K. S. Masters, and K. B. Carey. 2014. "Multidimensional Assessment of Religiousness/Spirituality and Health Behaviors in College Students." *International Journal for the Psychology of Religion* 24(3): 228–240.

Klempel, M. C., C. M. Kroeger, and K. A. Varady. 2013. "Alternate Day Fasting (ADF) with a High-Fat Diet Produces Similar Weight Loss and Cardio-Protection as ADF with a Low-Fat Diet." *Metabolism* 62(1): 137–143.

Koenig, H. G. 2003. "Health Care and Faith Communities." *Journal of General Internal Medicine* 18(11): 962–963.

Koenig, H. G., ed. 1998. *Handbook of religion and mental health*. Amsterdam: Elsevier.

Koenig, H. G. 2012. "Religion, Spirituality, and Health: The Research and Clinical Implications [review article]." *ISRN Psychiatry* (2012), Article ID 278730. doi:10.5402/2012/278730

Margolin, I., J. Pierce, and A. Wiley. 2011. "Wellness through a Creative Lens: Meditation and Visualization." *Journal of Religion & Spirituality in Social Work: Social Thought* 30(3): 234–252.

Mattson, M. P., V. D. Longo, and M. Harvie. 2016. "Impact of Intermittent Fasting on Health and Disease Processes." *Ageing Research Reviews* 31: S1568–1637.

McKinney, J. P., and K. G. McKinney. 1999. "Prayer in the Lives of Late Adolescents." *Journal of Adolescence* 22(2): 279–290.

Miendlarzewska, E. A., and W. J. Trost. 2014. "How Musical Training Affects Cognitive Development: Rhythm, Reward and Other Modulating Variables." *Frontiers in Neuroscience* 7: 279. doi:10.3389/fnins.2013.00279

Mottaghi, M. E., R. Esmaili, and Z. Rohani. 2011. "Effect of Quran Recitation on the Level of Anxiety in Athletics." *Quran and Medicine* 2011(1 Summer [Eng.]): 1–4.

Newberg, A., and M. R. Waldman. 2010. *How God Changes Your Brain: Breakthrough Findings from a Leading Neuroscientist*. New York: Ballantine Books.

Pajević, I., M. Hasanović, and A. Delić. 2007. "The Influence of Religious Moral Beliefs on Adolescents' Mental Stability." *Psychiatria Danubina* 19(3): 173–183.

Paul, G., B. Elam, and S. J. Verhulst. 2007. "A Longitudinal Study of Students' Perceptions of Using Deep Breathing Meditation to Reduce Testing Stresses." *Teaching and Learning in Medicine* 19(3): 287–292.

Pearsall, P., G. E. R. Schwartz, and L. G. S. Russek. 2000. "Changes in Heart Transplant Recipients that Parallel the Personalities of Their Donors." *Integrative Medicine* 2(2): 65–72.

Qujeq, D., K. Bijani, K. Kalavi, J. Mohiti, and H. Aliakbarpour. 2001. "Effects of Ramadan Fasting on Serum Low-Density and High-Density Lipoprotein-Cholesterol Concentrations." *Annals of Saudi Medicine* 22(5–6): 297–299.

Rana, S. A. and A. C. North. 2007. "The Effect of Rhythmic Quranic Recitation on Depression." *Journal of Behavioural Sciences* 17(1–2): 37.

Reza, M. F., Y. Urakami, and Y. Mano. 2001. "Evaluation of a New Physical Exercise Taken from *Salat* (Prayer) as a Short-Duration and Frequent Physical Activity in the Rehabilitation of Geriatric and Disabled Patients." *Annals of Saudi Medicine* 22(3–4): 177–180.

Saedeghi, H., M. S. Omar-Fauzee, M. K. Jahromi, M. N. Abdullah, and M. H. Rosli. 2012. "The Effects of Ramadan Fasting on the Body Fat Percent among Adults." *Annals of Biological Research* 3: 3958–3961.

Salahuddin, M., A. S. Ashfak, S. Syed, and K. Badaam. 2014. "Effect of Ramadan Fasting on Body Weight, Blood Pressure (BP), and Biochemical Parameters in Middle Aged Hypertensive Subjects: An Observational Trial." Journal of Clinical and Diagnostic Research 8(3): 16–18.

Sayeed, S. A., and A. Prakash. 2013. "The Islamic Prayer (Salah/Namaaz) and Yoga Togetherness in Mental Health." *Indian Journal of Psychiatry* 55(Suppl. 2): S224.

Schimmel, A. 2011. *Mystical Dimensions of Islam* (2nd ed.). Chapel Hill: University of North Carolina Press.

Schneider, S., P. W. Schönle, E. Altenmüller, and T. F. Münte. 2007. "Using Musical Instruments to Improve Motor Skill Recovery Following a Stroke." *Journal of Neurology* 254(10): 1339–1346.

Seaward, B. L. 2009. *Managing Stress: Principles and Strategies for Health and Well-Being*. Boston: Jones & Bartlett.

Sezer, F. 2012. "The Psychological Impact of Ney Music." *The Arts in Psychotherapy* 39(5): 423–427.

Soliman, H., and S. Mohamed. 2013. "Effects of *Zikr* Meditation and Jaw Relaxation on Postoperative Pain, Anxiety and Physiologic Response of Patients Undergoing Abdominal Surgery." *Journal of Biology, Agriculture and Healthcare* 3(2): 23–38.

Spaulding, S. J., B. Barber, M. Colby, B. Cormack, T. Mick, and M. E. Jenkins. 2013. "Cueing and Gait Improvement among People with Parkinson's Disease: A Meta-analysis." *Archives of Physical Medicine and Rehabilitation* 94(3): 562–570.

Thaut, M. H., A. K. Leins, R. R. Rice, H. Argstatter, G. P. Kenyon, G. C. McIntosh, ... M. Fetter. 2007. "Rhythmic Auditory Stimulation Improves Gait More than

NDT/Bobath Training in Near-Ambulatory Patients Early Poststroke: A Single-Blind, Randomized Trial." *Neurorehabilitation and Neural Repair* 21(5): 455–459.

Thaut, M. H., G. C. McIntosh, and V. Hoemberg. 2015. "Neurobiological Foundations of Neurologic Music Therapy: Rhythmic Entrainment and the Motor System." *Frontiers in Psychology* 5: 1185. doi.org/10.3389/fpsyg.2014.01185

Uyar, M., and E. A. Korhan. 2011. "Yogun bakim hastalarinda muzik terapinin agri ve anksiyete uzerine etkisi [The Effect of Music Therapy on Pain and Anxiety in Intensive Care Patients]." *Agri: The Journal of The Turkish Society of Algology* 23(4): 139–147.

Vanderbilt Health. n.d. "The Transplanted Heart." Retrieved from https://www.vanderbilthealth.com/transplant/11399

Vickhoff, B., H. Malmgren, R. Åström, G. Nyberg, S.-R. Ekström, M. Engwall, . . . R. Jörnsten. 2013. "Music Structure Determines Heart Rate Variability of Singers." *Frontiers in Psychology* 4: 334.

Virji, S. K. 1991. "The Relationship between Alcohol Consumption during Pregnancy and Infant Birthweight: An Epidemiologic Study." *Acta Obstetricia et Gynecologica Scandinavica* 70(4–5): 303–308.

Wachholtz, A. B., and K. I. Pargament. 2005. "Is Spirituality a Critical Ingredient of Meditation? Comparing the Effects of Spiritual Meditation, Secular Meditation, and Relaxation on Spiritual, Psychological, Cardiac, and Pain Outcomes." *Journal of Behavioral Medicine* 28(4): 369–384.

Wang, T.-H., Y.-C. Peng, Y.-L. Chen, T.-W. Lu, H.-F. Liao, P.-F. Tang, and J.-Y. Shieh. 2013. "A Home-Based Program Using Patterned Sensory Enhancement Improves Resistance Exercise Effects for Children with Cerebral Palsy: A Randomized Controlled Trial." *Neurorehabilitation and Neural Repair* 27(8): 684–694.

Wolf, S. L., H. X. Barnhart, N. G. Kutner, E. McNeely, C. Coogler, and T. Xu. 1996. "Reducing Frailty and Falls in Older Persons: An Investigation of Tai Chi and Computerized Balance Training." *Journal of the American Geriatrics Society* 44(5): 489–497.

World Health Organization (WHO), Expert Committee on Problems Related to Alcohol Consumption. 2007. "WHO Expert Committee on Problems Related to Alcohol Consumption. Second Report." *World Health Organization Technical Report Series* 944: 1.

Yeh, G. Y., M. J. Wood, B. H. Lorell, L. W. Stevenson, D. M. Eisenberg, P. M. Wayne, . . . R. B. Davis. 2004. "Effects of Tai Chi Mind-Body Movement Therapy on Functional Status and Exercise Capacity in Patients with Chronic Heart Failure: A Randomized Controlled Trial." *American Journal of Medicine* 117(8): 541–548.

Chapter 10

Lesser Known Spiritualities: Bahá'í', Rastafari, and Zoroastrianism

*Holly Nelson-Becker, Leanne Atwell,
and Shannan Russo*

This chapter discusses three lesser known, and thus less well understood, faith traditions that have distinct but significant views on health and health practices. Each section addresses brief historical elements and core beliefs, discusses beliefs that affect preferred health practices, and identifies the limited research available related to the particular faith. Although these spiritualities may be less well-known, each has had major influence on sizeable groups of people, some residing in particular geographic places and some worldwide. Their views on the interrelationships of faith and healing are consistent with the origins of Hippocratic medicine that adhered to worship of the Greek god of medicine, Asclepius (Nelson-Becker 2017). Fundamentally, these spiritualities are presented for the benefit of those who wish to understand what clinical interventions might enhance, and also what might impair, medical treatment with and for believers of these groups.

BAHÁ'Í'

History and Practice of the Faith

The Bahá'í' faith emerged in 1860 out of the earlier Babi movement of 1840. The latter arose in a context that was somewhat isolated in contrast to the Bahá'í' faith, which benefited from the more cosmopolitan environment of Iran during that period (McMullen 2015; Smith 2008). Iran was a monarchy with local governors, landowners, and nomadic tribes, all of whom held power. Traditional Islamic religious leaders—mostly Shia in Iran—were also influential in the developing Bahá'í' faith. However, other branches of Islam such as Sufis, Christian and Jewish minorities, and Zoroastrians were accepted in Iran. The origin of the Bahá'í faith was influenced by the religious and cultural context of Iranian Shi'a Islam.

Babi Movement   The Babi movement was founded on a local holy man, Siyyid 'Alí Muhammad (1819–1850), also known as the *Báb* (meaning gate or door in Arabic), who presented revelatory writings in the style of the Qur'an that secured his claim to authority as the Mahdi (the rightful ruler, similar to a messiah) and summoned all human beings to believe (Smith 2008; Stockman 1985). Similar to the Shi'a Islamic religion, the followers of the Báb believed in divine guidance and return of a messiah. Unsurprisingly, clerics of the time saw this movement as heretical. The Báb wrote more than 20 major works, including prayers, homilies, and letters (Smith 2008). His revelatory verses were viewed as proof of his divinity. The movement expanded rapidly. Accused of insurrection due to the unyielding declaration of their mission, they likely fought for their beliefs, but only defensively (Mihrshahi 2015). In a culture that glorified martyrdom, the Báb and thousands of followers were executed, leading to near-annihilation of the movement (Mihrshahi 2015). One of the remaining leaders, who also was imprisoned himself for many years, was Mírzá Husayn-'Alí, who had the religious title of *Bahá*. He later became known as *Bahá'u'lláh* ("Glory of God" in Arabic), and founded the Bahá'í' religion.

Bahá'u'lláh, Founder of the Faith   Bahá'í' members follow the teaching of Bahá'u'lláh, who lived from 1817 to 1892. An Iranian of noble birth, Bahá lived much of his life exiled in the Ottoman Empire. He declared himself God's messenger—the one foretold by the Báb—in 1863 (Smith 2008). He had gained approval as a practical organizer and then a religious leader. For a time he lived as a religious hermit, but returned after two years to provide direction to the Báb movement, writing with spiritual authority. When he professed to be the messianic savior expected by many religions, he was largely accepted by the Bábís. He determined that both Islamic law and mysticism carried moral weight, and that following the law alone would not lead to religiousness. He called on humanity to unite and establish a millennial peace promised by all religious faiths. Bahá'u'lláh faced harsh persecution by the Ottomans, Persian clergy, and the Islamic government. He spent much of his time in prison or in exile and died near Akka in Israel. With a strong leaning toward interfaith acceptance, Bahá'í's today regard major world religions as expressing aspects of the same truth. This open religious stance, a fundamental aspect of the faith, is all but unique among religions.

Bahá'u'lláh is seen as the most recent in a line of messengers of God referred to as "Manifestations of God"; this includes the founders of major world religions such as Zoroaster, Buddha, Moses, Jesus, and Mohammed. These leaders guide humanity in a progressive evolutionary path that will ultimately lead to a peaceful and prosperous world community. Following Bahá'u'lláh's teachings will result in this community of peace. Even under persecution, Bahá'u'lláh' wrote and left a range of several hundred pages of various kinds of writings. These texts, together with writings of the Báb, constitute Bahá'í sacred texts, and are considered the revealed word of God (Mihrshahi 2015). Through instructions left in his will, Bahá'u'lláh appointed his oldest son, Abdu'l Bahá (Servant of the Glory) to be his successor. Abdu'l Bahá served in his capacity as world leader of the faith until his death in 1921. The movement was then led by his grandson, Shoghi Effendi, who was named Guardian of the Bahá'í faith from 1921 until he died in 1957. This orderly succession must have helped retain stability for this faith. Further establishing validity, both Abdu'l Bahá and Shoghi Effendi were authorized as interpreters of the faith through the writings of their predecessors.

There are no professional clergy in the Bahá'í faith. However, following the writings of Bahá'u'lláh and Abdu'l Bahá, democratically elected administrators form the Spiritual Assemblies locally and nationally. On an international level, the Universal House of Justice is the administrative body. A concern mentioned by several writers is that women are not yet allowed to serve in this group (MacEoin 2013; Sergeev and Swidler 2015; Smith 2008).

Bahá'í's refer to the sharing of their faith as *teaching* rather than missionary work (Mihrshahi 2015). Traveling to teach others about the faith is referred to as *pioneering*. Teaching the Bahá'í faith is done by either direct or indirect teaching. Direct teaching includes assuring the fundamental truths of the Cause; indirect teaching is usually focused on the principles of the faith rather than the person of Bahá'u'lláh (McMullen 2015). Teaching the faith is considered a duty, the most meritorious of deeds, and a source of blessings (McMullen 2015). However, independent investigation of beliefs is primary and coercion of any kind is discouraged. Believers are exhorted to behave kindly toward all. Teaching has the potential to turn people towards God and is viewed as a sacred act. Teachers are cautioned to act in accord with their beliefs, to be humble, and not to worry about their faults or inadequacies. Teaching is viewed as a means of spiritual growth and of serving God and humanity.

The Bahá'í believe that divine revelation occurs every 500 to 1,000 years through manifestations of God to reaffirm eternal truths in world religions as well as provide guidance for societal needs at a given time (Smith 2008). The philosophies of major world religions are viewed as being in agreement rather than divergent or incompatible; Bahá'í interpretations seek to reconcile or harmonize world religion beliefs. Shoghi Effendi, the third leader of the faith, anticipated that the faith would grow through diffusion, penetration, and suffusion, increasing levels of development as more individuals were exposed to it (MacEoin 2013). In the 1960s, the Bahá'í faith was established in nearly every nation, and the goal of diffusion was largely completed. Current growth demonstrates penetration; suffusion will have been fulfilled when the Bahá'í religion is accepted by all peoples. Rather than assimilation, the goal is to celebrate diversity, leading to universal participation and a world civilization founded on principles of social justice.

Core Beliefs

Bahá'í members take an expansive approach to their faith that has implications for greater interreligious understanding. They believe that science and religion have many points of compatibility (International Teaching Centre 2011). They believe in one universal God and the essential unity of religions as well as of humanity. Prejudice should be relinquished, men and women are equal in worth, universal education should be available, and extreme poverty as well as extreme wealth should be eradicated. They also support the individual's search for truth: the "independent investigation of truth" as discussed earlier (International Teaching Centre 2011; Maloney 2006). The goal is to establish a spiritually wealthy world order that unites all humanity. In this model, no one is left out, and peace is the outcome. Beliefs of Bahá'í followers can be characterized as the oneness of God—where God is beyond understanding, the oneness of religions—where all religions are different expressions of unfolding understanding appropriate to their time and location, and the oneness of humanity (Kourosh and Hosada 2007). The oneness of humanity suggests that people are first world citizens and secondly, members of their nation, tribe, or cultural group.

A fundamental concept in the Bahá'í faith is that revealed divine knowledge was limited only by the capacity of people to understand at the time, not by the capacity of the prophet. Interracial and intercultural marriages are common and supported by the faith (Jenkins 2003). The ideals of the Bahá'í faith are aligned with those of many international organizations, such as the United Nations. Service to humanity is a primary goal and so believers support many grassroots efforts to achieve social and economic development.

Recent Growth

By 1963, the number of national Spiritual Assemblies had increased from 12 to 56 and the first Universal House of Justice was established. The House of Justice had been envisioned by Bahá'u'lláh and was the supreme global institution for the faith. Although the faith was largely constituted of Iranian members in the 1950s, by 1988 the numbers of adherents from other parts of the world was about 94% (Smith and Momen 1988). Because there had been rapid expansion in Third World countries, there was a need for greater understanding of the faith beyond initial conversion. The challenge was to build capacity of believers rather than ask them to rely on current teachers alone. Effective service is built on attitudes, spiritual qualities, and intellectual capacity. Teaching is refined through the interrelated processes of acting, reflecting, and consulting with others (International Teaching Centre 2011).

The Bahá'í faith has grown and established itself in nearly every country. There are about 5 to 7 million adherents globally (Mihrshahi 2015). However, the Bahá'í's themselves do not keep statistics on numbers of adherents, and many people follow Bahá'í teachings who may never have formally joined the religion. The geographic diversity makes estimates uncertain. The Association for Religion Data Archives suggest that there were about 7.3 million followers in 2010 (Bahai Teachings.org).

Beliefs and Practices That Influence Health-Related Behaviors

Holistic Health Philosophy   Consistent with belief in the compatibility between science and religion, Bahá'í's also believe in the value of seeking medical treatment. The entire accumulated body of scientific knowledge should be used as a guide to treatment of disease. The power of the intellect is one of God's greatest gifts to people (Smith 2008). "Resort ye, in times of sickness, to competent physicians" (The Kitáb-i-Aqdas [*Book of Laws*], available at http://www.bahai.org/bahaullah/articles-resources/from-kitab-i-aqdas). The advice of physicians should be heeded and they should heal in the name of God. "Whatever competent physicians or surgeons prescribe for a patient should be accepted" and followed (Bahá'u'lláh, from a tablet translated from the Persian). It is important for people to recognize that healing is in God's domain, but they are still encouraged to seek opinions from physicians. However, individuals should also not overtreat their illnesses, halting treatment when health is restored and not using a compound treatment when one herb or medicine may be enough. Diet is the preferred treatment approach (Esslemont 2006, p. 106). However, the healing of the body is secondary to the healing of the spirit. Thus, if the body is healed and the spirit continues to suffer, then the healing is not complete.

Illness may be healed through either physical or spiritual means. The physician will assist in healing the body, while those who are spiritual may heal through prayer. Each type of condition has its own province; for instance, fear and anxiety are more likely to be healed through spiritual treatment. Both types of healing are important and they do not contradict each other. However, the deep remedy for every ailment is to be found in the teaching of God. The purpose of health is to serve the Kingdom of God rather than to engage in sensual or evil everyday pursuits. The spirit is in a state which can neither be directly affected by illness nor directly cured. Although the spirit is viewed as separate, stronger than the body, and eternal, ill health may compromise the spirit and cause it to be diminished. The best method for healing is through an integrated approach of healing body and spirit. Spiritual healing alone is not a substitute for physical healing (Research Department of the Universal House of Justice 1990, letter written on behalf of Shoghi Effendi, 12 March 1934). However, physical healing will only endure if it is aligned with and reinforced by spiritual healing.

Physicians should be aware that when they undertake physical healing, they also have some capacity to influence spiritual healing. They should understand that the condition of the spirit influences the body, so in sharing joy and comfort, people may return to health more quickly. Ill health is not completely preventable; good health is a gift. Physicians, when they bring their hearts to the encounter with patients, are more likely to achieve healing. Their work, which is also their service, is a form of praise.

The soul is above and functions apart from all illnesses related to the body or the mind. There is recognition that illness is distracting and prevents one from sharing one's inherent light and power. "Bahá'í's also believe in the integration of the body and spirit, so both require treatment" (Kourosh and Hosada 2007, p. 446). "When the material world and the divine world are well co-related . . . this power [shall] produce a perfect manifestation. Physical and spiritual diseases will then receive absolute healing" (Zohoori 1985, p. 3). Ultimately, although patients and their physicians will do their best to comply with and provide protocols for healing, the ultimate outcome is not in the hands of people but rather God. Although the idea of miracles is accepted, magical or folk worldviews are not.

Healing Acts   The Bahá'í' members are encouraged to do healing work, but are cautioned against calling themselves healers. They are advised in this manner to avoid confusion with how this term is used by other religious groups. Healing is understood differently by various faith traditions, such as those who are Christian Science. Instead, adherents of the faith are to consider themselves both members of the Bahá'í' faith and also healers, which are two distinct but related roles.

Prayer as Health Practice   Members are asked to recite an obligatory prayer each day. Saying a prayer is powerful enough to make a space sacred in this low-ritual religion. Members should read from scriptures of the faith each morning and evening. Although the best medical treatment known may be sought, prayer is a support to medical treatment for illness. Remembering God can lead to healing of all ills. It is also important to know, however, that in some cases, healing of one illness might lead to other ailments, so not everything may be healed through prayer. By means of the holy spirit, good people who pray with desire can bring about healing in other places, even when they do not know the person who is ill. When a member is dying, the practice may continue and should be respected. Family members may also have a need to pray with the dying person.

Nutritional Beliefs   Nutritional and lifestyle choices are considered the optimal way of coping with illness, especially for the future (Smith 2008; Zohoori 1985). Food should be taken in moderation and should be of good quality. Although meat is not proscribed and is sometimes required for restoration of health, vegetarian diets (cereal and fruit) are preferred over meat. Augmenting or eliminating certain components of diet, when skillfully done, can lead to a return to health. Achieving equilibrium through diet is the preferred approach to healing. If done on a population level, the presence of certain chronic diseases may be reduced. It is believed that in the future the science of medicine will understand relationships between illness and food such that treatment will occur through prescribing certain foods and hot and cold drinks. Thus, eventually people will voluntarily give up eating meat in favor of a vegetarian diet.

Fasting is viewed as discipline for the soul. Self-restraint from physical appetite allows individuals to concentrate on their spirituality and draw closer to God. Abstaining from food is thus a symbol and not a goal in itself. A 19-day fast is done each year immediately before the Bahá'í' New Year (Metropolitan Chicago Healthcare Council 2002). Thus, it serves as spiritual preparation for the coming year. People who are ill, older adults, and very young children are not required to fast, as in Islam. Neither travelers nor those who are pregnant or nursing need fast.

Avoidance of smoking, alcohol, and opium leads to "strength and physical courage, for health, beauty, and comeliness" (Research Department of the Universal House of Justice 1990, Selections from the Writings of Abdu'l-Bahá, secs. 129, 150). When people are not under the control of these substances they are able to be "among the pure, the free, and the wise" (Research Department of the Universal House of Justice 1990, sec. 150).

The value of social support is also mentioned in Bahá'í religious texts. People are enjoined to visit those who are sick. "Happiness is a great healer to those who are ill" (Esslemont 2006, p. 204). An individual who visits people who are ill should do so with great compassion for their suffering.

Birth Control, Abortion, Artificial Insemination　Individual couples make their own decisions in matters of parenting based on Bahá'í teachings and medical advice. Birth control is permitted to manage the number of births, but similar to many faiths, avoidance of birth would be against a primary belief in the purpose of marriage for procreation (Kourosh and Hosoda 2007). Similarly, abortion is acceptable for medical reasons, such as to prevent a child being born with severe birth defects or to protect a mother's health. However, abortion to avoid unwanted children disturbs the sacredness of conception where the human soul first appears. Artificial insemination and in-vitro fertilization are permitted, but surrogacy is not due, to complex social and spiritual implications (Smith 2008, p. 167).

Organ Transplantation and Donation, and End-of-Life Concerns　Organ transplant is not prohibited; in fact, it is deemed "a noble thing to do" (Zohoori 1985, p. 4). When a body part is donated at the death of an individual, the rest of the body should not be cremated but buried. This is consistent with standard end-of-life practice.

There is no religious objection to a postmortem examination of the body. When a person dies, Iranian Bahá'í may want to be present for or wash the body, as is common in the largely Muslim culture. There are no specific Bahá'í end-of-life rituals (Ellershaw and Wilkinson 2011). Embalming is not allowed and the body should be buried within an hour's journey away geographically. Cremation is not acceptable in the faith. Advance care planning is likely acceptable to most people who follow the Bahá'í faith, because they do believe in an afterlife. Bahá'í's respect life and also believe that the soul continues to progress after death and to attain divine attributes (Ellershaw and Wilkinson 2011). The soul does not reside in the body, but is nonmaterial and connected with the body in a manner that remains mysterious. The soul is the essential inner reality that is formed at conception. The light of the soul is reflected in the mirror of the body. At death it continues on with a new existence (Smith 2008). Infants who die are held in God's mercy.

Mental Health   The material self, in contrast to the spiritual self, sometimes experiences emotions such as jealousy, greed, deception, and hypocrisy (Maloney 2006). The material self is considered the natal self and is referred to as Satan in older sacred writings. One can be imprisoned by these lower emotions, but is capable of transcending them through focus on one's higher nature. Happiness supports health, but depression can engender illness (Zohoori 1985). The rational soul is seen as a bridge between the two. Tension between the lower and higher selves leads to continuing opportunities for growth. Knowledge of self is gained through intuition and divine love. Greater knowledge leads to greater capacity of love for self and others. The energy freed by love leads to greater will and sense of direction.

Cognitive therapy is viewed as a useful approach, but is limited by the absence of recognition of the capacity of intuition. Behavioral approaches are also seen as limited, but humanistic and existential approaches to treatment highlight the need for courage and the development of authenticity (Maloney 2006). Sacred writings and prayer are seen as valuable methods for psychotherapeutic healing. Cultural values of Mideastern Bahá'í's would vary from those of American Bahá'í's and lead to different preferences for therapeutic interventions. The Bahá'í' worldview suggests that members benefit from dynamic processes of growth, but are not necessarily expected to achieve perfection and thus should not criticize themselves for presumed failures. Therapy should be nonjudgmental and explore thought distortions. Familiarity with Bahá'í' elements of faith may be helpful if included in treatment. Use of the nine-pointed star might bring comfort to those facing health and mental health challenges, as it symbolizes spiritual completion. Each point represents one of the messengers of God.

Suffering   Some causes of suffering occur as a result of individual choices. For instance, when someone overeats consistently, that person will become overweight and unhealthy. In these situations, obedience to the will of God and such activities as fasting may end such suffering. Attachment to the material world can be a source of suffering, but detachment leads to contentment which can be associated with good health. Emotional conditions such as anxiety and depression can also lead to poor physical health (e.g., poor sleep, under- or overeating, and lowered functioning of the immune system).

Suffering is both a reminder and a guide. It stimulates us to better adapt ourselves to our environmental conditions, and thus leads the way to self-improvement. In every suffering one can find a meaning and a wisdom. But it is not always easy to find the secret of that wisdom. It is sometimes only when all our suffering has passed that we become aware of its usefulness. (Research Department of the

Universal House of Justice 1990, letter written on behalf of Shoghi Effendi, 29 May 1935)

People should take precautions against adversity, but not seek to avoid death. This is consistent with the Bahá'í belief in an afterlife. Along with its social justice mission, Bahá'í's are invited to work to find solutions to poverty and disease and other forms of suffering.

Health-Focused Research

Little research is available that demonstrates effects of worldviews on health practices significant to the Bahá'í faith. A search was conducted in Medline in 2016 related to terms such as Bahá'í and medicine, Bahá'í and health practices, and Baha'i' religion and health. Research related to the Baha'i' faith was very sparse. Graham and Shier (2009) included research about the Bahá'í religion in an exploration of research articles related to religion and social work. None were located in any social work search engines. One study detailed views of religious leaders regarding UK organ donation policy, which was considering a change from an opt-in to an opt-out approach (Randhawa, Brocklehurst, Pateman, Kinsella, and Parry 2010). The individual who represented Bahá'í views had no concerns with either the current or the proposed policy. A study of the views of subgroups of religious faiths on respectful medical treatment identified the Bahá'í faith as a target group, but they were not mentioned specifically in the sample, leaving open the question of whether any participated (Davidson, Boyer, Casey, Matzel, and Walden 2008). An article explaining support for breastfeeding in the Bahá'í faith was one of the few located that addressed health issues and the Bahá'í faith specifically (Setrakian, Rosenman, and Szucs 2011). A few articles were located that provided general background on tenets of the faith related to health beliefs and practices, but they were conceptual instead of research oriented (Kourosh and Hosoda 2007; Metropolitan Chicago Healthcare Council 2002).

Professor Faraneh Vargha-Khadem, a Bahá'í, is Head of Section for Cognitive Science and Neuropsychiatry at the University College London Institute of Child Health, Head of Clinical Neuropsychology at Great Ormond Street Hospital for Children, and Director of the UCL Centre for Developmental Cognitive Science (https://www.ucl.ac.uk/centre-develop mental-cognitive-neuroscience). She was part of the team that identified the *FoxP2* gene, the so called "speech gene" responsible for speech difficulties. (A genetic mutation leads to underdevelopment of the circuit that coordinates movement and produces articulate speech.) Her family has always practiced the Bahá'í' faith; in fact, her great-great grandfather was one of the earliest believers in the Bahá'í' faith. He was imprisoned with her great-uncle (his son) and both were killed because they would not recant their faith.

Of her work as a scientist and a Bahá'í' Vargha-Khadem says, "It is the light within each of us that motivates us to realize our human potential, our spiritual endowment, and . . . use it for the good" (Vargha-Khadem 2013). Her faith believes there is harmony between science and religion: she indicated that a belief system that does not lead to harmony is "better not to have." Scientific principles must be used to improve the material well-being of humanity. However, a system of science that becomes so materialistic that it denies the existence of what is the essence of humanity is better not to have either. The goal of both science and religion is to understand truth. Scientific truth is not that different from the understanding of faith. We can have unlimited knowledge, but unlimited knowledge without context is a dictionary. She clearly links the foundation of her success to the teachings with which she was raised. Compassion and understanding are both required to guide action.

Influences on Health and Disease Risk

The Bahá'í' faith makes no demands in many areas of healthcare practice, leaving followers to make their own decisions on what practices to follow. Vaccination is left to individual choice, as is circumcision. Sterilization is generally not encouraged except in cases of medical need. Abortion as well is acceptable, but only if done for health reasons and not for reasons of an unwanted child. The faith remains neutral on organ donation, though it is described in sacred writings as a noble act. Breastfeeding is encouraged.

Followers of the faith are invited to consult with physicians when they are ill, so there is no suggestion at all that those who use medicine would be contravening their faith. A decision on removal or withholding of life support in medical cases where intervention prolongs life in disabling illnesses is not addressed in sacred texts. Therefore, decisions are left to those responsible, including the patient (Zohoori 1985). Moderation in diet is considered a positive health practice, as is avoiding tobacco and alcohol. Social support is encouraged when people become ill. Adherents of this faith would likely feel decreased stress, because beliefs of the faith do not contradict use of medical approaches to care. In general, there seems to be nothing about these faith beliefs that would increase any risk for disease. On the contrary, the faith seems well aligned with what is known to lead to more positive health behaviors and health outcomes.

Care for Patients

Bahá'í' patients are positively disposed toward seeking medical care, as this aligns very strongly with their favorable view of science and physicians' skill. Their belief in independent investigation of truth would likely mean that they would act as ideal patients, assisting in their own care by seeking out the latest research and sharing this with their physicians. They would be compliant with prescribed medical protocols. At the same time, they would make use of prayer, good nutrition, and social support. They would understand that healing is in the hands of God, but would view their physician as a partner of God.

RASTAFARIANISM

Rastafarianism is variously identified as a way of life, a religion, a cult, a movement, and a culture (Baxter 2002; Edmonds and Gonzalez 2010; Edmonds 2003). The labels vary much as the concept itself. In fact, many who follow this faith—an estimated 1 million worldwide—prefer to remove the "ism" because it is the "isms" that box those into what they are trying to avoid. Thus, the term *Rastafari* will be primarily used in this chapter (Edmonds 2003; "Rastafarianism" n.d.).

History and Practice of the Faith

Originating in Jamaica, Rastafari grew from opposition to the colonization that was taking place in the early 1930s (Chevannes 1994, 1998). Society at that time was controlled by a small group of wealthy white elite citizens at the top, and racism was evident everywhere. Some of the roots of this faith lie in Marcus Garvey's Universal Negro Improvement Association (UNIA) established in 1914 in Jamaica. He sought to have the British government repatriate African Americans to Africa, which he saw as the spiritual home of all blacks and a place of early civilizations (Chevannes 2011). Many former slaves had identified with Ethiopia mentioned in the Bible and with the oppression of Israelites. They believed in a mystical return to Africa.

Edmonds and Gonzalez (2010) provide insight demonstrating the complexity involved. "Rastafari shows us the manner in which Afro-Jamaicans sought to articulate a sense of African religion and identity while still being influenced by and struggling against the legacy of European colonialism" (Edmonds and Gonzalez 2010, p. 177). Several prominent members of the new religion separately identified Haile Selassie (Ras Tafari) as the promised Messiah (Chevannes 2011).

With roots in Christianity, there are some philosophical similarities as well as areas where Rastafari has created its own direction (Baxter 2002). Rastafari believe in God, whom they refer to as *Jah* (Baxter 2002) who is also black (Chevannes and Institute of Social Studies 1998). While Christians continue to wait for the second coming of Christ, many Rastas believe that Haile Selassie of Ethiopia was the second Christ (Dorman 2013; Edmonds and Gonzalez 2010). Haile Selassie, whose birth name was *Ras Tafari Makonnen*, was crowned Emperor of Ethiopia in 1930. The meaning behind Haile Selassie's name, which includes *King of Kings* and *Lord of Lords*, as well as suggestion of the lineage of David, parallels references in the Bible to the names referred to for Jesus Christ (Christensen 2014; Edmonds and Gonzales 2010, p. 184; Chevannes and Institute of Social Studies 1998). Though there is not agreement as to how, or if, his lineage connects him to Jesus Christ, there is conviction that Haile Selassie plays a significant role in Rastafari, representing a divine figure (Bedasse 2010). The divinity of Haile Selassie was largely promoted through Leonard Howell, one of the Rastafari originators (Erskine 2007). Other founding leaders included Joseph N. Hibbert, Archibald Dunkley, and Robert Hinds (Erskine 2007). Each had his own direction for the movement; however, the expectation that Haile Selassie was the divine one to deliver Jamaicans from oppression is common.

Perhaps as an example of the rebellion against conformity, there are many facets of Rastafari, and indeed inconsistencies within the faith. Through the years, different forms of expression evolved, some including a more defined lifestyle or organizational gathering. Three specific groups or *mansions* include the Nyabinghi Order, the Bobo, and the Twelve Tribes of Israel (Christensen 2014). The Nyabinghi Order emerged out of the Youth Black Faith reform movement of the 1940s. It includes descriptive requirements about dress and diet among other elements. "When one identifies with Rastafari as a Nyabinghi, one makes a strict commitment to codes of dress, dietary restrictions, gender roles, and various ritual observances" (Christensen 2014, p. xi). Another mansion or group, the Ethiopia Africa Black International Congress, popularly known as the *Bobo*, began during the 1950s and was led by Prince Emmanual Edwards. The Bobo Rastas are more structured, much like an organized church. Additionally, they identify primarily with a communal style of living (Christensen 2014). Members also are distinguished through wearing a tightly wrapped turban over their dreadlocks, rigid confinement of menstruating women for 21 days, and sale of brooms in remembrance of the children of Israel. In 1968, the Twelve Tribes of Israel arose. An order with strong connections to reggae musician Bob Marley, the Twelve Tribes of Israel provides opportunities for others outside of the Jamaican community to become members (Christensen

2014). This group is recognized for order and discipline and has been attractive to middle-class individuals and professionals.

Core Beliefs and Worldviews

For many Rastafari, no matter what mansion or order is followed, there are similar beliefs or worldviews that are common. As mentioned above, the belief in one god, *Jah,* is a common worldview (Baxter 2002). Other distinctive worldviews include the role of women as subject to the men who are also called Rasta or *king men* (Chevannes 1994). Though there appears to be some indication of change in women's roles, as some are taking leadership roles or choosing to express themselves through looser interpretation of dress codes, there are still some who hold to tradition. Ironically, some younger women feel inferior to or pressure from the older generations, which imposes additional oppression—something that Rastafari was founded to contravene (Julien 2003).

One of the most prominent characteristics of Rastafari was wearing dreadlocks. This was introduced by Youth Black Faith, a militant arm of the group, who thought this would link them to Maasai warriors in Kenya who also stood against colonialism (Chevannes 2011). However, in their own country, this, plus dressing in burlap used for produce, caused them to be seen as outcasts instead. A unique form of language known as *dreadtalk* was also developed. In this invented speech, the first person pronoun was used to replace both singular and plural pronouns. *I an' I* replaced "we," "you," and "us," for example. Other kinds of word inversions were also invented, such as *over* for *under*stand. These patterns of speech also led to a new way of understanding self and community.

The Rastafari lifestyle, represented by the term *Livity,* embraces adherence to the natural or organic. It is, in a sense, rebellion against artificiality and is demonstrated through living communally, growing food without the use of pesticides, using herbal remedies to treat physical and spiritual needs, and living simply (Johnson-Hill 1995; Chevannes and Institute of Social Studies 1998). *I-tal,* an expression of livity meaning "vital," often includes a vegetarian diet that involves eating foods in their natural state without additives such as salt or sugar. Processed foods are avoided. Additionally, alcohol and caffeine are seldom part of the diet. Illnesses are treated primarily with herbs and natural remedies (Chevannes and Institute of Social Studies 1998).

Beliefs and Practices That Influence Health-Related Behaviors

Just as there are differences in the practice of Rastafari, the role of women is also dependent on evolving philosophies. Generally speaking, Rastafari was originally patriarchal in nature: women were accepted as Rastafari through the husband or male partner, referred to as their *Kingman* (Christensen 2014; Chevannes and Institute of Social Studies 1998). Subordination of women is demonstrated through the lack of leadership roles, the requirement to cover the hair, and the stigma of uncleanliness that is forced upon them specifically during menstruation and childbirth. The times when women are deemed unclean requires them to wash their clothes separately from the men's garments, and women do not cook during this time (Chevannes and Institute of Social Studies 1998; Erskine 2007). Though not all groups adhere to these rules, many still do. The number of days included in the restriction range from 7 to 21. Women of the Nyabinghi mansion are not allowed to attend ceremonies for seven days during menstruation. For Bobos, "strict dress codes, long isolation periods during menstruation, and tight control by male members restricted equal access for women" (Christensen 2014, p. 61).

The role of women and the striving for equality has evolved to a point where in some circumstances such as gatherings or conferences, women have been able to speak, celebrate, or hold positions similar to men, though this is not yet the norm (Chevannes 1994, Christensen 2014). What does seem to hold true to many is the respected role of motherhood and caring for children. "On the one hand, women are respected, perhaps even feared, for their powers of fertility and command greater allegiance and love from males and females alike than do their male counterparts" (Chevannes 1994, p. 28). Chevannes (1994) further describes motherhood as "the highest fulfillment of womanhood" (p. 28).

Health-Focused Research

Adherence to the strict vegetarian lifestyle, specifically vegan which eliminates processed foods, has caused concern regarding the potential for vitamin deficiency. Campbell, Lofters, and Gibbs (1982) reported findings of the vegan syndrome that results from a deficiency of vitamin B_{12} (cobalamin) in those identifying as Rastafari. The deficiency has been seen not only in women, but also in their babies. "Infants breastfed by vegan mothers can develop vitamin B_{12} deficiency between the age of 2 and 12 months due to their limited body reserve at birth even in the absence of signs of the deficiency in the mother" (Winckel, Velde, Bruyne, and Biervliet 2011, p. 1490).

Research reports only a small number of cases of this deficiency and, as Yntema and Beard (2000) point out, many foods are now fortified with vitamins, including B_{12}. Awareness of and follow-up for the possibility of deficiency of B_{12} in infants, especially those breastfed by a mother who follows a strict vegan diet, are important. "Vegetarians, particularly women during pregnancy and lactation, should be knowledgeable about the cobalamin content of their food or seek nutritional advice" ("Neurologic Impairment" 2003, p. 63). Visible symptoms of this deficiency include irritability, failure to thrive, apathy, anorexia, refusal of solid foods, megaloblastic anemia, and developmental regression (Dror and Allen 2008).

Influences on Health and Disease Risk

Reasoning Ceremonies and Marijuana   Biblical scripture is used to reinforce many of the symbolic elements of Rastafari, including the use of cannabis (Gibson 2010). Rastafari provide biblical references such as Genesis 1:12, Genesis 1:29, Revelation 22:2, and Psalm 18:18 to justify the use of cannabis for spiritual and healing purposes (Erskine 2007). Gibson (2010) states that believing it is sanctioned in the Bible "adds scriptural force to Rastafari claims that cannabis aids reflection, meditation, wisdom and scriptural insight" (p. 326).

Cannabis or *ganja* is used during ceremonies such as *Reasoning*. Rastafari Reasoning is a ceremony of varying degrees of formality in which participants access the spirit through the ritual smoking of herb (ganja) and the use of word/sound/power for the purpose of gaining clarity about spiritual, philosophical, political and social truth claims. (Christensen 2014, p. 62)

Relationship to Research on Medical Marijuana   Use of marijuana for medical treatment is on the rise, but the actual value of its use for medical reasons is contested (Malec 2016). There are at least 38 medical diagnoses that are considered qualifying conditions for which marijuana may be dispensed after physical observation by a physician (Malec 2016). Physicians may not legally help patients obtain marijuana or direct its usage. Differences in metabolism lead to wide interindividual variation in the effects of this drug, which is classified as a Schedule I drug in the United States. Clinically significant benefits for pain and for some conditions warrant further study (Whiting et al. 2015). As Rastafari already use marijuana for religious purpose, they could experience a dual effect for some medical concerns.

Care for Patients

Within Rastafari, differing beliefs or customs are held depending on the person and his or her interpretation of the context (Baxter 2002). It is important to understand and treat a patient as an individual, making no assumptions, creating a safe environment, communicating thoroughly, and providing information as well as alternatives in order to demonstrate respect for the person's beliefs but also for the person as an individual. A specific example, drawn from the I-tal living described earlier, may come as a request for dietary exceptions when in a hospital setting. Medications may be refused by those who prefer herbal remedies. Honoring and educating without judgment may help bridge the relationship between a health professional and patient practicing Rastafari.

There are many ways to embrace the Rastafari movement. Ideologies seem to be evolving as women take ownership of their personal interpretation of the movement, and participate as individuals rather than subjects of the Rastaman. For those within and outside of the community, recognizing the benefits of a faith is important. Through structure within a faith, whether limited or stringent, there are opportunities to bring people together for support, for guidance, and for providing a way of perceiving and dealing with issues such as life, illness, and personal struggles. As healthcare professionals, spiritual advisers, or simply respectful human beings, acceptance of an individual provides an opportunity to build a relationship that will be beneficial to the encounter. MacKenna (2007) points out, "What we need to avoid, if we can, is either just ignoring the patient's spiritual communications, or, ponderously rephrasing them in our own psychological or psychiatric language; reactions which may well be experienced as rejection, or as desecration" (p. 254).

ZOROASTRIANISM

History

Zoroastrianism originated in the nation of Persia, now Iran. Specific dates ascribed to the founding vary. The religion's prophet, Zoroaster (known also as Zarathustra in Iran), is known to have lived and taught in Persia before the Achaemenid dynasty, which has roots in the year 550 BCE, and thus Zoroaster may have founded the religion around 600 BCE (Nigosian 1993). Greek scholars and resources place Zoroaster at 6350 BCE, 6,000 years before the death of Plato; in contrast, Chinese archaeological resources place Zoroaster's birth at 1767 BCE (Contractor and Contractor 2003). Other scholars place his birth between 1500 and 1200 BCE (Contractor and Contractor 2003). There is no clear agreement on the founding of the religion by scholars, but there is general consensus that it was founded before Christianity.

Though this monotheistic religion came into being before the birth of Christ, it is noted by scholars as having a great deal of influence on other monotheistic religions, including Judaism, Christianity, and Islam (Occhiogrosso n.d.). Some historians credit Zoroastrianism and the cults that came from it with introducing concepts commonly known to Western religions: immortality and the concept of the soul, the Last Judgment, belief in a future state of rewards and punishments, the transformation of the Earth after a long struggle, and a Satan-like figure (Occhiogrosso n.d.). It is also suspected that the idea of the guardian angel in Christianity and Judaism was inspired by the *fravashi*, the divine guardian-spirit of each individual human being in the Zoroastrian faith (Shapero 1997).

According to the Zoroastrian Association of Metropolitan Chicago, there are between 200,000 and 250,000 Zarathushti in the world; this number dwindles to 20,000 when looking at the United States, and dwindles even further when one looks at a city like Chicago, which houses a population of 700. The majority of this religious population is still located in India and Iran, their places of origin (Metropolitan Chicago Healthcare Council 2002). A subgroup identifies as the Parsis (or Parsees, *Persians*), descendants of Iranian refugees who brought Zoroastrianism to India beginning in the 10th century (Occhiogrosso n.d.).

Zoroastrians call their ancient text the *Avesta;* it is written in the Avestan language. The Avesta was scribed in the 4th or 5th centuries CE. Their divine hymns are called the *Gathas*, and are the words of the Prophet Zarathustra (Metropolitan Chicago Healthcare Council 2002). They are the only words formally attributed to the prophet of the religion. The religion has other specific religious texts that are of import: *Vendidad* (statutes regarding purity), *Siroza, Yashts* (hymns to each of 21 deities), and *Hadhoxt Nask* (Sayings) (Occhiogrosso n.d.).

Zarathustra, the Prophet, is considered a *saoshyant*, or savior to the faith tradition, similar to the idea of Jesus in Christianity. Zarathustra, or Zoroaster, is credited by the Greeks and Romans as being a founder of the Magi tradition. The Magi were sorcerer priests skilled in interpretation of dreams and prophecy. Zoroastrian faith teaches that Zoroaster had a vision at age 30 of facing Ahura Mazda (God), in which he was instructed to found a new religion.

Health and Basic Cosmology

The Zoroastrian cosmology comprises the dual aspects of good and evil. According to classic Zoroastrian thought, the natural human condition is a state of perfection and good health. Factors that cause poor health statuses—such as pain and fever—are considered unnatural; mortality itself is also perceived as an abnormal condition. Disease is considered the work of the devil figure Ahriman (Hinnells 1999). Illness was created when Ahriman, the devil or the Destroying Spirit, saw the entire good that God—called Ohrmazd or Ahura Mazda—had created. His jealousy and destructive instincts took over and he attacked the world, inflicting destruction and suffering on man, plants, and the entire Earth (Hinnells 1999). This concept of good versus evil, found in the majority of religions in the world, is the explanation for sickness.

To Zoroastrians, the belief in responsibility for one's own words and actions—at the behest of the deity—may translate into illness caused by personal failures or infractions in life. This provides the opening for demonic and evil forces to attack people (Metropolitan Chicago Healthcare Council 2002). Feelings of guilt could lead to decreased self-worth; low self-worth could potentially interfere with recovery from illness, substance abuse, and mental health concerns.

Health and Demonology   Demons play a pivotal role in the idea of health for Zoroastrians. Human beings should be allies to Ohrmazd, and should annihilate Ahriman in order to restore and renovate the world (Hinnells 1999). This can be accomplished simply by living a virtuous life under the ideals that the religion promotes; this leaves no space for Ahriman to exist in body or soul. Denying the devil Ahriman entry to one's body is cited in a Pahlavi text: "When he [Ahriman] will have no dwelling in people's bodies, he will be annihilated from the whole world" (Hinnells 1999, p. 11). Ejecting Ahriman can be done by ejecting other demons: Violence, Greed, Wrath, Sloth, Fury, and the essence of all evil, the Lie (Hinnells 1999). Adding to this, Ohrmazd sent 9,999 medicinal herbs to counter that exact number of diseases that Ahriman had sent to destroy humanity. "One ought to be diligent and eager to know each medicinal plant, for . . . one may abolish ailments and disease in the world against which there is no [other] stratagem" (p. 12).

Furthermore, Zoroastrians believe that concepts of purity and pollution are important; dead matter—such as corpses—draws out evil. They believe that the demon *Nasu* can bring forth diseases, distress, and destruction, and she can be strengthened by anything considered dead; she can be drawn out from her home through the presence of corpses, and comes from the north when someone has died. Anything that is dead, or decaying, is considered a pollutant. Zoroastrians also consider anything that leaves the body—including nail clippings, cut hair, excrement, and blood—a pollutant that draws forth evil and should be dealt with quickly (Hinnells 1999).

Holistic Views in Zoroastrianism

Zarathustra's teachings, in general, exhorted followers to lead an industrious, honest, and charitable life (Metropolitan Chicago Healthcare Council 2002). Zoroaster also focused on three main beliefs that every person of the faith should do their best to embody:

- *Humata*: good thoughts
- *Hukhta*: good words
- *Huvereshta*: good deeds (Metropolitan Chicago Healthcare Council 2002)

Zoroastrians also hold other specific views that have a holistic quality. These views do not merely touch on spiritual aspects of life, but also physical aspects. Named the *Amesha Spenta*, these views are:

- *Vohu Mano* is the good mind. People must think for themselves, and be able to choose between good and evil. No matter their choice, persons are responsible for the consequences that result from their choice.
- *Asha* is principled, honest, beneficent, ordered, lawful living—for some, righteousness and piety. It is the Divine Law and focuses on truth and wisdom and justice. All Zoroastrians do their best to follow the path of Asha.
- *Khshathra* is having dominion and sovereignty over one's life. It promotes the need to fight evil while also doing good or kind acts.
- *Armaiti* is serenity. It is also considered purity and devotion to Ahura Mazda.
- *Haurvatat* is about living in a holistic and healthy manner. It concerns seeking excellence in all we do.
- *Amertat* involves transcending mortal limitations through good health, by handing down the spiritual flame, and building an enduring, undying spirit. Both of these traits are the rewards of a righteous life.

The Amesha Spenta are considered the attributes of Ahura Mazda, and are the grandest ideals for persons to emulate (Metropolitan Chicago Healthcare Council 2002; Eduljee 2014b).

Healing Roles in the Faith

Zoroastrian texts mention five different kinds of healing roles that can be embodied by all believers. These five different types are roles people play in their lives in order to encourage healing in themselves and others. The name in parentheses is considered the name of the healer in the Avestan language (Eduljee 2014b). They are labeled as:

1. One who heals with goodness and care (*Asho-Baeshazo*)
2. One who heals with justice (*Dato-Baeshazo*)

3. One who heals with surgery (*Kareto-Baeshazo*)
4. One who heals with plants (*Urvaro-Baeshazo*)
5. One who heals with the *manthra*, or meditations (*Mathro-Baeshazo*)

The first type of healer is someone who embodies the previously listed Amesha Spenta values in his or her life and heals others through having a good mind, being righteous, and being lawful. Those who heal with justice are mentioned in two different ways in Zoroastrian faith. First, healing is done through the Dastur, a type of high priest whose duty is to defend the law. These priests conduct ceremonies, are high in status, and function as spiritual guides (Eduljee 2014c). Second, those who heal with justice may also be involved in conflict resolution and ensure that the faith's moral and ethical code is followed. Typically, they were older priests who knew the community well (Eduljee 2014c).

Those who heal with surgery and plants are mentioned in ancient Zoroastrian texts. The father of the ancient Zoroastrian King Jamsid was the first person to prepare and use haoma juice, a plant-based healing substance that is used in drinks; this tradition of using haoma was eventually passed down to Zarathustra's father (Eduljee 2014d). Also in the Zoroastrian texts, the Vendidad (20.2) credits the man named Thrita as the first holistic physician (Eduljee 2014d). These examples show that the importance of health is intertwined with the Zoroastrian faith, because some of their most influential figures were either physicians, or healers, or descended from healers and physicians.

Thrita's work was important for both surgical need and plant-based healing. During Thrita's time, "many hundreds and thousands of healing plants were identified," and cures for diseases and ailments were found and applied according to the Vendidad texts in the Avesta (Eduljee 2014c). Conditions treated included pain, fever, rot, and infection; other conditions may have been successfully treated then as well, but this information, along with many Zoroastrian texts, is missing. It is also noted that Thrita the healer developed a steel surgery knife that was bound in gold, at the time the preferred metal for surgery and sterilization.

Thrita was not the only surgeon of note in the ancient texts. Per the *Shahnameh* (stories of heroes), the famed Rustam, a mythological figure who became a full-grown man in mere weeks and possessed supreme physical strength, was born through caesarian section. A healing drink of milk and plants was given to his mother Rudabeh to calm her through the surgical process (Eduljee 2014d). Thus, surgical processes were important in Zoroastrian times; caesarian sections were encouraged to help mothers through the birthing process. This example provides evidence that Zoroastrianism focuses on physical and spiritual healing. In sum, Zoroastrianism's mythology is directly connected to improving health; historical and mythological figures of the faith emphasized a holistic, healthy life which influences Zoroastrians to this day.

The final category of those healers includes those who use the manthra. The manthra consists of insightful thoughts that focus on reflection, contemplation, and meditation on God's work, as well as personal spiritual growth (Eduljee 2014b). The manthra can also be used to focus on personal goals and recommit to the faith. Reciting manthras allows one to refocus his or her mind and could be considered a type of mindfulness. Zarathustra reportedly meditated in a cave before beginning his journey, so a focus on healing the mind and spirit through meditation is consistent with religious teachings (Eduljee 2014b). Daily prayers encourage serenity and can occur in any space. Orthodox adherents usually face a light source when praying, such as a sunrise or sunset. Light in itself is a symbol of healing and insight (Eduljee 2014b).

Prayers for Health

Zoroastrians engage in prayers to help with ailments. Because they may find comfort in usage of these prayers, patients should be encouraged, if comfortable doing so, to use prayer while managing any illness or strain. There are prayers for specific health issues, but also general prayers for mental health, childbirth, marital peace, and success.

Many of the prayers can be used for more than one ailment. For example, both childbirth and chest pains are ailments that may lead Zoroastrians to use the Ava (or Aban) Niyayesh, a litany directed to water. The healing or purifying elements of this litany are directed to healthy children. A few of the lines of this prayer include: "And (the outflow) of this one water of mine, flows continuously, both summer and winter. She purifies my waters, she (purifies) the seed of males, the wombs of females, the milk of females" (Khorda Avesta n.d.).

While water is revered in the religion, fire is even more so (see "Reverence for Fire" section). There is a litany to fire as well, called the *Atash Niyayesh*, that can be used during sacrifices, and to imbue oneself with strength: "Give me, O Fire, son of Ahura Mazda! well-being immediately, sustenance immediately; life immediately, well-being in abundance; sustenance in abundance, life in abundance; knowledge, holiness, a ready tongue, understanding for (my) soul; and afterwards wisdom (which is) comprehensive, great, imperishable" (Khorda Avesta n.d.).

Hymns may surface that give Zoroastrians strength, and those in the health fields should recognize the importance of these hymns. Another common hymn sung in Zoroastrian faith is the *Hom Yasht*. The Hom

Yasht is a prayer that is commonly used for heart problems, headaches, reproductive health, and overall health improvements (Khorda Avesta n.d.). The Hom Yasht includes the following lines:

I make my claim on thee for strength; I make my claim on thee for victory; I make my claim on thee for health and healing (when healing is my need); I make my claim on thee for progress and increased prosperity, and vigor of the entire frame, and for understanding. (Khorda Avesta n.d.)

In addition to the foregoing, there are three basic prayers that Zoroastrians use to symbolize lessons for good living: *Ashem Vohu* (to do good for the sake of doing good), *Yatha Ahu Vairio* (to be of service) and *Yangahe Atam* (a lesson for good living) (Metropolitan Chicago Healthcare Council 2002). The first prayer is considered an invocation of Asha related to righteous and devout living.

Finally, there is one more important prayer that clinicians and health personnel should take note of: the Benediction, or Prayer for Health. This prayer, called the *Tan-Dorosti,* includes the following lines:

May there be health and long life, complete Glory giving righteousness! . . . May this household be happy, may there be blessing! . . . We beseech you, Lord, to grant to the present ruler, to all the community, and to all those of the Good Religion, health and fair repute . . . Keep them long happy, long healthy, and long just! (Boyce 1990)

Reverence for Fire

In many religions, the symbol of fire is very important in praise and worship, but none more than Zoroastrianism. Zoroastrians are known for their worship of fire, considering it sacred and a type of illumination (Occhiogrosso n.d.). To Zoroastrian adherents, fire is the son of Ahura Mazda and the most important gift their creator bestowed upon them. Sacredness is shown through praying to fire in order to ask it to imbue them with strength. Zoroastrian texts discuss many types of fires, and also refer to fires as *energies*. *Athra, Atarsh*, and *Atash* are all different words used in texts for fires; other fires are considered cold to the touch or are contained in objects (Eduljee 2014a). Zoroastrianism also refers to a type of spiritual fire, called the *mainyu athra* (Eduljee 2014a). This spiritual fire is what leads Zoroastrians to *Asha,* referenced earlier as piety and devout living that is lawful. The eternal flame in Zoroastrianism is reinforced when one person passes Zoroaster's teachings to others and on down through generations.

In regards to energies, there are five different fire-associated energies referenced in the Avestas. They are:

1. *Barezi-Savangh* (ultimate purpose): The energy or fire of original creation that is self-sustaining.
2. *Vohu-Frayan* (good propagator): The fire or energy found in human and animal bodies. It requires both food and water to be sustained.
3. *Urvazisht* (most useful): A fire or energy that is found in plants and needs only water to be sustained.
4. *Vazisht* (most supporting): Found in clouds (manifests as lightning) and requires neither food nor water to be sustained.
5. *Spenisht* (most brilliant and beneficent): Found in temporal fires and requires fuel but no water to be sustained (Eduljee 2014a).

The concept of fire is intricately connected to the spiritual and physical health of the Zoroastrian people. It provides them with energy to live, is a religious representation very much like Christianity's Holy Spirit, and exists all through the entire universe.

Nutrition

Nutrition and food guidance are another area important to Zoroastrians. Many Zoroastrians see their diet as a way of restoring balance to their bodies. In orthodox Yazdi communities, healing foods such as aush stew are cooked to restore what the Zoroastrian people refer to as a hot and cold balance (Eduljee 2014b). Foods are classified as either hot or cold, and healers will specifically select foods for individuals to restore their balance and health. Herbal remedies work in a similar way, and herbs are essential ingredients in Zoroastrian food in Iran.

Women's Health

Normal female health processes such as the menstrual cycle can carry a particular connotation. Blood loss is considered an act of pollution and can invite evil to oneself. In Zoroastrian faith, the womb is considered a focal point for the daily struggle between good and evil because of the menstrual cycle (Hinnells 1999). Both this monthly flow of blood, and the fact that death was common in ages past during childbirth, have commonly been viewed as assaults of evil, in this case on women. Women are considered unfortunate victims who are impure during their menstrual cycles and after childbirth. Furthermore, menstruation is the main reason that women are prohibited from being priests in the Zoroastrian faith.

Family Life, Birth, and Contraception

Zoroastrians are encouraged to marry within the religion; this is described as an obligation. Zoroastrians commonly do not accept interreligious marriages, nor do they accept children of mixed marriages (Foltz 2011). Zoroastrians do not typically have many children; the average Zoroastrian couple is likely to have only one child. Furthermore, marriage is respected in Zoroastrianism and those who go against the tradition—such as through divorce, remaining unmarried, or practicing polygamy—are seen as committing acts that are big errors (Halvaei, Khalili, Ghasemi-Esmailabad, Nabi, and Shamsi 2014).

Specific rituals are associated with the birth of a child. First, a traditional ritual is to light a lantern of clarified butter at the completion of the fifth and seventh months of pregnancy. This lamp also burns for three days after the child is born (Nigosian 1993). The lantern is noted to discourage evil spirits, but with less availability of lanterns this ritual is likely less often practiced currently. Births through caesarian sections were not considered impure or inappropriate, but were life-saving tools to make the birth easier. Abortion and contraception are not distinctly mentioned and are thus regulated as personal decisions (Metropolitan Chicago Healthcare Council 2002).

Organ Donation and End of Life

Zoroastrian faith does not have any specific religious instruction on organ and tissue donation. Many faith traditions in the United States favor the practice and have expressed desire to donate (Metropolitan Chicago Healthcare Council 2002). Disposal of the dead body must occur within 24 hours of death. The funeral ceremony for a Zoroastrian should occur within 6 hours of the death. The ceremony is called *one gah* (Metropolitan Chicago Healthcare Council 2002). Quick disposal of bodies, according to Zoroastrian cosmology, prevents attraction of evil. The urgency of the burial could interfere with autopsies for any Zoroastrian patient. Although there is no religious instruction on autopsies for Zoroastrians, they still must occur within the 24-hour time threshold. Autopsies are considered a personal issue for family members and should be explained thoroughly to the family decision makers.

HEALTH-FOCUSED RESEARCH

Studies have focused on Zoroastrian healthcare beliefs (Halvaei et al. 2014). One study considered beliefs, attitudes, and knowledge among

Zoroastrian participants on embryo donation and oocyte donation. In 2012, 318 Zoroastrian persons from two cities in Iran (Yazd and Kerman) were selected to answer a questionnaire handed out in person. The participants were split up into groups that focused on oocyte donation (OD) and embryo donation (ED) as well. In both groups, the majority of participants were female, and 65% of all participants were married (Halvaei et al. 2014). Regarding treatment for infertile patients, 69.7% of participants noted support for OD, whereas 71.3% of participants noted support for ED (Halvaei et al. 2014). Less than the majority (40% for OD and 42% for ED) supported these methods in comparison to adopting children, which was the preferred approach to childlessness. One-third of participants reported belief that Zoroastrianism accepts these methods, but more than half did not know. Overall, the majority of Zoroastrian people in the study accepted these fertility methods and agreed that they should be used. However, moral and ethical issues could arise in individual cases. Respondents supported psychological counseling for both donors and recipients (Halvaei et al. 2014). More than 80% of respondents also believed that discussions of OD and ED infertility treatment should be kept between couples and doctors; 70% of respondents believed that the child should not be informed of how he or she was conceived (Halvaei et al. 2014). This study could be used as a primer for those who need to have discussions with Zoroastrian couples about fertility.

Another health condition studied was diabetes (Khalilzadeh, Afkhami-Ardekani and Afrand 2015). Type 2 diabetes mellitus is very prevalent in Middle Eastern countries, and these countries will have the largest increase in diabetes cases by 2030. Undiagnosed Type 2 diabetes can lead to more serious conditions, such as mortality due to cardiovascular problems. The Zoroastrian minority has lived in isolation for a great deal of the time due to persecution. Isolation and limits on genetic variability—since Zoroastrians do not typically marry outside the religion—provided opportunity to study their risk factors for Type 2 diabetes (Khalilzadeh et al. 2015). Using systematic random sampling, a cross-sectional study of the Zoroastrian population in Yazd, Iran, led to a sample of 406. Ages ranged from 30 to 88. Diabetes was found in 26.1% of the subjects, and the prevalence of diabetes was found to be higher in women than men (28% of women to 22% of men). One-third of those found to have diabetes had been previously undiagnosed. According to this study, the prevalence of diabetes is four times higher than previously reported (Khalilzadeh et al. 2015). The authors proposed many reasons for why the subjects above 70 years of age could have a higher prevalence for diabetes than their younger counterparts; this included malnutrition, insufficient care, and socioeconomic status of the subjects. Health factors can vary from country to country and cohort to cohort, but they are important in all health settings. Finding those previously undiagnosed could represent lack of access to health care for the Zoroastrian population in different parts of the world, or in all parts of the world. It could represent modernization of society, in that factors that lead to diabetes are now reaching more isolated populations, such as Zoroastrians. Finally, it could represent specific healthcare beliefs of the Zoroastrians, in that they do not see certain health conditions as requiring treatment.

Finally, one should take into account mental health research for the Zoroastrian population. Mental health and physical health needs are intricately intertwined and should both be considered; one can suffer emotionally or mentally due to physical ailments. Furthermore, mental health needs may also be underdiagnosed or undiagnosed, just like health needs. Bakhtiari and Plunkett (2015) focused on anxiety, self-esteem, quality of family interactions, and other factors in Zoroastrian adolescent mental health. Self-report survey data was collected from 209 Zoroastrian young adults through online surveys; ages ranged from 18 to 30 and most were single college students who lived with parents. This study found that most of the Zoroastrian respondents reported positive mental health (i.e., positive self-esteem and happiness) while at the same time reporting infrequent symptoms of depression (Bakhtiari and Plunkett 2015). Young men reported significantly higher levels of happiness than did young women. Women reported significantly higher levels of depressive symptoms, and also reported meeting parental dating expectations significantly more often than men. Overall, stress levels of the respondents averaged 61 on a scale from 0–100, where 100 means extreme stress. Zoroastrian young adults reported infrequent cultural/ethnic discrimination. Finally, Zoroastrian young adults characterized their families in these ways: relatively high parental support and family cohesion, low to moderate parental psychological control (guilting and shaming the child), and low to occasional parent-child conflict. These studies provide a guide to mental health services with a relatively small religious population.

CARE FOR THE ZOROASTRIAN PATIENT

The Zoroastrian patient in traditional settings could wear a loose white cotton shirt called the *Sudreh*, and a wooden girdle or cord that circles the waist three times called the *Kushti*. These clothes traditionally provide comfort to the patient, and neither should be cut or disposed of nonchalantly; this is especially important for those in hospital and emergency room settings, as spontaneously cutting the garment could cause distress to the patient (Metropolitan Chicago Healthcare Council 2002). The garment can be removed during surgery or other procedures, but professionals should understand its significance and the patient should be permitted to re-don it as soon as possible.

Body fluids and anything else eliminated from the body can be considered impure and attractive to evil. Thus, personal hygiene remains extremely important in any health setting for a Zoroastrian patient. Bodily excretions should be disposed of immediately (Metropolitan Chicago Healthcare Council 2002).

Many Zoroastrians live connected to Earth and identify with it. Eduljee (2014b) spoke of an interview with a village of nomadic people. They had a Zoroastrian heritage and took care of livestock. They hiked and exercised daily; they collected herbs such as rosemary, cumin, and fennel, and nuts such as almonds and walnuts. Their diet was often vegetable stew. Previously, they worshiped the sun as well. Thus, encouraging those of Zoroastrian heritage to participate in activities in natural settings could be useful therapeutically. This could assist Zoroastrians to live a holistic lifestyle even in metropolitan cities. Furthermore, yoga and tai chi would be well-received for healing. These activities would correspond well with Zoroastrian principles and could help a Zoroastrian gain serenity, stability, and balance.

COMMONALITIES SHARED WITH OTHER WORLDVIEWS

Bahá'í'

Beliefs about following a moderate diet and aiming for complete vegetarianism (although those who eat meat are not discouraged from it) place Bahá'í's in line with the worldview of many other religions. Seventh-day Adventists are vegetarians and that practice, along with their faith and sense of community, have made their locale in Loma Linda, California, one of the "Blue Zones" where people are more likely to age into centenarians. The Bahá'í's also have a strong sense of community, perhaps partly because of early persecution of religious leaders and a theology that practices tolerance of other religions and embraces historical divinity in leaders of many world faiths. Overall, Bahá'í' is seen as a syncretic faith that encompasses all of the great religions of both past and present. Bahá'í's have a millennial focus, defined as having prophets who give instructions about how to live to bring about a divinely inspired plan that will utterly transform life on earth (Wessinger 2011). This they share with Christianity. Like Zoroastrianism, though not ancient, the Bahá'í' movement developed in the Middle East, in the area now known as Iran, formerly Persia. Influenced by Islam, Bahá'í's also practice a fast somewhat like Ramadan, and have daily obligatory prayer. Their sense of harmony, even unity, between science and religion, is quite unusual; many religions view their particular religion and religious beliefs as superior to any materialistically oriented science.

Rastafari

Similar to the Bahá'í faith, Rastafari is considered a millennial religion. One key difference is that Rastafari is centrally practiced in Jamaica, whereas followers of Bahá'í exist throughout the world. Both emerged out of oppression, and thus share some elements; however, while early Rastafari members often were defensive and militant, evolving into three subgroups with a doctrine that led to oppression, the Bahá'í chose an expansive, inclusive, and tolerant view as their response. Following a vegetarian diet is the preferred approach in all three spiritualities of Bahá'í, Rastafari, and Zoroastrianism. Each espouses a holistic approach toward health, though the Bahá'í and Zoroastrian faiths offer greater coherence in their teachings than Rastafari.

Zoroastrianism

Zoroastrianism is one of the most ancient spiritualities, even beyond the origins of the three monotheistic religions of Judaism, Christianity, and Islam. The general geography of its origins are shared with the much later millennial faith of Bahá'í. Because of its early historical foundation, it contains some beliefs which could be regarded as more mythical within its cosmology, such as reverence for fire. The duality of good versus evil, however, is shared by primary monotheistic religions. Sin is seen as creating vulnerability to illness, a concept from which liberal components of modern monotheistic faiths have moved away. The concept of anything emanating from the body (such as blood or fluid of any type) being a pollutant has roots in this faith and seems somewhat unique to it, though other faiths do have the concept of impurity, often applied to women undergoing the normal menstrual cycles. This tradition also has a very well delineated cosmology in the Amesha Spenta; this shows some coherence with Hindu beliefs about fire through the god Agni, the Hindu god of fire, which can purify. Like many other religions, this faith promotes holism through understanding the need for balance in living and good nutrition. Reciting specific prayers is a practice leading to health. Overall, unlike the Bahá'í, this spirituality has a defined view and would have less acceptance of the teachings and health practices of other faiths.

CONCLUSION

The medical and philosophical traditions of lesser-known religions such as Bahá'í, Rastafari, and Zoroastrianism are crucial to advancing our knowledge base as practicing clinicians, educators, researchers, and policy influencers. Because the numbers of adherents of each are small, it is less likely that healthcare or mental health professionals would frequently interact with patients from one of these faiths. However, equally likely is that a health or mental health professional would be less prepared to work with a believer concerning health issues. Understanding the ideologies of these religions allows medical providers and others to enhance their cultural competency, facilitating more appropriate, respectful, and effective treatment modalities. Further, implementation of coordinated interventions can serve to enhance meaning, ethical practice, hope, and identity. This chapter has sought to provide some knowledge to further that purpose.

ACKNOWLEDGMENT

Thanks to Marissa Marshak-Krol, PhD, for her assistance in researching these topics and providing some initial thoughts.

REFERENCES

Bakhtiari, F., & S. Plunkett. 2015. "Family Qualities and Mental Health of Zoroastrian Young Adults (A Lab Report No. 1)." Northridge, CA: Adolescent & Adult Adjustment Research Lab, California State University Northridge. http://parsikhabar.net/wp-content/uploads/2015_Bakhtiari_Plunkett_Zoroastrian_Report_PK.pdf

Baxter, C. 2002. "Nursing with Dignity. Part 5: Rastafarianism." *Nursing Times* 98(13): 42–43.

Bedasse, M. 2010. "Rasta Evolution: The Theology of the Twelve Tribes of Israel." *Journal of Black Studies* 40(5): 960–973.

Boyce, M. 1990. *Zoroastrianism: Textual Sources for the Study of Zoroastrianism.* Chicago: University of Chicago Press.

Campbell, M., W. S. Lofters, and W. N. Gibbs. 1982. "Rastafarianism and the Vegans Syndrome." *British Medical Journal* (Clinical Research Edition) 285.6355 (1982): 1617–618. Print.

Chevannes, B. 1994. *Rastafari: Roots and Ideology* (1st ed.). Syracuse, NY: Syracuse University Press.

Chevannes, B. 2011. "Millennialism in the Caribbean." In C. Wessinger, ed., *The Oxford Handbook of Millennialism,* ch. 21. New York: Oxford University Press. doi:10.1093/oxfordhb/9780195301052.003.0021

Chevannes, B., and Institute of Social Studies. 1998. *Rastafari and Other African-Caribbean Worldviews.* New Brunswick, NJ: Rutgers University Press.

Christensen, J. 2014. *Rastafari Reasoning and the Rasta Woman: Gender Constructions in the Shaping of Rastafari Livity* (Critical Africana Studies: African, African American, and Caribbean Interdisciplinary and Intersectional Studies). Lanham, MD: Lexington Books.

Contractor, D., and H. Contractor. 2003. "Zoroastrianism: History, Beliefs, and Practices." *Quest* 91(1) (Jan.-Feb. 2003): 4–9. Retrieved from https://www. theosophical.org/publications/quest-magazine/42-publications/quest-mag azine/1231-zoroastrianism-history-beliefs-and-practices

Davidson, J. E., M. L. Boyer, D. Casey, S. C. Matzel, and D. Walden. 2008. "Gap Analysis of Cultural and Religious Needs of Hospitalized Patients (Clinical Report)." *Critical Care Nursing Quarterly* 31(2): 119–126.

Dorman, J. S. 2013. *Chosen People: The Rise of American Black Israelite Religions.* New York: Oxford University Press.

Dror, D. K., and L. H. Allen. 2008. "Effect of Vitamin B 12 Deficiency on Neurode-velopment in Infants: Current Knowledge and Possible Mechanisms." *Nutrition Reviews* 66(5): 250–255.

Edmonds, E. B. 2003. *Rastafari: From Outcasts to Culture Bearers.* New York: Oxford University Press.

Edmonds, E. B., and M. A. Gonzalez. 2010. *Caribbean Religious History: An Introduction.* New York: New York University Press.

Eduljee, K. E. 2014a. "Fire, Light & Zoroastrianism." Zoroastrian Heritage. Retrieved from http://www.heritageinstitute.com/zoroastrianism/worship /fire.htm

Eduljee, K. E. 2014b. "Zoroastrian Healing Concepts: Holistic Wellness and Healing." Zoroastrian Heritage. Retrieved from http://www.heritageinstitute. com/zoroastrianism/healing/

Eduljee, K. E. 2014c. "Zoroastrian Priesthood—Dastur." Zoroastrian Heritage. Retrieved from http://www.heritageinstitute.com/zoroastrianism/priests/ index.htm#dastur

Eduljee, K. E. 2014d. "Zoroastrianism Heroes—Shahnameh." Zoroastrian Heritage. Retrieved from http://www.heritageinstitute.com/zoroastrianism/shahnameh /heros.htm

Ellershaw, J., and S. Wilkinson. 2011. *Care of the Dying: A Pathway to Excellence* (2nd ed.). New York: Oxford University Press.

Erskine, N. L. 2007. *From Garvey to Marley: Rastafari Theology* (1st paperback ed.). History of African-American Religions series. Gainesville: University Press of Florida.

Esslemont, J. E. 2006. *Baha'u'llah and the New Era.* Wilmette: Bahá'í' Publishing Committee.

Foltz, R. 2011. "Zoroastrians in Iran: What Future in the Homeland?" *Middle East Journal* 65(1): 73–84.

Gibson, M. 2010. "Rastafari and Cannabis: Framing a Criminal Law Exemption." *Ecclesiastical Law Journal* 12(3): 324–344.

Graham, J. R., and M. Shier. 2009. "Religion and Social Work: An Analysis of Faith Traditions, Themes, and Global North/South Authorship." *Journal of Religion & Spirituality in Social Work: Social Thought* 28(1–2): 215–233.

Halvaei, I., M. A. Khalili, S. Ghasemi-Esmailabad, A. Nabi, and F. Shamsi. 2014. "Zoroastrians Support Oocyte and Embryo Donation Program for Infertile Couples." *Journal of Reproduction and Infertility* 15(4): 222–228.

Hinnells, J. R. 1999. "Health and Suffering in Zoroastrianism." In J. R. Hinnells and R. Porter, eds., *Religion, Health and Suffering*, pp. 1–22. London: Kegan Paul International.

International Teaching Centre. 2011. *The Five Year Plan 2006–2011: Summary of Teaching and Achievements.* Haifa, Israel: Haifa Bahá'í' World Center.

Jenkins, K. E. 2003. "Intimate Diversity: The Presentation of Multiculturalism and Multiracialism in a High-Boundary Religious Movement." *Journal for the Scientific Study of Religion* 42(3): 393–409.

Johnson-Hill, J. A. 1995. *I-sight: The World of Rastafari: An Interpretive Sociological Account of Rastafarian Ethics* (ATLA Monograph Series; No. 35). Metuchen, NJ: American Theological Library Association/Scarecrow Press.

Julien, L.-A. 2003. "Great Black Warrior Queens: An Examination of the Gender Currents within Rastafari Thought and the Adoption of a Feminist Agenda in the Rasta Women's Movement." *Agenda* 17(57): 76–84.

Khalilzadeh, S., M. Afkhami-Ardekani, and M. Afrand. 2015. "High Prevalence of Type 2 Diabetes and Pre-Diabetes in Adult Zoroastrians in Yazd, Iran: A Cross-Sectional Study." *Electronic Physician* 7(1): 998–1004. doi:10.14661/ 2015.998-1004

Khorda Avesta. n.d. "Book of Common Prayer." Retrieved from http://www.avesta .org/ka/ka_tc.htm

Kourosh, A., and E. Hosoda. 2007. "Eye on Religion: The Bahá'í' Faith (Special Section: Spirituality/Medicine Interface Project)." *Southern Medical Journal* 100(4): 445–446.

MacEoin, D. 2013. "Making the Invisible Visible: Introductory Books on the Bahá'í' Religion (the Bahá'í' Faith)." *Religion* 43(2): 160–177.

MacKenna, C. 2007. "A Plea for Broad Understanding: Why Mental Health Practitioners Need to Understand Spiritual Matters." In P. Gilbert, V. Nicholls, and M. E. Coyte, eds., *Spirituality, Values and Mental Health: Jewels for the Journey*, pp. 246–255. London/Philadelphia, PA: Jessica Kingsley Publishers.

Malec, M. 2016. *Medical Marijuana: Hype versus Evidence.* Paper presented at Coleman Interprofessional Palliative Medicine Winter Conference, Chicago, IL, September 16, 2016.

Maloney, M. 2006. "Toward a Bahá'í' Concept of Mental Health: Implications for Clinical Practice (Counseling Research)." *Counseling and Values* 50(2): 119–130.

McMullen, M. 2015. *The Bahá'í's of America: The Growth of a Religious Movement.* New York: New York University Press.

Metropolitan Chicago Healthcare Council. 2002. "Guidelines for Healthcare Providers Interacting with Patients of Bahá'í' Religion and their Families." Retrieved from https://www.advocatehealth.com/documents/faith/CGBahai.pdf

Metropolitan Chicago Healthcare Council. 2002. "Guidelines for Health Care Providers Interacting with Patients of the Zoroastrian/Zarathushti Religion and Their Families." Retrieved from http://www.kyha.com/docs/Preparedness Docs/cg-zoroastrian.pdf

Mihrshahi, R. 2015. "The Bahá'í' Faith." In A. J. Ghiloni, ed., *World Religions and their Missions*, pp. 48–88. New York: Peter Lang, 2015.

Nelson-Becker, H. 2017. *Spirituality, Religion, and Aging: Illuminations for Therapeutic Practice*. Thousand Oaks, CA: Sage.

"Neurologic Impairment in Children Associated with Maternal Dietary Deficiency of Cobalamin—Georgia, 2001." 2003. *Morbidity and Mortality Weekly Report* 52(4): 61–64.

Nigosian, S. A. 1993. *The Zoroastrian Faith: Tradition and Modern Research*. Quebec, Canada: McGill-Queen's University Press.

Occhiogrosso, P. n.d. "Zoroastrianism." Free Resources—World Religions. Retrieved from https://www.myss.com/free-resources/world-religions/zoroas trianism/

Randhawa, G., A. Brocklehurst, R. Pateman, S. Kinsella, and V. Parry. "'Opting-in or Opting-out?'—The Views of the UK's Faith Leaders in Relation to Organ Donation." *Health Policy* 96(1): 36–44.

"Rastafarianism." n.d. ReligionFacts. Retrieved from http://www.religionfacts.com /rastafarianism

Research Department of the Universal House of Justice. 1990. *Extracts from The Writings Concerning Health, Healing, and Nutrition*. Also published in Compilation of Compilations vol. I, pp. 459–88. n.p.: Bahá'í' World Centre. Retrieved from http://bahai-library.com/pdf/compilations/health_healing _nutrition.pdf

Sergeev, M., and L. J. Swidler. 2015. *Theory of Religious Cycles: Tradition, Modernity, and the Bahá'í' Faith* (Value Inquiry Book Series 284). Leiden, Netherlands: Brill.

Setrakian, H. V., M. B. Rosenman, and K. A. Szucs. 2011. "Breastfeeding and the Bahá'í' Faith." *Breastfeeding Medicine* 6(4) 4: 221–25.

Shapero, H. M. G. 1997. "Zoroastrianism, Judaism, and Christianity." Retrieved from http://www.pyracantha.com/Z/zjc3.html

Smith, P. 2008. *An Introduction to the Bahá'í' Faith*. New York: Cambridge University Press.

Smith, P., and M. Momen. 1988. "The Bahá'í' Faith 1957–1988: A Survey of Contemporary Developments." *Religion* 19: 63–91.

Stockman, R, H. 1985. *The Bahá'í' Faith in America*. Wilmette, IL: Bahá'í' Publishing Trust.

Vargha-Khadem, F. 2013. "The Ideas that Make Us" (interview with Bettany Hughes). *BBC Radio* (September 16 and 18).

Wessinger, C. 2011. *The Oxford Handbook of Millennialism*. New York: Oxford University Press.

Whiting, P. F., R. F. Wolff, S. Deshpande, M. Di Nisio, S. Duffy, A. V. Hernandez, . . .
   J. Kleijnen. 2015. "Cannabinoids for Medical Use: A Systematic Review and
   Meta-analysis." *JAMA* 313(24): 2456–2473.
Winckel, M., S. Velde, R. Bruyne, & S. Biervliet. 2011. "Clinical Practice." *European
   Journal of Pediatrics* 170(12): 1489–1494. doi:10.1007/s00431-011-1547-x
Yntema, S., and C. Beard. 2000. *New Vegetarian Baby*. Ithaca NY: McBooks Press.
Zohoori, Elias. 1985. *The Throne of the Inner Temple: A Compilation*. n.p.: Univer-
   sity of the West Indies.

Chapter 11

North American Indigenous Spiritualities

Jeff King

The purpose of this chapter is to share the unique knowledge held by North American indigenous peoples[1] in regard to worldview and spirituality and their associated dynamics that have preserved their lifeways and healing traditions for thousands of years. Congruent with Native storytelling and teaching, I will first provide a broader context in which these can be better understood. Demographic information is discussed first, followed by an historical framework for the American Indian/Alaska Native experience. This context will be referred to throughout the chapter, as it provides greater insight into the strength of these beliefs and practices. The major components within a Native worldview are then presented, with the related wisdom and benefits that emerge from each of them.

The focus of the chapter is primarily, though not exclusively, on mental health and well-being, since I draw not only from research and indigenous narratives, but also my experience as a Native clinical psychologist. Overall, this chapter links how Native communities understand what it means to be healthy, to achieve wellness through spirituality and traditional culture, and how to make sense of and engage with the realities of living in a neocolonial society.

DEMOGRAPHICS

The 2011 American Community Survey (U.S. Census Bureau 2011) reported the nation's population of American Indians and Alaska Natives, including those of more than one race. They made up 1.6 percent of the total population of the United States. Of this total, about half were American Indian and Alaska Native only, and about half were American Indian and Alaska Native in combination with one or more other races (Science Daily 2004). If past trends continue, more than 72% will live in urban, off-reservation, rural locations. Of the more than 200 major Native/indigenous American languages that existed prior to European contact, about 150 are still spoken, excluding hundreds of dialectal variations. At present, there are more than 560 federally recognized tribal entities, an additional 100 or so that have been afforded tribal status by the states in which they reside, and several dozen that are not formally recognized by any governmental entity.

Depending on who you read, scientists have estimated that American Indians/Alaska Natives have inhabited North America for the past 15,000 up to 60,000 years. They may often refer to themselves as "Native"; however, this can be complicated because many people born in the United States of European descent refer to themselves as Native as well. (On previous U.S. Census reports, many non-Natives marked "Native American," assuming that because their families have been here for such a long time, they were Native Americans.)

Geographical regions tend to designate tribal characteristics, albeit there are many exceptions. For example, tribes from similar regions such as Northeast Woodland, Northern Plains, Southwest, or Northwest Coast typically share common backgrounds and languages. However, even within these categories one finds substantial variation in language and cultural tradition. Currently, American Indians and Alaska Natives live in all areas across the United States. The nine largest populations are located in California, Oklahoma, Arizona, Texas, New York, New Mexico, Washington, North Carolina, and Florida (U.S. Census Bureau 2011). Currently, up to 67% of American Indians and Alaska Natives who solely identify as American Indians and Alaska Natives live outside of American Indian and Alaska Native reservations or territories. For example, as part of the "Indian Relocation Act," many American Indians and Alaska Natives were relocated to cities. Currently, the cities with the five largest populations of American Indians and Alaska Natives are New York, NY; Phoenix, AZ; Oklahoma City, OK; Anchorage, AK; and Tulsa, OK, all primarily due to the Indian Relocation Act of 1956 (Robbins 1992).[2]

Historically, the U.S. government tried to wipe out Native spiritual and healing practices through legal suppression; the establishment of reservations; missionaries; elimination of tribal languages, customs, rituals, ceremonies; and use of boarding schools for "killing the Indian and saving the person." It was thought that as long as traditional spirituality and healers existed, Native people would resist conversion to Christianity and full assimilation into White society.

However, the 1970 Indian Policy Statement reversed this trend and called for Native self-determination and tribal control of federal programs, which was one of the first marks of this policy shift (Rhoades 2000, p. 69). In 1975, the Indian Self-Determination and Education Assistance Act followed, directing the Bureau of Indian Affairs (BIA) and Indian Health Service (IHS) to turn over to the tribes management of most of the services administered by these agencies upon formal request by the various tribes (Rhoades 2000, p. 70).

During this same period, government policies toward American Indian religious freedom also changed. As mentioned previously, the federal government had outlawed Native religious practices, suppressing Native traditions through imprisonment, restriction of rations, and military force. These policies remained in effect until the Wheeler Howard Act of 1934 (which allowed, to some degree, freedom in religious expression), the American Indian Religious Freedom Act of 1978, and finally the Religious Freedom Restoration Act of 1993 (GovTrack 1993). Native communities are now increasingly taking control of their resources and social services, and are drawing upon traditional cultures, oral traditions, symbol systems, and relational networks.

Regarding health, research has indicated that even with the paucity of data on American Indians and Alaska Natives, the consistent finding is that they show poorer health outcomes across most health indicators. Native people born today have a life expectancy 4.4 years fewer than the U.S. "all races" population. They continue to die at higher rates than other Americans in many categories, including chronic liver disease and cirrhosis, diabetes mellitus, unintentional injuries, assault/homicide, intentional self-harm/ suicide, and chronic lower respiratory diseases. Many of these outcomes are related to unmet medical needs (in particular, due to cost). Furthermore, it is thought that other factors such as inadequate education, disproportionate poverty, discrimination in the delivery of health services, and cultural differences are related to these health problems. Despite dismal outcomes in a variety of physical and mental health domains, it is necessary to understand the unique strengths and belief systems of American Indians and Alaska Natives that support their lifeways despite living with these formidable challenges. It is imperative for those wanting to understand and/or work with American Indians and Alaska Natives to understand these strengths, which stand in contrast to an extensive, violent, oppressive history as well as ongoing disparities in all areas of health care and national social support.

Given what American Indians and Alaska Natives have faced in the past and continue to face today, much work has focused on the construct of *historical trauma*. Duran, Duran, Yellowhorse, and Yellowhorse (1998) have referred to historical trauma as "soul wound." Despite genocide and efforts under a "eugenics"(Lawrence 2000) paradigm held by leaders in U.S. government and the medical establishment to eliminate them, as well as forced boarding school attendance that sought to wipe out any trace of traditional culture, American Indians and Alaska Native cultures continued to survive due to their resilience and perseverance (Whitbeck, Adams, Hoyt, and Chen 2004). Although no discussion of Native peoples is complete without acknowledging the unimaginable horrors they have endured, this chapter focuses on the spirituality that has made them so resilient. Most of the time, they kept their beliefs hidden from their oppressors. When their spiritual practices were outlawed, they took them underground and/or interwove them into the oppressor's religion forced upon them. This genius provided a strength that endured the severest of hardships.

Although the resilience of Native people is quite remarkable and profound, the current difficulties indigenous communities are facing cannot be overlooked. Thus, while this chapter focuses on the strengths and positive aspects of Native spirituality, it is also important to understand the Native predicament in a broader context. The issues mentioned earlier in terms of health problems, psychological distress, suicide, PTSD, substance abuse, violence, and so forth can be seen as the result of social conditions, both current and historical. Globally, we see the same manner of negative impacts in communities, countries, cultures, and societies that have essentially been deprived of access to resources that are vital to growth and health. For example, these same patterns are evident among the Baltic nations that were colonized by the former U.S.S.R., where their language was stripped from them, their names were changed, their educational systems highlighted the dominant culture and minimized their original culture, families were separated, and so on (Helasoja et al. 2006). This same pattern and outcome has repeated itself in poverty-stricken barrios and inner cities within the United States (Pappas 2006), with the aboriginal peoples of Australia and New Zealand (BigFoot and Funderburk 2011), the Pacific Islander nations (Australian Indigenous HealthInfoNet 2015), and the indigenous peoples of Central and South America (Asian and Pacific Islander American Health Forum 2010).

WORLDVIEWS

For the purposes of this chapter I will use the sociocultural definition of worldview: *worldview* refers to the outlook or image we have concerning the nature of the universe, the nature of humankind, the relationship between humanity and the universe, and other philosophical issues or orientations that help us define the cosmos and our place in it. These orientations are tied directly to the ideological, historical, philosophic, and religious dimensions of a culture. Thus, key elements of the Native worldview are provided here with descriptions of how each is viewed and how each plays out in all manners of living. Within the Native worldview, it is extremely difficult to isolate individual worldview components because they are interwoven and not seen as separate. The reader will notice the necessary overlap of concepts in the descriptions that follow.

Centrality of Spirit

Contextually, and as mentioned previously, it is essential to understand the extraordinarily diverse demographic and individual identity characteristics of the groups that make up North America's indigenous populations. In fact, these populations are considered more diverse than the ethnic groups comprising European countries. It is unclear how many follow traditional lifestyles compared to those who hold to the values and lifestyles of mainstream North American culture. As a result of centuries of colonization, much of "Indian country"—a general euphemism for describing where Native people live—has become Christianized, with multiple variations in how this has played out both between and within tribes. For example, among the Cherokee (as well as other tribes), there are the "traditionals" and the "church-goers." However, among the church-goers, there is a further divide: those who still practice the traditional ways along with their Christianity and those who practice Christianity exclusive of their tribal beliefs. One Cherokee elder exclaimed to me, "Oh, yeah! They [Cherokee Christians] believe in the little people (spirit entities) and in the Bible. They believe in both just as strongly" (Stewart, personal communication/interview, May 26, 1991). Thus, there is disagreement between Traditional medicine men and women and Native Christians as to whether these beliefs are compatible.

Furthermore, there is considerable variation in lifestyle and physical appearance among Native populations. This presents a daunting challenge for those who typically view North American Indians as a homogeneous group. The tendency of non-Natives to group American Indians and Alaska Natives in such a collective manner has been a source of considerable concern among scholars. This type of categorization may be the reason so many non-Natives have difficulty understanding the complexity of the lives and spiritual beliefs of Native Americans. However, beneath this variability there is a shared theme: it is the conviction that all things have *spirit*.

The term for *spirit* in the English language is what the Lakota call *wakan.* Wakan means both mystery and holiness, and is used by the Lakota to designate all that is sacred, mysterious, spiritual, or supernatural. The Muscogee Creek use the term *boea fikcha/puyvfekcv,* which encompasses "all my relations, male, female, human and non-human, known and unknown, all . . . part of a continuum of energy that is at the heart of the universe (Chaudhuri and Chaudhuri 2001, p. 2). Numerous tribes such as the Navajo, Hopi, Tlingit, Ojibwe, Mohawk, Anishinaabe, Cheyenne, Arapahoe, Kiowa, and Osage have similar words to convey *spirit.*

North American Indian spirituality is centered on the belief in a Creator and human beings' unique, personal relationship with the Creator. Creator's spirit is everywhere, imbued in all of life (earth's beings, rocks, trees, animals, wind, etc.). This is not to be confused with animism, in which all entities are considered part of the Creator; rather, it holds that the sacredness of Spirit permeates all things. Spirit encompasses human relationships with all beings. Spirituality is not seen as just at the core, but rather infused throughout all ways of life. These sacred teachings come from oral traditions, some recognized as more than 8,000 years old (King and Trimble 2013).

Unlike the predominant Western worldview, there is not a separation of the physical from the spiritual, mind or body. Attaining and maintaining a sense of physical, emotional, and communal harmony is central in the belief of relationship to Creator and the need to be in balance with all things.

Vine Deloria, Jr., a renowned Native scholar, articulated this fundamental difference between Western and indigenous ways of life: "Indians experience and relate to a living universe, whereas Western people—especially scientists—reduce all things, living or not, to objects" (Jensen 2000, pp. 5–8). Tewa scholar Philip Duran speaks similarly, "Our ancestors lived in a spiritual universe. We are still conscious of it but many immigrants from Europe do not experience it because they do not see that all things are imbued with spirit. The world that the Indian knew was changed after two waves of immigrants, first from Spain then England, brought another culture and disregarded Indian ways that respected Creator's Earth. The [system] that now governs us has no relationship to the land that sustains us" (Duran n.d.).

In Native thought, spirituality is everywhere, imbued in all of life (earth's beings, water, rocks, trees, wind, etc.). While historically this view was seen as primitive and animistic, by simply substituting the word "energy" for the word "spirit" we have quantum physics' definition of energy/matter. In fact, Chaudhuri and Chaudhuri (2001) offer a modern interpretation of Muscogee concepts of the spiritual: "There is, however, a single, unifying principle in the universe that links every manifestation of body, mind and spirit. This unifying principle is energy . . . [It is termed] *Ibofanga* [italics added], which covers everything and within which both rest and motion exist" (p. 23).

Many tribal terms of spirituality (encompassing health, well-being, and social responsibility, etc.) embrace this idea. *Mitakuye Oyasin* is Lakota for "all my relations," implying a responsibility to all that is in the world. *Hózhó*[3] is Diné (Navajo) for the responsibility to live in balance with all of life. Thus, the main purpose in life is for people to take care of the earth and to serve others. Peace and wholeness come through living in balance. Personal well-being cannot be separate from this purpose. In this context of all things related, Native American Indians' spirituality also encompasses the healing ways in overcoming colonization.[4]

Looking deeper into how these spiritual traditions (see Table 11.1 for a brief description) were retained, the Muscogee Nation of Oklahoma possess a "sacred fire" which was given to them in the beginning and has been

Table 11.1 Native American Spiritual Traditions

Sweat Lodges: The Native American sweat lodge has been used for many purposes. It is typically a small, dome-like structure in the center of which are placed heated stones. The leader of the sweat lodge pours water on the stones to create an intense steamy atmosphere, which when followed with the proper mindset can lead to acute focus and openness on the part of the participants. It has been used for purification, healing, blessing, renewal, personal growth, and intense prayer. The ritual cleans and heals the body, mind, and spirit. It can also bring in entities from the spirit world responding to the specific needs of the participants.

Smudging: The smoke from burning sweet grass, cedar, white copal, or sage is used for purification and is part of many Native American tribal traditions. It can allow the individual or group to feel purified and gain a sense of being part of the sacred. Smudging can be used by itself for entering into sacred discussion or a sense of being centered. It can also be a first step for other ceremonial/healing activities, as cleansing is necessary for involvement in these practices. Smudging is also used to cleanse objects, rooms, and to rid places of negative energy or spirits.

Medicine Wheel: The medicine wheel is used among many tribes for numerous purposes. Although tribes vary on the colors and dimensions, the core lesson of the wheel is harmony with all the elements of the universe. The medicine wheel is a circle divided into quadrants, most often corresponding to the four directions, and each direction representing life dimensions (e.g., east represents renewal). These are further broken down into various areas of life issues that correspond with the central meaning within the quadrant. The colors are also associated with these core meanings.

(continued)

Table 11.1 Native American Spiritual Traditions (*continued*)

Talking Circle: The talking circle is a group process that involves passing the talking stick (or feather) from speaker to speaker as a respectful way to communicate and share opinions. Often this involves initial smudging with sweet grass, cedar, or sage; the group leader opens the discussion by sharing a personal experience, and then the group members talk about their own experiences and feelings. Only one person speaks at a time, and there is no cross-talk or questioning.

Vision Quest: The vision quest has been part of many tribal practices for centuries. The core of the vision quest is receiving a vision from the spirit world. Some tribes have used this as a rite of passage for youth, whereas others have used it as part of a journey toward maturity. The "vision" quest is a bit of a misnomer in that it is not in the seeking that the vision comes. Rather, the individual makes himself or herself available through the ritual, but the vision comes from the spiritual world.

Smoke House: The Smoke House is practiced by Native people along the coast and Puget Sound in the Pacific Northwest. Actual practices are sacred and cannot be documented.

Tribal Journey: Tribal Journey was practiced for thousands of years prior to being outlawed and has been in resurgence since 1989. Native communities from Alaska, Canada, Washington, Oregon, California, Hawaii, New Zealand, Japan, and other indigenous communities travel via canoe for up to three weeks. Protocol, ceremony, and "work" take place each night upon landing, and teachings are passed via traditional oral practices.

Rites of Passage: These ceremonies have been practiced by indigenous cultures since time immemorial. They offer collective support, accountability, recognition, visibility, and community acknowledgment. While spiritual in meaning, they also provide a manner in which the community acknowledges the child or adult as he or she transitions into a new life stage. These may include the Cradle Ceremony, acknowledging a child's birth; First Laugh Ceremony, celebrating a child's first laugh; vision quests, which can begin as early as age five; puberty rituals; kiva practices for learning traditional sacred teachings, the ancient language, and transition to manhood; naming ceremonies; and adopting-into-family rituals.

kept throughout time. The fire was and is regarded as an essential part of all life. The fire supplied heat and light for both the households and the community ceremonies, just as the sun supplied the same so that all living things might flourish. For the Muscogee, the sun and the sacred fire within the ceremonial ring (*paskofv*, where ceremonial stomp dances are held) are the same. The fire, like an ancestor or tribal elder, must be treated with respect. When the United States government forced the tribe's removal from the southeastern part of the United States, their homeland for centuries, the Muscogee brought the embers of the sacred fire all along the way of the Trail of Tears into their new settlements in what is now Oklahoma. They used these embers to light the fire of their new paskofv. This story metaphorically highlights what many or most tribes have done over the centuries. They have maintained their spiritual and cultural essence as a people—in spite of forced relocations, invasions, betrayal, the forced separation of children from families, death, poverty, disease, and genocidal attempts.

For many Native communities, spirit and spirituality are "reawakening" after being forced underground (as described earlier). For example, in the Pacific Northwest, the annual Tribal Journey is experiencing a strong resurgence since being reinstituted in 1989 with "Paddle to Seattle," during which a few canoes/communities participated. By 2016, with "Paddle to Squaxin," more than 100 canoes and more than 15,000 indigenous people participated, representing the re-emergence of traditional spiritual beliefs and practices. It is not appropriate to share the protocols in a written document, but the journey is a sacred practice that involves intense spiritual and physical preparation, and during which specific protocols are shared by and with each Tribe/community until the destination is reached. A week of cultural and spiritual protocol is shared and preparation begins for the next journey. During the closing ceremonial times, many will share the personal and collective healing they experienced by participation in the journey.

Others have ingeniously interwoven their spirituality into the fabric of the religion that was forced on them. For example, the Picuris Pueblo have their Feast Day on August 10th, honoring the Catholic Saint Lawrence. Lawrence was known for his care for the poor and oppressed, so this day has a double meaning for the Picuris. Deeper still, this day is also the anniversary of the Popé (Pueblo) revolt that drove the Spanish out of the land for more than 13 years. Hence, the strength and essence of the Pueblo are celebrated and kept alive in the midst of oppression.

Needless to say, Native spirituality has been vibrant, powerful, life-giving, and culture-preserving for thousands of years and has withstood the fiercest forms of oppression, genocide, and hardship. Yet, given these examples, it is still important to avoid any stereotype of North American indigenous peoples in a manner that locks them into a certain time frame, for this has never been the case. One must understand that Native people have always been cultivating change and adaptation, and continue to do so today despite pressure from Western society to "freeze" indigenous people in time in "romantic" or "savage" notions of what it means to be Native.

Relatedness and Balance

Most tribes have traditionally believed that humans and the natural world are inextricably linked in a manner quite different from Western European views. Indeed, in contrast to the Western view, in which humans are viewed as superior to and separate from creation, American Indians and Alaska Natives view themselves as an integral part of all creation. "*Mitakuye oyasin!*" meaning "all my relatives," or "we are all related," is a Lakota expression that exemplifies this worldview, meaning all other aspects of nature are as relatives and should be treated respectfully (O'Brien 2008). This primary view forms an integral part of their health beliefs. Mentioned previously, Navajos call this worldview of everything in life being interconnected *hózhó* meaning "walking in beauty." Sickness, according to this belief, results from the various influences becoming out of balance (Alvord and Van Pelt 1999). Thus, the healthy "individual" among many tribes is not viewed in isolation from family, community, or even the land. Among the Muscogee the words for a healthy individual are *heyv este hermemahet omet, cemvnice tayet omes*, meaning, "This person is there, a person of good repute, around and available to help . . . ," implying that one cannot be healthy without a spirit of generosity toward others. Lakota terminology for well-being is *tiwahe eyecinka egloiyapi nahan oyate op unpi kte*, meaning "the family moving forward interdependently while embracing the values of generosity and interdependence always with the community in mind." In Tewa (Pueblo), the term is *ta e go mah ana thla mah*, translated "This person is of good demeanor, kind and empathetic to the people and generous to those in need, including the animals" (King 2012).

The Western concept of the individual self has made it difficult for clinicians and others to perceive a construction of the self that includes aspects of family, community, and nature (e.g., plants, animals, rocks, and spirit guides). Leroy Little Bear, a Blackfoot elder, has commented, "You psychologists talk about identity crisis. I'll tell you what an identity crisis is. It is when you don't know the land, and the land doesn't know you" (Little Bear, personal communication/interview, June 16, 2008). What is implied in this statement is that self is not an individuated entity among the Blackfoot (or many other tribal communities). Rather, the self is construed as family, community, and even the land. One's "self" is not distinguished apart from these. Interestingly, Abraham Maslow, famous for his hierarchy of needs framework, was greatly influenced by the Blackfoot worldview. What he found during his time there was a highly sophisticated society organized by principles and practices he could barely comprehend. It was a community whose members functioned as a collective, exhibited high levels of well-being and assuredness, interacted altruistically, and discouraged internal competition. In this world, Maslow quickly learned that it was his assumptions, and the systems of thought and practice they derived from, that were truly deviant (HeavyHead 2016).

Another example of the understanding that comes with relatedness is portrayed within the Iroquois spiritual worldview. Their cosmology recognized that corn, squash, and beans were the Three Sisters of the Earth. Because they were compatible spirits and inhabited a certain place and order in this world, they were always planted together. Only recently has Western science discovered that planting these three together produces a natural nitrogen cycle that keeps the land fertile and productive (Deloria Jr. and Wildcat 2001). Certainly, appreciating the sacred and spiritual allows and fosters a breadth of perspective that the conventional scientific model does not. There are countless examples where solutions to a multitude of problems were discovered and woven into the fabric of the village's or tribe's lifeways and thoughtways (O'Brien 2008). Furthermore, this relatedness, as demonstrated by the Iroquois, is not separate from tribal life. The planting pattern is interwoven with its social, cultural, political, and economic realms (Lewandowski 1987). Agronomist Jane Mt Pleasant remarks:

The Three Sisters are prominent in Iroquois oral texts including the creation story and the thanksgiving address, and they continue to play important roles in the ceremonial life of Iroquois communities today. Referring to the cropping complex as "our sustainers" suggests an Iroquoian view of agriculture quite different from that of Euro-Americans. Furthermore, women's prominent role in cultivating these crops and controlling their distribution has had profound effects on Iroquoian social, political, and economic structures. The Three Sisters Mound System can be recognized as a complex knowledge system, which enabled Iroquoian farmers to develop an extensive, productive, and stable agricultural system. As an agronomist, I find that a careful analysis of the Three Sisters reveals a crop and soil management system that is surprisingly sophisticated and rational. (Mt Pleasant 2006, p. 530)

Still, many contemporary scientists continue to think that Native (and other non-Western) cultures have not been sophisticated enough in scientific inquiry regarding the specific problems they encounter, and thus have not been able to make effective strides to address those, and/or that the traditional, religious, or spiritual approaches are inferior (Warber and Irvine 2008). The notions of scientific supremacy within conventional science are displayed when scientists suggest that they must go into these communities and conduct research with predetermined research protocols focused on real or imposed "problems" in order to determine what are being referred to in modern medicine and treatment as "best practices." In fact, this is what has been happening over the decades, with little to show in terms of improving health services to Native communities (President's New Freedom Commission on Mental Health 2003).

Unlike Western science, traditional Native American Indians tend to be more open to the spiritual, and thus pay more attention to and assign meaning to dreams, have visions, see spirits, and interpret synchronicities and other life events as nonrandom (Deloria 2006; Mehl-Madrona 1997; Schwarz 2008). However, they may be reluctant to reveal these experiences to outsiders, especially health workers. Admitting these experiences on some psychological tests can lead to misdiagnosis and/or elevated psychosis scores (King and Fletcher-Janzen 2000). Yet, often these experiences define the individual's current health status, and much will be missed and overlooked without this valuable information. Once again, this speaks to the great need for cultural sensitivity and competence among practitioners.

Well-Being

Balance or harmony are key concepts for well-being among Native peoples. For the Inupiat Eskimo, *ahregah,* or "well-being," is a state of being in which one experiences a healthy body, inner harmony, and "a good feeling within" oneself. For the Ojibwe, the Seven Council Fires of Life mark significant transitions through life stages. These transitions are focused on how to maintain harmonious relationships throughout life's journey. Locust points out that "Native American Indians believe that each individual chooses to make himself well or to make himself unwell. If one maintains harmony by living by both tribal and the sacred laws, one's spirit will be strong and negativity will not be able to affect it. If harmony is broken, then the spiritual self is weakened and one becomes vulnerable to physical illness, mental and/or emotional upsets, and the disharmony projected by others" (Locust 1988, p. 325). This predates Western medical approaches to understanding the effects of well-being and self-efficacy, as well as negative stressors, on the immune system. This way of life provides the individual with traditionally grounded directions and guidelines for living a life free of emotional turmoil, confusion, animosity, unhappiness, poor health, and conflict-ridden interpersonal and intergroup relations. The goal of traditional spiritual beliefs and practices is to provide assistance for the individual to once again find the "straight path."

For many North American indigenous cultures, the goal in life is to live life in a good way. To "live life well" embodies difficult experiences and encourage one to face them with courage and integrity. The Mohawk teaching regarding living a good life is to strive for *Skennen* (Peace based on both social and political consciousness) and *Kariwiio* (Good Mind by getting rid of prejudice, privilege, and superiority) with the outcome of *Kastasensera* (Strength) (Morse, McIntyre, and King 2016). Crazy Horse, a Lakota holy man, is recognized for the saying, "Today is a good day to die!" This statement encapsulates the view that one should never live a moment of one's life with any regrets, or tasks left undone. For the Native person, the goal in life is not the pursuit of happiness, a construct often cited in the literature and seen as a universal (Wong 2013), but rather to live life well—through good times and bad times. Similarly, Pacific Northwest Coast tribal peoples viewed pain as something to be endured and/or overcome through spiritual strength. The predominant theme of well-being associated with happiness may be misleading within traditional Native values. Living life well does not solely include positive emotion for Native American Indians. Among the Lakota, early childhood training as well as the various ceremonies focus on enduring hardship as a means to living life well (Eastman 1922; Strickland 2001). Many tribal rites of passage emphasize perseverance through suffering, which could include days of separation and isolation, fasting, running long distances, and waiting for a vision (Mehl-Madrona 2011).

A brief case study can highlight this dynamic. A Lakota grandmother was raising 11 grandchildren. A local social services agency was called in by the administration of the school that the older children attended because the grandmother was thought to be "depressed" and thus her ability to care for the children was called into question. Fortunately, a local Native American Indian family organization was consulted concerning the family and its closeness to the community. The Native organization arranged for a culturally sensitive evaluation by a Native American Indian psychologist. As there are no culturally congruent psychological measures, the psychologist used a number of standardized tests as well as an extended interview with the grandmother. Although on their face the test scores indicated depression, chronic stress, and poor coping skills, the psychologist reframed the score outcomes by deeming this grandmother as overwhelmed with responsibility, struggling, appearing to be depressed—yet at her core maintaining a deep fortitude learned through her life that despite significant difficulties, one can still persevere. Recognizing the impact of tribal values lived out over a lifetime allowed for a reinterpretation of test data that could easily have been misunderstood. Such a misunderstanding could have resulted in outcomes vastly different for this grandmother and her grandchildren.

While mainstream psychology acknowledges the value of addressing difficulty and trauma in life by embracing positive attitudes of fortitude, perseverance, and growth after adversity (Hall, Langer, and McMartin 2010), most therapies and the psychological literature tend to portray suffering as an anomaly rather than an integral part of life (Miller 2008). This view makes it difficult to address critical issues such as historical trauma from a Native perspective (Gone and Alcántara 2007; Whitbeck et al. 2004). An embracing of suffering or difficulty as an integral part of life develops the kind of character that embraces life when pain is evident, whereas viewing pain or suffering as interfering with our pursuit of happiness invokes a very different attitude that typically involves distancing behavior. A friend of mine whose son died of cancer at age 11 stated, "When I tell about the loss of my son, those who know pain move closer, while others change the subject."

Time

One's perception of time is also shaped by one's worldview. In the view that seeks mastery, control, and domination, time becomes something to be managed and used to our benefit. A Pueblo elder once asked Carl Jung about the White man, stating "they are always seeking something . . . they were always wanting something . . . always uneasy and restless [to get to the next thing]" (Jung 1961, p. 248). The elder was trying to understand the Western relationship to time, where it is viewed in a linear progressive mode, as compared to Native views where time is not a possession, nor does it operate in a linear fashion. In the present time, Native people have of necessity learned to operate within the Western linear time frame, yet there is still a sense or connection to a nonlinear time. The degree to which this connection exists for Native people depends on their level of acculturation. The more traditional the person, the more the connection to nonlinear time.

For traditional Native people, past and future exist in the present. This is not just a concept or a way of viewing life. It is a psychic and experiential reality for the Native. There are many stories and experiences where deceased ancestors manifest themselves to a group or individual. Thus, "the past" is part of the present. The implications for providing help are many, including the Native patient's ability/openness to access the past, and healing from past wounds is made more accessible within this viewpoint. A Native patient will more easily be able to psychologically and emotionally access past experiences because time is not perceived to be linear. However, for the non-Native, linear time may present a block to accessing past psychological and emotional wounds, as it conveys the notion that the traumatic event happened a long time ago and a large gap of time exists between the present and the past. For Native clients with a nonlinear connection to time, the event can be brought into the present more readily. One patient of mine could not remember her childhood because of early abuse in her life. Through visualization, we were able to connect to herself as the little girl who existed before the abuse occurred. She had a very vivid, realistic encounter with her childhood self which included such detail that it brought back images long forgotten. This encounter brought about a renewed hope for healing and reconciliation within herself. For her, the communication she had with herself as a child was very real and very present. Powerful elements of healing emerged for her through this merging of time and place and her life began to blossom. One of the most essential parts of this healing process was the ease with which she was able bring her past into the present and vice versa.

Another facet of "Native" time is that it is seen in a more circular fashion, where things of the past and the future have life, meaning, and obligations in the present as well. Native people embrace ancient wisdom and teachings as well as contemporary approaches to life. It should come as no surprise that a medicine woman would not only have knowledge of her tribal ways, but also perhaps acupuncture or Ayurvedic medicine, and possibly a doctorate in cell biology as well. This intersectionality of traditions and time is evidenced by a Dakota medicine man who told me that in his visits to various traditional healers in Africa, there was a shared understanding of the spirit world and that his visits were full of exchanges of knowledge. It is also demonstrated by the fact that tribal people who have been cured of disease in ceremony will often go to allopathic doctors for confirmation of the healing (Schwarz 2008).

Person

I was once asked to write an article about supervision of counselors in Indian country. The theme throughout the edited volume was "the self in multiple roles/identities." While the editors were well-meaning in their intent, I found it difficult to try to write an article on this theme. Frustrated, I telephoned a Native American colleague (Lakota) and asked, "What is the term for 'self' in Lakota?" He replied, "There is none." Hence, my frustration and difficulty! The concept of self, individuation, autonomy, and self-identity are foreign concepts for many tribes and tribal languages. Yet, the Western system of psychology has defined psychological health as one based on autonomy and individuality. It is this Western concept of self that has made it difficult for clinicians and others to perceive a construction of the self that includes aspects of family, community, and nature (plants, animals, rocks, spirit guides, and so forth).

Clearly, the implications for the focus of understanding Native people are vastly different from a typical Western approach. It is not uncommon for the focus to be on the community rather than the individual. Other themes in therapy may be on teachings from the elders, recognizing what the spirits are saying, determining what may be going on with a patient in the context of his or her cycle of spiritual growth based on time of year and messages received or prayers offered during ceremony.

Maslow commented on what he observed during his time among the Blackfoot at the Siksika Reserve, in Alberta, Canada:

From childhood the individual is made to feel the warm emotional ties uniting him to the rest of his society. He can rely on the help of his associates and is sure of their affection. Discipline is not lacking in childhood, but it is never understood as involving the loss of love. The individual thus begins life surrounded by a basically friendly world in which he is expected to take his place, extending the same warmth to those children who will follow him . . . The personality that emerges can be described as secure, in the sense of feeling safe in an all-friendly world. (Maslow and Honigmann n.d., pp. 21–22)

Psychology has long understood the role of social support across dimensions of coping, mental health, stress reduction, recovery from illness or trauma, performance, childhood development, ethnic identity, and physiological processes (Cohen 1985). Here we see interwoven in the Native worldview these very principles.

UNDERSTANDING NATIVE SPIRITUALITY

The ability to understand North American indigenous perspectives and experiences with spirituality, religion, healing, and psychology begins with a recognition of the limitations of Western science. Staying within the contemporary and conventional scientific grid can hinder one's capacity to see or understand Native American spiritual ways of being. Yet, allowing ourselves to move outside this perspective can open up dimensions of knowing and relating that have previously been hidden from the scientific mind. Charles Eastman (1911/1980, p. *i*), Santee Sioux, echoed these sentiments when he wrote, "The religion of the Indian is the last thing about him that the man of another race will ever understand."

In thinking through the various worldviews present among Native American Indians, consider the following comments and observations. Donald Fixico, a Native scholar and Distinguished Foundation Professor of History, points out that "[f]or Indian people who are close to their tribal traditions and Native values, they think within a Native reality consisting of a physical and metaphysical world." He goes on to maintain that "[f]or the present, the indigenous way of seeing things like traditional Indians is becoming increasingly incongruent with the linear world [of science]. The linear mind looks for cause and effect, and the Indian mind seeks to comprehend relationships" (Fixico 2003, p. 8). These three American Indian and Alaska

Native culturally sensitive statements are echoed by numerous researchers/ scholars who have worked among Native peoples. Former Harvard psychiatrist Robert Coles, in his book, *The Spiritual Life of Children* (1990), tells of meeting a young American Indian (Hopi) girl who explained to him why he wasn't getting much response from the Pueblo people to his inquiries: "My grandmother says they [you] live to conquer the sky, and we live to pray to it, and you can't explain yourself to people who conquer—just pray for them, too" (p. 26). Robert Bergman, a psychiatrist who worked among the Diné (Navajo) has stated that "some familiarity with Navajo tradition has helped me to focus my dissatisfaction with the way we [psychiatrists] organize our work and to see alternatives to our methods that I wouldn't have seen otherwise" (Bergman 1973, p. 8). Some of his early experiences with the Diné may have helped his understanding. For instance, he met medicine men who were able to provide types of healing that Western medicine could not and still cannot provide, including the healing of schizophrenia. He mentions one case in particular:

a woman who had been hospitalized several times as a schizophrenic. A social worker and I set out to track her down to see how she was. We found her father first. He agreed to take us to see her but said that maybe we wouldn't be interested anymore because now she was perfectly well. We said that if she was perfectly well, we were even more interested in seeing her. She was at home taking care of several very active, healthy-looking children and weaving a rug at the same time. After a visit of several hours, we agreed that she was indeed well again. (Bergman 1973, p. 8)

Numerous Native American clients and acquaintances of mine have, over the years, reported visions, contact with spirits (including deceased relatives), and experiences of entering into the spirit world—sometimes voluntarily, other times not. As Bergman has stated, if we do not open ourselves to "see alternatives to our methods" we will not perceive the world in which Native people move and exist.

Many non-Native people view this type of worldview as at best confusing and, at worst, dismissible as animistic, ethereal, and lacking in "demonstrable" evidence. Thus, to discern what is spiritual and sacred among North American indigenous people, the reader must be willing to set aside the Western worldview that divides the world into physical and spiritual and the subject from the object. As stated, for many Native indigenous people there is no divide or separation: all is an integral part of life.

For non-Native practitioners who will be working with Native people, it is of central importance to understand and acknowledge the spiritual realm, ceremony, and sacred quality of places, persons, and life and to do so with the utmost respect and cultural humility. Although traditional healing has been passed down through the generations; not all choose or have opportunity for participation. Individual Native people may be active participants in these practices, but look to traditional healers—not counselors—for this knowledge. Choice of a mental health provider apart from traditional healers is a choice potentially associated with distrust, misunderstanding, apprehension, and the possibility that mental health practitioners may be ignorant of or insensitive to the cultural backgrounds, worldviews, and historical experiences of Indian and Native clients. Clients' presenting problems may be misunderstood, misinterpreted, and/or distorted by Western protocol, resulting in diagnoses and misdiagnoses guided by a different cultural worldview. In addition, a worldview and acceptance that the Creator has purpose for each of us, and that challenges and difficulties are presented by the Creator for a reason, may be misunderstood by a clinician as lack of engagement or resistance to the therapeutic effort, rather than a belief that things will work out as they are intended to. Finally, the mere assumption that the appropriate place for therapy is in a room within a clinic may be difficult for non-Native clinicians to consider, as may be the understanding that credentials or degrees, so valued by Western psychology, mean very little compared to the genuineness and quality of the relationship that the clinician offers. Traditional Native people are likely to be assessing counselors in light of whether they speak truthfully and whether they can connect spiritually or not. It is not necessary for the counselor to embrace the specific beliefs of the tribal person. However, it is extremely important that the counselor hold the sacred and spiritual in highest regard, with respect and cultural humility. Anything less will hinder the therapeutic relationship.

Although incorporating traditional spiritual and healing methods (see Table 11.1) such as the sweat lodge and talking circles can facilitate counselor effectiveness, patient retention, and progress under controlled circumstances, decisions to use such techniques must be made with a strong degree of caution, respect, and humility. LaDue (1994) strongly recommends that non-Indian counselors abstain from participating in and using such practices, asserting that they should not promote or condone the stealing, appropriation, and inappropriate use of Native spiritual activities. Doing so may invoke ethical considerations, as Native spiritual activities and practices are the sole responsibility of recognized and respected Native healers and Elders. Indeed, there is currently high interest in spirituality worldwide, and part of this growing interest involves the exploitation and appropriation of traditional Indian and Native ceremonies without the consent of indigenous healers. Matheson (1986) maintains that non-Native individuals who use traditional Native American Indian spiritual healing practices are under mistaken—even dangerous—impressions, and as a consequence are showing grave disrespect for the indigenous origins, contexts, and practices of these traditions by Native peoples. Furthermore, many tribes believe that using sacred medicine or teachings without full knowledge will bring harm to the individuals and to the tribe. If the essence of a counseling relationship is built on trust, rapport, and respect, then the exploitation and appropriation of indigenous traditional healing ceremonies and practices for use in counseling sessions will undoubtedly undermine a counselor's efforts to gain acceptance from the Indian community and the patient.

SUMMARY AND CONCLUSIONS

This chapter presented important elements and dynamics related to American Indian spirituality and worldview. Spirituality encompasses all of traditional North American Indian culture. It is the organizing principle from which all community activities, knowledge, identification, relationships, practices, and religions are derived. Spirituality is not seen as just at the core, but rather infused throughout all ways of life.

The processes by which traditional Native peoples go about relating to life are drastically different from the processes utilized by Western science and psychology. In fact, knowledge of these traditional ways cannot be obtained through the scientific method or grid. Furthermore, a different attitude and mindset toward the universe in which we live, including living and nonliving entities; obligations to past and future generations; toward one's position in life, power, space, and time are necessary before one can begin to grasp Native American Indian traditional knowledge. Furthermore, Native spirituality and religion are not static, but are, and are expected to be, continually evolving. Tribal or community understanding may deepen and/or change over time and religious practices may undergo transformation. Yet, the essence of tribal spirituality remains the same, the essence containing that of change and transformation.

Native traditional ways and spirituality can be unique to an individual, but in saying this it must be understood that the *individual* is not construed in the same way as Western European culture construes the individual. Rather, the individual is seen as part of the community, and his or her purposes and gifts are directly tied to community functioning. An individual spiritual experience (such as a vision during a vision quest) is not solely for the person, but for the whole community. In light of this, tribal religious practices are recognized as an outward ritual of the communally shared essence of spirituality. This, too, is not person-centric, as many of the religious practices honor the animals, plants, and land that share and contribute to our life together.

It has been acknowledged that there is tremendous diversity among individuals, tribes, and communities in terms of both spirituality and religion, yet common themes exist across these groups. Tied into the cosmology of most, if not all, North American Indian tribes is the importance of harmony, balance, vision, relationship, transcendence, connectedness, humility, respect, obligation, and mystery. While there is no denying the schisms and conflicts that exist within and between tribes regarding spirituality and religious practices, it is remarkable that these values have endured. Further complications have been introduced by colonization, oppression, disease, relocation, the maintenance (or not) of tribal language, acculturation, and the degree to and way in which Christianity has had its impact upon Native peoples.

It cannot be underscored enough how remarkable it is that the essence of tribal spirituality has survived holocaust conditions and assimilation policies. Not only has there been survival, but there has been a growing momentum among Native peoples to thrive and reclaim and allow this essence to flourish and inform our tribes and communities. It is now recognized that the introduction of traditional teachings and spirituality improves treatment strategies in the areas of both mental health and substance abuse. Furthermore, traditional teachings and spirituality have been demonstrated to serve as protective factors in these same areas.

NOTES

1. Throughout this chapter, different terms are used to refer to the indigenous peoples of North America; these terms include American Indians, Alaska Natives, First Nations peoples, Native American Indians, Native Americans, Indians, North American indigenous peoples, and Natives. The briefest of these terms is frequently used for ease of reading and to make the best use of our limited space. Though all these terms have historical and sociopolitical value, in fact the indigenous peoples of the Americas generally prefer to be referred to by the names of their tribes or village affiliations.

2. It is interesting that Central American Indians are not included as part of North American indigenous cultures, as if there were some magical line that separated them from other tribal peoples. Indeed, that line does not exist.

3. In its essence, *hózhó* reflects the imperative of respect and reciprocity as a way of life. When this is attained, there is Beauty and harmony—within the individual, within the community, and within the cosmos. For the Diné (Navajo), Beauty is a word of power as well as a descriptor (Bernstein 2010).

4. Though there is no English translation to fully explain it, the concept of *sa'ah naaghaii bik'eh hózhó* is more commonly known as *hózhó* in the shorthand. *Sa'ah naaghaii bik'eh hózhó* consists of two distinct phrases that together form a unity. The whole phrase exemplifies a model of balance in living. At the core of its

meaning, *hozho hózhó* is about balance. It is about health, long life, happiness, wisdom, knowledge, harmony, the mundane and the divine. For the Navajo people, *hozho hózhó* represents a synthetic and living description of what life on the surface of planet Earth should be, from birth until death at an old age (Drake 2004).

REFERENCES

Alvord, L. A. and E. C. Van Pelt 1999. *The Scalpel and the Silver Bear. The First Navajo Woman Surgeon Combines Western Medicine and Traditional Healing.* Des Plaines, IL: Bantam Books.

Asian and Pacific Islander American Health Forum. 2010. "Native Hawaiian and Pacific Islander Health Disparities." Retrieved from http://www.apiahf.org /sites/default/files/NHPI_Report08a_2010.pdf

Australian Indigenous HealthInfoNet. 2015. "Summary of Aboriginal and Torres Strait Islander Health." Retrieved from http://www.healthinfonet.ecu.edu.au /health-facts/summary

Bergman, R. L. 1973. "Navajo Medicine and Psychoanalysis." *Human Behavior* 2: 9–15.

Bernstein, J. 2010. *The Borderland Patient: Reintroducing Nature as the Missing Dimension in Clinical Treatment: What I've Learned from Navajo Medicine Men.* Paper presented at the 18th International Association of Analytical Psychology Conference, Montreal, Canada, August 2010.

BigFoot, D. S., and B. W. Funderburk. 2011. "Honoring Children, Making Relatives: The Cultural Translation of Parent-Child Interaction Therapy for American Indian and Alaska Native Families." *Journal of Psychoactive Drugs* 43: 309–318.

Chaudhuri, J. and J. Chaudhuri. 2001. *A Sacred Path: The Way of the Muscogee Creeks.* Los Angeles, CA: UCLA American Indian Studies Center.

Cohen, S. 1985. *Social Support and Health.* Orlando, FL: Academic Press.

Coles, R. 1990. *The Spiritual Life of Children.* Boston: Houghton-Mifflin.

Deloria, V. 2006. *The World We Used to Live In.* Golden, CO: Fulcrum.

Deloria, V. Jr., and D. R. Wildcat. 2001. *Power and Place: Indian Education in America.* Golden, CO: Fulcrum Resources.

Drake, R. S. 2004. *Hozho: Diné Concept of Balance and Beauty* (unpublished manuscript). Arizona State University.

Duran, E., B. Duran, M. Yellowhorse, and S. Yellowhorse. 1998. "Healing the American Indian Soul Wound." In Y. Danieli, ed., *International Handbook of Multigenerational Legacies of Trauma*, pp. 341–354. New York: Plenum Press.

Duran, P. n.d. Retrieved from http://www.philliphduran.net

Eastman, C. A. 1911/1980. *The Soul of the Indian: An Interpretation.* Lincoln: University of Nebraska Press.

Eastman, C. A. 1922. *Indian Boyhood* (1st ed.). Boston: Little, Brown.

Fixico, D. L. 2003. *The American Indian Mind in a Linear World: American Indian Studies and Traditional Knowledge.* New York: Routledge.

Gone, J. P., and C. Alcántara. 2007. "Identifying Effective Mental Health Interventions for American Indians and Alaska Natives: A Review of the Literature." *Cultural Diversity & Ethnic Minority Psychology* 13: 356–363.

GovTrack. 1993. "H.R. 1308—103rd Congress: Religious Freedom Restoration Act of 1993." Retrieved from https://www.govtrack.us/congress/bills/103/hr1308/text

Hall, E. L. M., R. Langer, and J. McMartin. 2010. "The Role of Suffering in Human Flourishing: Contributions from Positive Psychology". *Journal of Psychology and Theology* 38(2): 111–121.

HeavyHead, R. 2016. "Abstract for Symposium: North American Indigenous Influences on Psychology." American Psychological Convention, Denver, Colorado, August 4–7.

Helasoja, V., E. Lahelma, R. Prättälä, A. Kasmel, J. Klumbiene, and I. Pudule. 2006. "The Sociodemographic Patterning of Health in Estonia, Latvia, Lithuania and Finland." *European Journal of Public Health* 16: 8–20.

Jensen, D. 2000, July. "Where the Buffalo Go: How Science Ignores the Living World—An Interview with Vine Deloria." *Sun Magazine:* 5–8.

Jung, G. C. 1961. *Memories, Dreams, Reflections.* New York: Random House.

King, J. 2012. "A Critique of Western Psychology from an American Indian Psychologist." *Spring Journal* ("Native American Culture and the Western Psyche: A Bridge Between" theme issue) 87: 37–59.

King, J., and E. Fletcher-Janzen. 2000. "Neuropsychological Assessment and Intervention with Native Americans." In E. Fletcher-Janzen, T. L. Strickland, and C. R. Reynolds, eds., *Handbook of Cross-Cultural Neuropsychology,* pp. 105–122. New York: Springer.

King, J., and J. E. Trimble. 2013. "The Spiritual and Sacred among North American Indians and Alaska Natives: Synchronicity, Wholeness, and Connectedness in a Relational World." In K. I. Pargament, J. Exline, J. Jones, A. Mahoney, and E. Shafranske, eds., *Handbook of Psychology, Religion, and Spirituality,* pp. 565–580. Washington, DC: American Psychological Association.

LaDue, R. 1994. "Coyote Returns: Twenty Sweats Does Not an Indian Expert Make." *Women and Therapy* 5(1): 93–111.

Lawrence, J. 2000. "The Indian Health Service and the Sterilization of Native American Women." *American Indian Quarterly* 24: 400–419.

Lewandowski, S. 1987. "Diohe'ko, the Three Sisters in Seneca Life: Implications for a Native Agriculture in the Finger Lakes Region of New York State." *Agriculture and Human Values* 4 (2–3): 76–93.

Locust, C. 1988. "Wounding the Spirit: Discrimination and Traditional American Indian Belief Systems." *Harvard Educational Review* 58: 315–331.

Maslow, A. H., and J. J. Honigmann. n.d. "Northern Blackfoot Culture and Personality." Psychology Department Brooklyn College (unpublished draft).

Matheson, L. 1986. "If You Are Not an Indian, How Do you Treat an Indian?" In H. P. Lefley and P. B. Pedersen, eds., *Cross-Cultural Training for Mental Health Professionals*, pp. 115–130. Springfield, IL: Charles C Thomas.

Mehl-Madrona, L. 1997. *Coyote Medicine: Lessons Learned from Native American Healing*. New York: Scribner.

Mehl-Madrona, L. 2011. "Sundance No. 2." Retrieved from http://www.futurehealth .org/articles/Sundance-No-2-2011-by-Lewis-Mehl-Madrona-110904-227 .html

Miller, A. 2008. "A Critique of Positive Psychology—or 'The New Science of Happiness.'" *Journal of Philosophy of Education* 42: 591–608.

Morse, G. S., J. G. McIntyre, and J. King. 2016. "Positive Psychology in American Indians." In E. A. Chang, C. C. A. Downey, J. K. Hirsch, & N. J. Lin, eds., *Positive Psychology in Racial and Ethnic Minority Groups: Theory, Research, Assessment, and Practice*, pp. 109–127. Washington, DC: American Psychological Association. http://dx.doi.org/10.1037/14799-000

Mt Pleasant, J. 2006. "The Science Behind the 'Three Sisters' Mound System: An Agronomic Assessment of an Indigenous Agricultural System in the Northeast." In *Histories of Maize: Multidisciplinary Approaches to the Prehistory, Linguistics, Biogeography, Domestication, and Evolution of Maize*, pp. 529–538. Burlington, MA: Academic Press.

O'Brien, S. J. C. 2008. *Religion and Healing in Native America: Pathways for Renewal*. Westport, CT: Praeger.

Pappas, G. 2006. "Geographic Data on Health Inequities: Understanding Policy Implications." *PLoS Med* 3(9): e357. doi:10.1371/journal.pmed.0030357

President's New Freedom Commission on Mental Health. 2003. *Achieving the Promise: Transforming Mental Health Care in America, Final Report* (Pub. No. SMA-03-3832). Rockville, MD: U.S. Department of Health and Human Services.

Rhoades, E. R., ed. 2000. *American Indian Health: Innovations in Heath Care, Promotion and Policy*. Baltimore, MD: The Johns Hopkins University Press.

Robbins, R. L. 1992. "Self-Determination and Subordination: The Past, Present, and Future of American Indian Governance." In M. A. Jaimes, ed., *The State of Native America*, pp. 87–122. Boston: South End Press.

Schwarz, M. T. 2008. "Lightening Followed Me: Contemporary Navajo Therapeutic Strategies for Cancer." In S. J. C. O'Brien, ed., *Religion and Healing in Native America: Pathways for Renewal*, pp. 19–42. Westport, CT: Praeger.

Science Daily. 2004. "New Evidence Puts Man in North America 50,000 Years Ago." Retrieved from www.sciencedaily.com/releases/2004/11/041118104010.htm

Strickland, J. C. 2001. "Pain Management and Health Policy in a Western Washington Indian Tribe." *Wicazo Sa Review* 16(1), Native American Health in the 21st Century, 17–30.

U.S. Census Bureau. 2011. "2011 American Community Survey." Retrieved from http://factfinder2.census.gov/bkmk/table/1.0/en/ACS/11_1YR/S0201//pop group~009

Warber, S. L., and K. N. Irvine. 2008. "Nature and Spirit." In D. Goleman & Assocs., eds., *Measuring the Immeasurable: The Scientific Case for Spirituality*, pp. 135–182. Boulder, CO: Sounds True.

Whitbeck, L. B., G. W. Adams, D. R. Hoyt, and X. Chen. 2004. "Conceptualizing and Measuring Historical Trauma among American Indian People." *American Journal of Community Psychology* 33(3/4): 119–130.

Wong, P. T. P. 2013. "Cross-Cultural Positive Psychology." In *Encyclopedia of Cross-cultural Psychology*. Oxford, UK: Wiley Blackwell. Retrieved from http://www.drpaulwong.com/cross-cultural-positive-psychology

Chapter 12

The Spirituality of the Eastern Cherokee and Ani'-Yun-Wiya Shamanistic Medicine

Kevin A. Harris

"The branch will tell me how to carve it . . .
Each piece of wood has its own shape, which you must respect . . .
In each olive branch lies a flute; (my) job is to find it."
 —*Native American flute carver/artist* (Thomas 1994, p. 11)

The Cherokee, or the Ani'-Yun-wiya, as they call themselves, are one of the largest Native American tribes in the United States today. There is some contention as to whether they are the largest (Ogunwole 2002; Robbins, Stoltenberg, Robbins, and Ross 2002; Sutton 2004) or second-largest (French and Hornbuckle 1997) Native American tribe in the United States. There were perhaps 281,000 Cherokee as of the year 2000 (Sutton 2004), roughly 280,000 Cherokee as of the year 2010 (U.S. Census Bureau 2015), and another 448,000 people who report Cherokee and at least one other ethnicity (Ogunwole 2002), which would make them the largest Native American tribe (Ogunwole 2002; Sutton 2004). Even if more stringent membership criteria are used, however, they are still one of the three largest groups of American Indians today (French and Hornbuckle 1997). Principally, they are concentrated in two areas of the United States today: a small Eastern band in North Carolina, the remnants of the Cherokee who have remained living on their traditional lands, and a larger Western band in Oklahoma, the descendants of the Cherokee who were forcibly marched halfway across the country in a tragic relocation that has become known as the Trail of Tears (French and Hornbuckle 1997; Sutton 2004). They have a rich and varied cultural tradition: an Earth-based spirituality and cosmology that stresses balance and harmony above all else. This worldview typically contributes to a sense of well-being and promotes mental health.

Cherokee culture, however, has come under serious attack. Some Ani'-Yun-wiya traditions have been lost or forgotten forever, while others have been fundamentally altered in response to White cultural influences (Fazel, Wheeler, and Danesh 2005; Garrett and Myers 1996). Throughout history, the Cherokee have been displaced, pursued, assimilated, split up, forcibly marched across the country, crowded into tiny reservations, or simply killed—occasionally by other Native American tribes, but mostly by the dominant White culture. They have become refugees in their own land. A 2005 meta-analysis of 7,000 refugees resettled in Western countries revealed that approximately 1 in 10 refugees has experienced some form of posttraumatic stress disorder, 1 in 20 has experienced major depression, and roughly 1 in 25 has experienced some form of anxiety disorder (Fazel et al. 2005). Similarly, Native American groups have experienced a variety of problems as a result of their historical treatment and the destruction of their culture, including unemployment rates from three to eleven times higher than that in the general population, high school dropout rates higher than 60% in some areas, a median income only half that of the general population, and arrest rates three times higher than those of African Americans (Garrett and Myers 1996).

By far, however, the most serious health problem today among Native Americans in general—and the Cherokee in particular—is alcoholism (Komro et al. 2015; Lynne-Landsman, Komro, Kominsky, Boyd, and Molina 2016). Native Americans have the highest rates of alcoholism in the United States (French 2002)—fully twice that of the general population (Garrett and Myers 1996). Alcoholism and alcohol use disorders account for the four leading causes of death among the Cherokee: homicide, suicide, cirrhosis, and accidents (French 2002). In traditional Ani'-Yun-wiya culture, alcohol was much less potent and was only used in specific social situations, usually as a part of ceremonies, rituals, and celebrations. Moreover, there were social proscriptions against excessive drinking and public drunkenness that prevented alcoholism from being a significant issue traditionally. With the breakdown of traditional Ani'-Yun-wiya culture, however, these customs and social proscriptions have broken down. Much stronger and more potent alcohol is available today, and many Native Americans—including both the

Eastern and Western bands of Cherokee—have turned to alcohol as a way of coping with the breakdown of their culture, their status as "refugees" in their own homeland, and the other economic, health, and social problems they currently face (French 2002).

In traditional Ani'-Yun-wiya culture, shamans or spiritual healers heal the sick, addressing both their spiritual and physical ailments at the same time, treating each person as a unified whole (J. T. Garrett and Garrett 1996). In contemporary American society, in contrast, the care of sick Cherokee is typically given over to secular doctors and mental health counselors, who treat the body but often ignore or leave aside the cultural and spiritual aspects of the ill and the illness (King, Trimble, Morse, and Thomas 2014; Trujillo 2000).

It is the purpose of this chapter to explore the role of traditional Ani'-Yun-wiya culture and spirituality among the Eastern band of Cherokee. It briefly explores the history of Cherokee culture, addresses the role that spirituality and shamanism have played in Ani'-Yun-wiya culture, and investigates how traditional Ani'-Yun-wiya shamanistic medicine has been incorporated into two modern Cherokee substance use treatment programs. The Eastern band is emphasized in preference to the Western band because a greater amount of literature is available on this group, and because three notable authors in the mental health literature—Laurence French (2002; French and Hornbuckle 1997), J. T. Garrett (J. T. Garrett and Garrett 1996), and Michael Garrett (1998; Garrett and Garrett 2002; Garrett and Myers 1996; Garrett and Wilbur 1999; Garrett et al. 2015)—are themselves Eastern band Cherokees. Also, the Eastern band has until recently lived in relative isolation, much less affected by interaction with other Native tribes than their Western counterparts, and thus represents a "purer" form of traditional Ani'-Yun-wiya culture (French 2002).

A BRIEF HISTORY OF CHEROKEE CULTURE

The Cherokee call themselves the Ani'-Yun-wiya (or Ani-Yun-Wiya), which means the "real people" or "principle people" (French and Hornbuckle 1997; Sutton 2004). Other Native American groups called them the Tsalagi or "cave people." The word *Cherokee* is an English translation of this word (French and Hornbuckle 1997), or a Portuguese-to-French-to-English mistranslation of the name of an Ani'-Yun-wiya village (Sutton 2004). The Cherokee are related to the Iroquois and to the Tuscarora American Indians, an unrecognized tribal confederation today located in North Carolina (French and Hornbuckle 1997). They spoke Cherokee, a language from the Southern Iroquoian language family which presently has three spoken dialects. After 1819, Cherokee was also a written language with 86 letters, thanks to the efforts of an Ani'-Yun-wiya man named Sequoyah, who devised the written characters from Cherokee spoken dialect (Sutton 2004). The Cherokee originally occupied 40,000 square miles in what are now eight Southeastern United States: West Virginia, Virginia, North Carolina, South Carolina, Georgia, Alabama, Tennessee, and Kentucky (French and Hornbuckle 1997). Their climate was temperate, with mild winters and warm summers. The landscape was covered with rolling hills, fertile valleys, and oak and hickory forests, and traversed by many rivers (Sutton 2004).

Dress and Appearance

The Cherokee had a light brown or olive complexion. Lieutenant Henry Timberlake wrote in the 1800s that the Cherokee were a people "both handsome and proud . . . they had erect posture and were well built with small hands and feet" (French and Hornbuckle 1997, p. 79). Men wore shirts, buckskin loincloths, moccasins, and belts and pouches for personal items. During the winter they wore leggings and bison skin cloaks for more protection from the elements. Women wore waistcoats or no top, buckskin skirts, leggings, and moccasins. During the winter they wore bison skin cloaks to keep warm. Children wore nothing until puberty, at which time they began dressing like the adults of their gender. Women wore their hair long, braided, or coiled. Men shaved their heads except for a small patch on the back of their scalps, where they wore a single feather to signify their clan affiliation. Both genders pierced their ears, wore jewelry, and got tattoos (French and Hornbuckle 1997; Sutton 2004).

Social Structure and Customs

Ani'-Yun-wiya society was composed of seven matrilineal clans: the Wolf, Deer, Bird, Red Paint, Blue Paint, Wild Potato, and Long Hair (Twister) Clans. Each clan had a mother village where the clan's ultimate matriarch lived. These clans lived in one of 60 permanent villages spread throughout what is now the Southeastern United States; most villages had members of all seven clans living within their borders. These 60 villages were divided into 4 districts, each with a *strong village* acting as its "capital." Each village had a Town House at its center. This was the largest structure in a village. It was either round or seven-sided to represent the seven clans (the number seven also figures prominently in Cherokee cosmology, as discussed later), was often elevated on a mound, and always had a flame burning inside that symbolized the heart of the village. Prior to contact, the two largest villages were Kituwah and Chota (French 2002; Sutton 2004).

Each village had a *White Chief* who oversaw domestic affairs and a *Red Chief* who acted as a War Chief. Chiefs were most often men, though women were sometimes White Chiefs. Women were rarely War Chiefs but were frequently *War Women* (or *Pretty Women*), sitting on war councils that determined battle strategies. All important matters were discussed publicly and decided by consensus. Each adult had an equal vote—men and women alike (French and Hornbuckle 1997). Prior to the devising of a written Cherokee language, agreements were often recorded on wampum belts (Sutton 2004).

In the summer, the Ani'-Yun-wiya lived in rectangular homes with wooden walls and gabled roofs, and in the winter they occupied round homes covered in dried mud. They were both farmers and hunters, but predominantly the former. They grew a white corn (for flour), a multicolored "hominy" corn, beans, and several other crops including squash, pumpkins, watermelons, sunflowers, and peas. They hunted for deer, bear, birds, rabbits, and fish. They used stone to fashion knives, arrowheads, pipes, and axes, and wood to construct bows and arrows, houses, and masks. The Ani'-Yun-wiya were prolific at basketry, pottery making, and gourdwork. As art, they enjoyed decorating ceremonial objects, body painting, tattooing, and wearing jewelry. As recreation, the Ani'-Yun-wiya enjoyed dancing and a variety of types of music, including drums, rattles, flutes, and singing (Sutton 2004). They also played several sports, including stick ball, foot races, a form of lacrosse using two sticks, and a game called *chunkey*—in which contestants rolled a stone down a hill and threw spears ahead of the stone, the object being to anticipate the stone's movements and get one's spear as close as possible to the place where the stone would come to rest (French and Hornbuckle 1997; Sutton 2004).

When a woman reached puberty and had her first menses, she was required to seclude herself from the rest of the village. After that, she was considered a woman and was allowed to marry, though she was required to seclude herself from the village during every subsequent menstrual cycle. Marriage among the Cherokee was traditionally regulated by women. Dowries were not typically exchanged. Both men and women could choose their mates freely, though a person was prohibited from marrying someone from their own or their father's clan, and people were often encouraged to marry within either of their grandfathers' clans (French and Hornbuckle 1997). A man required the permission of a woman's parents before he could marry her (Sutton 2004). After the marriage, living arrangements were matrilocal: men moved in with their wives' families (French and Hornbuckle 1997). A woman and her female relatives were the primary caretakers for children. Babies were delivered while the mother was standing or sitting—never lying down. New mothers were required to stay in seclusion for seven days after giving birth. While in infancy, children were placed in cradleboards to flatten the backs of their skulls, a trait that was considered to be attractive in a Cherokee (Sutton 2004). Most men and women were devoted to their children, though divorce was allowed. If a man sought to initiate a divorce, he simply had to move out of the house; if a woman desired a divorce, she placed her husband's belongings outside her house. In the case of the death of a spouse, men often married their late wives' sisters (the *sororate*), while women often married their late husbands' brothers (the *levirate*) (French and Hornbuckle 1997).

The Cherokee celebrated several rituals throughout the year. The first ritual of the year was the new year purification ritual, which involved drinking the *black drink*, a beverage that induced vomiting. This was believed to cleanse one's inside (French and Hornbuckle 1997). In late summer, when the corn ripened, there was the *Green Corn* ceremony, at which disputes were settled, debts were forgiven, and both nature and society were renewed. There were also many agricultural ceremonies, female puberty (first menses) ceremonies, and dances to purify people. Interestingly, there were no hunting ceremonies in Cherokee culture, further highlighting the importance of farming over hunting. Men and women conducted ceremonies separately (Sutton 2004).

A Brief Overview of Cherokee History Since Contact

The Cherokee had their first contact with Europeans in 1540, when the Spanish explorer de Soto visited one of their villages. Over the next 200 years, they also had contact with the English and French. By 1720, several trading posts had been established in Cherokee territory. The Europeans brought their diseases with them; a smallpox epidemic in 1738 wiped out a considerable number of Cherokee. Over the next 50 years, the Cherokee felt increased pressure from European settlers, who were competing with the Cherokee for land in the Southwest. In 1791, just a few years after the American revolution, the Cherokee signed a treaty with the U.S. government. That same year, in response to increasing U.S. pressure to assimilate or move, they established a Grand Cherokee National Council (see Table 12.1 for a timeline of Cherokee history; French and Hornbuckle 1997; Sutton 2004).

Over the next several years, the Cherokee made a considerable effort to "modernize" their customs in an effort to be recognized by the U.S. government as an independent nation. They founded the Cherokee Nation, establishing a "national" capital at New Echota, appointing Principal Chiefs as "Presidents," setting up both a bicameral legislature and a supreme court,

Table 12.1 A Timeline of Cherokee History

1540—First contact with Europeans: de Soto (Spanish)

1566—Pardo (Spanish)

1673—First contact with English

1682—First contact with French (La Salle)

1720—Several trading posts established in the region

1738—Smallpox epidemic

1791—Treaty with U.S. government

1791—Grand Cherokee National Council developed; Little Turkey appointed first Principal Chief

1817—New Echota founded

1817—Bicameral legislature established

1819—Some Cherokee moved to Texas (Spanish, then independent)

1819—Written language developed by Sequoyah

1823—Cherokee Supreme Court established

1827—Cherokee formed the Cherokee Nation

1827—Constitution adopted, New Echota established as a national capital, women and black mixed-bloods disenfranchised

1831—Supreme Court ruled that Indians were dependent nations

1830—Indian Removal bill passed

1831—Indian Removal Act enacted

1832—Supreme Court upheld Cherokee sovereignty, but federal government ignored ruling

1835—A few Cherokee signed the New Echota Treaty, agreeing to give up their lands and move to Indian Territory

1838—Trail of Tears: 12,000 Cherokee forced march to Indian Territory; 4,000 died

1839—Expelled from Texas

1887—Dawes Act abolished common (hence, tribal) ownership of lands

1889—Eastern Cherokee reservation established in North Carolina for descendants of 1,000 Cherokee who escaped removal

1890—Oklahoma became a Territory

1891—Federal government abolished Cherokee Nation in Oklahoma and began partitioning 19,500,000 acres of Cherokee land

1907—Oklahoma became a state

1971—Cherokee Nation reestablished with 150,000 acres of land

---

Sources: French and Hornbuckle 1997; Sutton 2004.

and adopting a constitution, all modeled on the U.S. government. In 1830 and 1831, however, the U.S. Supreme Court ruled that all Native Americans were dependent (not sovereign) nations, and Congress passed the Indian Removal Act, requiring all American Indians in U.S. states to move west to Indian Territory, in what is now Oklahoma. A later case involving the Cherokee Nation (*Worcester v. Georgia*), brought before the U.S. Supreme Court in 1832, upheld Cherokee sovereignty. Unfortunately, the executive branch of the federal government ignored this ruling. In 1838, 12,000 Cherokee were rounded up and forced to march nearly halfway across the continent, taking with them only what they could carry. Four thousand Cherokee died on this forced march, and hundreds more died of disease and starvation once they reached Indian Territory; for this reason, their journey has been dubbed the "Trail of Tears" (French and Hornbuckle 1997; Sutton 2004).

Slowly, the Cherokee began to rebuild their society in Indian Territory. By 1891, the Cherokee Nation held more than 19,500,000 acres of land, but the Dawes Act of 1887 abolished common (and hence tribal) ownership of land, and in 1891, the federal government abolished the Cherokee Nation and began partitioning its land and selling it to White settlers and developers. Not until 1971 was the Cherokee Nation formally reestablished and given 150,000 acres of land. Today, most Cherokee are affiliated with the Cherokee Nation in Oklahoma (French and Hornbuckle 1997; Sutton 2004).

Approximately 1,000 Cherokee escaped removal in 1838, and lived in hiding, or on lands purchased for them by sympathetic Whites. In 1889, an Eastern Cherokee reservation was established in North Carolina for their descendants. This reservation has remained in place ever since, even while the federal government was partitioning Western Cherokee lands. Today, there are more than 10,000 Eastern Cherokee. Though there are more than 27 times that number of Western Cherokee, the Eastern Cherokee were not forced to live in close proximity and cooperate with the many other Native American tribes in Indian Territory; thus, Eastern Cherokee culture was not as influenced by other Native American ways and customs, and has remained closer to traditional Ani'-Yun-wiya culture (French and Hornbuckle 1997; Sutton 2004).

The history of the Cherokee is not just of academic or historical interest: it is of direct relevance to health-related treatment. Their history has been characterized by *historical trauma*, "the impact of colonization, cultural suppression, and historical oppression of Indigenous peoples in North America" (Kirmayer, Gone, and Moses 2014). For example, Alex Trujillo (2000), in the first edition of the *Handbook of Psychotherapy and Religious*

Diversity, points out that historical challenges to the Native American way of life include multiple attempts to:

1. Exterminate the Native American people,
2. Relocate the Native Americans from their native land,
3. Use boarding schools to change the lives of Native Americans,
4. Destroy the Native American peoples' culture, and
5. Destroy the Native Americans' religion and spirituality (Beck, Walters, and Francisco 1977; Choney, Berryhill-Paake, and Robbins 1995; Trujillo 2000)

This historical trauma is a direct contributor to many of the current mental health problems experienced by the Ani'-Yun-wiya. Fortunately, spirituality and shamanism are sources of great resilience endemic to their culture which have helped the Cherokee cope with mental health problems.

SPIRITUALITY AND SHAMANISM

Cherokee Values

The Cherokee adhere to an ethic of harmony (J. T. Garrett and Garrett 1996; Garrett et al. 2015). Cherokee values include acceptance, sharing, cooperation, harmony, balance, noninterference, family, reverence for nature, awareness of relationship, immediacy of time, respect for elders, and the importance of contributing to the community (Garrett and Garrett 2002). Time is viewed as fluid; rigid punctuality is not expected. Group accomplishments are valued over the achievements of individuals. Cherokee values are family oriented, emphasizing the importance of tradition, sharing over materialism, and reverence for elders. Humility is highly respected; arrogance is disdained (Wetsit 1999). According to Garrett and Garrett (2002), a traditional Native corollary to the American ideals of "life, liberty, and the pursuit of happiness" would be the Cherokee ideals of "life, love, and the pursuit of harmony" (p. 150). The Cherokee emphasize cooperation in preference to competition. This involves showing deference to elders; performing ritual purifications of the body, mind, and spirit; and avoiding conflict with others through ostracism, disapproval, ridicule, and (in extreme circumstances such as murder, child abuse, and violation of mourning taboos) death to those who violated social norms (French and Hornbuckle 1997).

Central to Cherokee values are three life-principles: harmony with nature, connectedness, and maintaining the separateness of dichotomies. First, harmony with nature is a value that traditional Cherokee share with most other Native American cultures. Historically, the Cherokee depended on nature and lived off of it. They viewed themselves not as masters or conquerors or even stewards of nature, but as part of it: people were animals that were little different than deer or bears in that respect (Wetsit 1999). Second, connectedness—the power of relationship—is central to the Cherokee worldview. Not only do they view themselves as part of nature, but they also view themselves as part of their tribe, being depended on and depending upon their fellow tribespersons (Garrett and Garrett 2002). Though not Cherokee, a Rosebud Sioux once observed that "about the most unfavorable moral judgment an Indian can pass on another person is to say, 'He acts as if he didn't have any relatives'" (J. T. Garrett and Garrett 1996, p. 155); the same would apply to the Cherokee as well. Finally, Cherokee believe that it is important to maintain the separateness of dichotomies in order to ensure harmony. Nature is full of dichotomies: day and night, men and women, good and bad, war and peace, east and west, north and south, and the like. Therefore, in order to ensure balance and harmony, opposites should not be put together. By tradition, men and women were kept apart at most public functions. Wartime and domestic duties were given to different chiefs. Women who were giving birth or menstruating (whose blood was thus leaving its "natural" place in their body) were sequestered from the rest of the tribe. Most Cherokee taboos involved the violation of some boundary that kept apart two opposites (Sutton 2004).

Two other principles found in Cherokee values are worth mentioning: the Rule of Acceptance and the Rule of Opposites. The *Rule of Acceptance* is "the ability to accept anything said or done with the realization that it is what another says or does, not what we say or do" (J. T. Garrett and Garrett 1996, p. 23). In other words, Cherokee should accept the actions of others for what they are, rather than trying to change their minds, and learn how to listen without responding. The *Rule of Opposites* is the notion that whatever people do, there is always an opposite, and a person pursuing one extreme to the exclusion of the other may inadvertently end up doing the opposite of what he or she intended (J. T. Garrett and Garrett 1996).

The Sacred Circle

Also central to Cherokee spirituality is the concept of the sacred circle. The sacred circle is a circle drawn between the four cardinal directions: South, West, North, and East. Everything in Nature had four types of energy in it: physical, mental, spiritual, and natural energy. Each corresponded to one of the four cardinal directions: South to the natural environment, West to the physical body, North to the mind or mental, and East to the spirit or spiritual. When the sacred circle was used in the context of healing, it was called the Medicine Wheel (J. T. Garrett and Garrett 1996; Garrett and Garrett 2002).

South is the direction of the Natural, the path of peace. Its colors are white for purity or green for plants, and it is associated with innocence, friendship, and interdependence. Natural Medicines of the South include aloe, balm, burdock, comfrey or healing herb, cucumber, dandelion, garlic, ginger or wild ginger, mints, onion, plantain, and yellow root or goldenseal (J. T. Garrett and Garrett 1996).

West is the direction of the Physical, the path of introspection. Its color is black, and it is associated with adolescence; with the bear, buffalo, or wolf; and with helping those less fortunate. Physical Medicines of the West include alfalfa, aloe, blackberry, blue cohosh, cabbage, carrot, echinacea/purple cone flower, garlic, hawthorn, horehound, peppermint, oats, and the pine tree (J. T. Garrett and Garrett 1996).

North is the direction of the Mental, the path of quiet. Its color is blue or blue-white, like snow and cold wind, and it is associated with teaching, sharing, and creativity. Mental Medicines of the North include catnip, chamomile, fennel, feverfew, peppermint, mullein, passion flower, skullcap, valerian, yarrow, and wild cherry (J. T. Garrett and Garrett 1996).

Finally, East is the direction of the Spiritual, the path of the Sun. It is the most sacred direction (French and Hornbuckle 1997). Its color is red, and it is associated with the spirit path and the sacred fire, and with coming together and honoring the elders. Spiritual Medicines of the East include alfalfa, dock or yellow dock, ginseng, heal-all or self-heal, hawthorn, sage, and sunflower (J. T. Garrett and Garrett 1996).

The sacred circle delineates a space between the four cardinal directions. It represents a balance between East and West, North and South. Similarly, the Medicine Wheel describes a person as a whole. It represents a balance between the Spiritual and Physical, Mental and Natural. The Cherokee views life as a series of concentric circles. The first and innermost circle represents a person's inner spirit or essence of being—their self. The second circle represents a person's family or clan, including their extended family, community, and nation. The third circle represents the natural environment and the person's relationship with it. The fourth and outermost circle represents the spirit world. The Cherokee also believe that there are four stages of life: childhood, adolescence, adulthood, and Elder life. This is the significance of the number four (J. T. Garrett and Garrett 1996; Garrett and Garrett 2002).

The number seven is also significant to the Cherokee. There are seven matrilineal Cherokee clans. Beyond that, however, the *Sacred Seven* refer to the cardinal directions of South, West, North, and East, as well as to the Sun or Upper World, Mother Earth or This World, and the Sacred Fire at the center of the circle (J. T. Garrett and Garrett 1996; Garrett and Garrett 2002). These Sacred Seven form the *Sacred Circle of the Harmony Ethos*, sometimes depicted as a three-dimensional circle, or sphere: South, West, North, East, up (Upper World), down (This World), and center (Fire). In sweat lodge ceremonies, the Sacred Seven are often represented with seven stones (French and Hornbuckle 1997).

Cherokee Cosmology

According to Ani'-Yun-wiya cosmology, there are three levels of the cosmos: an Upper World, This World, and an Under World. The Upper World is a place of order and harmony, where the divine Beings live. The Under World is a place of chaos, populated by ghosts and mischievous Little People that are somewhat akin to the European troll. This World, Earth, is a great island floating in a sea of water, beneath a great Sky Vault made of rock. The island was created by mud scooped up out of the sea by Water-Beetle and shaped by Great Buzzard's wings, suspended from the Sky Vault by four cords attached to the four corners of the Earth, each corresponding to one of the cardinal directions. This World was created because the Upper World was getting crowded, so that Beings from the Upper World could live here. After some time here, the Beings returned to the Upper World, but left behind their images, which became the plants, animals, and people (French and Hornbuckle 1997; Garrett and Garrett 2002; Sutton 2004).

In general, the Cherokee spirituality is Earth-based and polytheistic. There is a Cherokee highest power, sometimes referred to as the *Great Spirit* (French and Hornbuckle 1997). Traditional ethnographic data predominantly described this highest power as female, though in more recent ethnographic research, the gender of this highest power is often not specified. Similarly, Sun is an ancient Cherokee deity with both positive qualities (such as giving people fire and energy and serving as the source of life on Earth) and negative qualities (causing drought, scorching/burning things, and sending heat—fever—into the body) (Irwin 1992). Sun is sometimes conflated with the Great Spirit, though more often they are referred to as distinct deities. In some writings (e.g., Irwin 1992), Sun is a female deity, whereas in other writings (e.g., J. T. Garrett and Garrett 1996) Father Sun is a male complementary deity corresponding to the female Mother Earth. In general, then, Cherokee spirituality refers to many different deities. It is polytheistic, or both polytheistic and monotheistic, depending upon whether the unity or the diversity of the divine is being emphasized (cf. Carpenter 1995).

The first Cherokee were Kana'ti and his wife Selu. Kana'ti kept animals in a cave, and killed one whenever they were hungry. Selu could make corn and beans grow overnight, so there was always an abundance of food. Their twin sons, however, were not very bright. One day, they accidentally let their father's animals out of the cave; now their descendants (the Cherokee) must hunt to get their meat. The sons also killed their mother because they thought she was a witch, so now Cherokee must work and wait a full season in order to grow corn and beans (Sutton 2004).

The early Cherokee hunted and killed animals without respect. The divine animals in the Upper World decided to punish the people by sending illnesses and diseases. Fortunately, the plants took pity on humans and agreed to help whenever people called on them. Now, Cherokee shamans mediate this fundamental tension between the plant and animal worlds. Cherokee people are now also required to show respect for the plants and animals they consume. Corn (a deity) willingly allows herself to die for people to eat, but requires reverence and special ceremonies in exchange. Similarly, Selu, the Corn Mother, allowed her twin sons to kill her, but demanded that they treat her reverently and observe all the proper procedures for fostering the growth of corn, which grew from her body (Irwin 1992). She warned them, however, that "should you forget to think of me and of these things which I enjoin, if you take no heed, but make use of me without remembering my words—I will fling among you Ool-skay-tah. What is Ool-skay-tah? It means disease, distress, anguish, the destroyer" (Payne 1838, p. 55, cited in Irwin 1992, p. 240).

Shamanism

Cherokee religious leaders are called *shamans*. Shamans formed a complex hierarchic priestly society in traditional times. After the invention of the written Cherokee language, many priests began to set down their clerical roles in writing—mostly in small, highly structured texts. Shamanic knowledge was considered to be a closely guarded secret, so few non-Cherokee people (or non-shamans) were able to look at these texts, and those who did found them to be highly structured and cryptic. Few of these texts have survived into the present day, so much of what is now known about traditional Cherokee religion came from Payne (1838), Mooney (1890, 1891, 1900a, 1900b; Mooney and Olbrechts 1932), and Olbrechts (1931), all cited in Irwin (1992).

Shamans preside at a variety of different Native healing ceremonies, including sweat lodges, vision quests, blessing-way ceremonies, clearing-way ceremonies, sunrise ceremonies, sundances, pipe ceremonies, and powwows. All shamans are involved with illness—either curing or causing it. Illness could be caused by ghosts, by failing to observe proper taboos, by failing to give respect to animals that one killed, or by bad dreams. Illness could also be caused by shamans (Irwin 1992).

There are four types of Cherokee shamans: Ada'nunwisgi, Adanisgi, Sunnayi Edahi or Tsikili, and Anidawehi. Ada'nunwisgi are healers or curers, who often specialized in one or more specific illnesses. Adanisgi are diviners who determined the cause of an illness, and who often take the sick to rivers to be treated. *Going to the water* is a common treatment for illnesses, because it was believed that (with the aid of a shaman) rivers would carry away a person's illness. Sunnayi Edahi ("night goers") or Tsikili ("horned owls") are bad shamans, witches or sorcerers who use their skills to cause illness or death. Finally, Anidawehi are master shamans (Irwin 1992).

Shamans seek to heal by restoring balance, using their knowledge and power to eliminate the cause of an illness or to transform a person's dream experience; dreams are believed to cause many illnesses. In fact, dreams are often interpreted as more important indications of the cause of an illness than physical symptoms. One traditional shamanic practice and belief was to gather plants, place them in a sacred hide or cloth, and set the bundle in a river. If the bundle floated, the medicine had been gathered properly and the cure would be successful; if not, the shaman has to start over. Sick people would commonly give shamans a cloth or hide, and often other items such as moccasins, to demonstrate their willingness to give up something to the sacred, thus demonstrating a reciprocal relationship—a balance—both between the sick person and the shaman, and between the world of people and the spiritual world. Shamans are also known to have sucked pebbles or splinters out of a person's body, or to blow medicine over a person's body through a blowing tube, or *go to the water* and let the river carry away a person's illness. A shaman's healing is centrally focused on helping the sick person restore balance to his or her life. In order for a shaman's work to be successful, certain taboos have to be observed. For example, most shamans cannot work in the vicinity of pregnant or menstruating women, since they are believed to have strong powers that could neutralize the shaman's powers (Irwin 1992).

Another characteristic to note is that shamans practice Medicine, as distinct from medicine. In modern terms, *medicine* refers simply to medications, pharmaceutical, herbal, or otherwise—in other words, pharmacology. In Cherokee spirituality, however, Medicine can include medicine, but it is also something much broader that reflects the person's connection to and involvement with a more powerful and transcending spiritual reality. Indeed, Medicine is the essence of a person's inner being and the source of his or her inner power. As Garrett and Garrett (2002) observed:

Medicine is in every tree, plant, rock, animal, and person. It is in the light, the soil, the water, and the wind. Medicine is something that happened 10 years ago that still makes a person smile when thinking about it. Medicine is that old friend who calls up out of the blue just because he or she wanted to. There is Medicine in watching a small child play. Medicine is in the reassuring smile of an elder. There is Medicine in every event, memory, place, person, and movement. There is even Medicine in "empty space" if one knows how to use it. There can also be powerful Medicine in painful or hurtful experiences. Even such experiences offer the opportunity to see more clearly the way things connect and disconnect in the greater flow of this stream called life. (Garrett and Garrett 2002, p. 153)

Thus, the purpose of shamanistic Medicine is to help people understand themselves, through helping them connect with their inner power or open themselves to the guidance of the spirits.

Finally, the shamanistic worldview has a unique and empowering way to reframe mental illness. In several Native American cultures, mental illness is not viewed as pathological, but instead signifies the emergence of a shaman or the birth of a healer (Marohn 2003, 2011). Marohn (2003) recounted a case study where a doctor took a patient with schizophrenia from the United States on a trip to a small village in Africa, where the patient not only lived normally but also became a healer. Bancarz (2014) observed:

Taking a sacred ritual approach to mental illness rather than regarding the person as a pathological case gives the person affected—and indeed the community at large—the opportunity to begin looking at it from that vantage point too, which leads to . . . a whole plethora of opportunities and ritual initiative that can be very, very beneficial to everyone present. (p. 189)

Marohn (2011) argued that mental disorders should be viewed as "spiritual emergencies, spiritual crises, and need to be regarded as such to aid the healer in being born" (p. 173). While this is an ancient viewpoint, it is nevertheless novel to the modern medical worldview in the United States and Western Europe, but it represents a powerful—and empowering—way to avoid cultural paternalism and apply ancient Cherokee views to the modern mental health treatment of the Ani'-Yun-wiya—particularly substance use disorder treatment.

MODERN CHEROKEE SUBSTANCE USE DISORDER TREATMENT

Traditional Ani'-Yun-wiya shamanistic Medicine has found its way into modern Cherokee substance use disorder treatment programs. Two examples are briefly reviewed here: a technique called *Ayeli* and a treatment program called the UNITY Regional Youth Treatment Center. Both were developed within the Eastern band of Cherokee by Cherokee counselors who are modern practitioners of shamanistic Medicine.

Ayeli

The Ayeli technique is a simple counseling technique based on the *Sacred Circle of the Harmony Ethos. Ayeli* is a Cherokee word that literally means "coming to center." This technique was developed by Garrett and Garrett (2002) and involves five steps:

Step 1: Prepare the client using psychoeducation. Discuss traditional Cherokee values. What creates balance and harmony in their lives? What are their goals?

Step 2: Clear a physical space. Have the client move to each of the four directions and answer the following four questions:

East (belonging): Where do you belong? Where do you not belong? Who is your family? Your clan? Your tribe?

South (mastery): What do you do well? What do you enjoy doing?

West (independence): What are your strengths? What are your sources of strength? What limits you?

North (generosity): What do you have to offer? What have you received from others?

Step 3: Have the client move to the center of the circle. Ask the client to think about belongingness and independence, and to move eastward or westward "to a place that represents the client's current state of balance between those two directions" (Garrett and Garrett 2002, p. 155).

Step 4: Have the client face east. Ask the client to think about mastery and generosity and move northward or southward to a place of balance between these.

Step 5: Have the client repeat steps 3 and 4 to represent where he or she would like to be—their ideal center.

As with any technique "borrowed" from Native cultural tradition, there is a danger that the client might see the use of this technique as inappropriate or exploitative of Native tradition. Hence, this technique should only be used with a Cherokee client who is receptive to its use and who can benefit therapeutically from it. Under the right circumstances, however, Ayeli can be a very useful technique to use with Cherokee clients, even if used by a non-Cherokee counselor, as long as it is used in a respectful and culturally sensitive manner (Garrett and Garrett 2002).

The UNITY Regional Youth Treatment Center

The UNITY Regional Youth Treatment Center (UNITY RYTC) is one of only ten Indian Health Service Youth Regional Treatment Centers in the United States—and the only center east of the Mississippi. Developed by French and Hornbuckle (2002), the UNITY RYTC is a 20-bed co-ed facility that provides a home-like environment that addresses the physical, mental, emotional, and spiritual needs of youth that require long-term, intensive residential treatment for alcoholism. Also based on the *Sacred Circle of the Harmony Ethos*, the UNITY RYTC is housed in an old Cherokee hospital in Cherokee, North Carolina, overlooking the scenic Oconoluftee River, and incorporates Native arts and crafts, traditional dancing, legend-telling, sweat lodge purifications, and a cultural/spiritual assessment with the traditional *Twelve Steps* to recovery, which have been modified for American Indians, using *Great Spirit* in place of the Judeo-Christian term *God* (French and Hornbuckle 1997).

Youths progress through five levels of treatment: Coyote, Deer, Wolf, Bear, and Eagle. Except for Coyote, each level was represented on a Cherokee Medicine Wheel—Deer was associated with South, Wolf with West, Bear with North, and Eagle with East. Coyote was left outside the Medicine Wheel, "indicating that Coyotes are marginal Indians who have not yet been integrated into the Circle of Harmony" (French and Hornbuckle 1997, p. 100). At the Coyote level, a client is introduced to the program. The theme for the Deer level is self-esteem and hope. The theme for the Wolf level is trust and care. The theme for the Bear level is gratitude and self-appreciation. The theme for the Eagle level is self-sufficiency as an American Indian. At each level, a client writes about the expectations of members of that level; how it feels to be regaining control; his or her understanding of the 12 Steps; daily journal entries; and specific experiences of trust, being loved, or gratitude. The client undergoes trust-building experiential activities, participates in "Feeling" and "Issues" groups, makes shields to depict what he or she is "shielding," participates in *Stump Therapy* (studying and removing the roots from an upside-down tree stump "to identify inner and outer conflicts among the roots" French and Hornbuckle 1997, p. 104), experiences vision quests, presents skits on specific issues and on how it feels to be a Native American, goes on trust-building outings and Trust Walks, does creative "how I feel about myself" activities, receives academic instruction, and takes communication skills classes. The client also prepares a meal for another group, does environmental activities, uses "Wolf Time" to focus on daily survival skills (taking care of basic needs in the wild), and takes individual outings alone in the woods to practice his or her survival skills (French and Hornbuckle 1997).

So far, the UNITY RYTC has been remarkably successful. Not only is it the only accredited Indian Health Service Regional Youth Treatment Center, it has also received "commendations" from its last two accreditation visits. As a result, out-of-region tribes, including the Navajo, Apache, Hopi, and other Pueblo Indians, often make referrals to UNITY RYTC (French and Hornbuckle 1997).

CONCLUSION

Spirituality is an important part of the worldview of the Cherokee, and hence a potentially important and invaluable part of treatment (King et al. 2014). Whereas Western scientific empiricism overvalues objectivity and devalues other epistemologies, Native American spirituality emphasizes harmony and spiritual balance, or the balance of physical, mental, and spiritual health. In Cherokee shamanistic medicine, spirituality is all-powerful, all-knowing, and all-present and binds the mind, heart, and body to the larger world, so King et al. (2014) noted that "it is extremely important that the counselor hold the sacred and spiritual in highest regard and with respect and cultural humility" (pp. 453–454).

Outcome studies of Cherokee mental health interventions are few and far between. Most published articles about counseling Native Americans, like the two just described, are conceptual articles, presenting conceptualizations and proposing interventions without empirical evidence (e.g., Garrett and Carol 2008). Of the articles that do present data, most are limited to case studies of treatment or program reviews (cf. Brennan 1995; Eason, Colmant, and Winterowd 2009; Lowe 2005). What few empirical reviews have been conducted (e.g., Blume 2016) suggest that "novel, culturally grounded interventions in partnership with communities, in addition to adaptive existing mainstream interventions for use by other cultures" (p. 47), are effective in treating substance use disorders. This would certainly include interventions that use spirituality.

Both the Ayeli technique and the program at the UNITY Regional Youth Treatment Center are excellent examples of traditional Ani'-Yun-wiya shamanistic Medicine developed by Cherokee counselors for Cherokee dealing with alcohol problems. They are both respectful cases of a tradition that seeks "to bridge the gap of intrapersonal, interpersonal, and environmental disharmony as a way of transforming 'disconnect' to 'connect'" for the purpose of "helping individuals make good choices for themselves towards harmony and balance of physical, mental, spiritual, and natural dimensions" (Garrett and Garrett 2002, p. 157). Though quite different from one anther, each represents how ancient Cherokee values, spirituality, and the Sacred Circle of the Harmony Ethos can be incorporated into modern therapy. Perhaps even more importantly, however, they each incorporate the Cherokee notion of Medicine into counseling—a concept which fits well with the overall philosophy of counseling. As one Cherokee Medicine Elder explains:

Your Medicine is your life, and your life is represented by all those things that you have said, that have been given to you, and that you have given others, and it is all that you are. Your Medicine is all the things that you "bundle" together in the form of objects that you hold sacred to the world. (J. T. Garrett and Garrett 1996, p. 11)

The incorporation of such wisdom into counseling could prove quite helpful, to both therapists and clients alike.

> *"If we were able to understand sickness and suffering as processes of physical and psychic transformation, as do . . . many tribal cultures, we would gain a deeper and less biased view of psychosomatic and psychospiritual processes and begin to realize the many opportunities presented by suffering."*
> —Holger Kalweit (1989, p. 80), psychologist and anthropologist

REFERENCES

Bancarz, S. 2014. "What a Shaman Sees in a Mental Hospital." Retrieved from http://thespiritscience.net/2014/06/16/what-a-shaman-sees-in-a-mental-hospital/

Beck, P. V., A. L. Walters, and N. Francisco. 1997. *The Sacred*. Tsaile, AZ: Navajo Community College.

Blume, A. W. 2016. "Advances in Substance Abuse Prevention and Treatment Interventions among Racial, Ethnic, and Sexual Minority Populations." *Alcohol Research: Current Reviews* 38: 47–58.

Brennan, J. W. 1995. "A Short-Term Psychoeducational Multiple-Family Group for Bipolar Patients and Their Families." *Social Work* 40: 737–743.

Carpenter, D. D. 1995. "Spiritual Experiences, Life Changes, and Ecological Viewpoints of Contemporary Pagans." *Dissertation Abstracts International, Section A: Humanities and Social Sciences* 55(9-A): 2866.

Choney, S. K., E. Berryhill-Paake, and R. R. Robbins. 1995. "The Acculturation of American Indians: Developing Frameworks for Research and Practice." In J. G. Ponterotto, J. M. Casas, L. A. Suzuki, and C. M. Alexander, eds., *Handbook of Multicultural Counseling*, pp. 73–92. Thousand Oaks, CA: Sage.

Eason, A., S. Colmant, and C. Winterowd. 2009. "Sweat Therapy Theory, Practice, and Efficacy." *Journal of Experiential Education* 32: 121–136.

Fazel, M., J. Wheeler, and J. Danesh. 2005. "Prevalence of Serious Mental Disorder in 7000 Refugees Resettled in Western Countries: A Systematic Review." *Lancet* 365: 234–239.

French, L. A. 2002. "Indians and Substance Abuse: The Major Clinical Issue." In L. A. French, ed., *Counseling American Indians*, pp. 1–25. Lanham, MD: University Press of America.

French, L. A., and J. Hornbuckle. 1997. "The Cherokee Cultural Therapy Model." In L. A. French, ed., *Counseling American Indians*, pp. 77–110. Lanham, MD: University Press of America.

Garrett, J. T., and M. Garrett. 1996. *Medicine of the Cherokee: The Way of Right Relationship*. Santa Fe, NM: Bear & Co.

Garrett, M. T. 1998. *Walking on the Wind: Cherokee Teachings for Healing Through Harmony and Balance.* Santa Fe, NM: Bear & Co.

Garrett, M. T., and J. J. Carol. 2008. "Mending the Broken Circle: Treatment of Substance Dependence among Native Americans." *Journal of Counseling and Development* 78(2000): 379–388.

Garrett, M. T., and J. T. Garrett. 2002. "'Ayeli': Centering Technique Based on Cherokee Spiritual Traditions." *Counseling and Values* 46: 149–158.

Garrett, M. T., and J. E. Myers. 1996. "The Rule of Opposites: A Paradigm for Counseling Native Americans." *Journal of Multicultural Counseling & Development* 24: 89–104.

Garrett, M. T., and M. P. Wilbur. 1999. "Does the Worm Live in the Ground?: Reflections on Native American Spirituality." *Journal of Multicultural Counseling and Development* 27: 193–206.

Garrett, M. T., C. Williams, R. Curtis, I. T. Brown, T. A. A. Portman, and M. Parrish. 2015. "Native American Spiritualities and Pastoral Counseling." In E. A. Maynard and J. L. Snodgrass, eds., *Understanding Pastoral Counseling*, pp. 303–325. New York: Springer.

Irwin, L. 1992. "Cherokee Healing: Myth, Dreams, and Medicine." *American Indian Quarterly* 16: 237–257.

Kalweit, H. 1989. "When Insanity Is a Blessing." In S. Grof and C. Grof, eds., *Spiritual Emergency: When Personal Transformation Becomes a Crisis*, pp. 77–98. New York: Jeremy P. Tarcher/Putnam.

King, J., J. E. Trimble, G. S. Morse, and L. R. Thomas. 2014. "North American Indian and Alaska Native Spirituality and Psychotherapy." In P. S. Richards and A. E. Bergin, eds., *Handbook of Psychotherapy and Religious Diversity* (2nd ed.), pp. 451–472. Washington, DC: American Psychological Association.

Kirmayer, L. J., J. P. Gone, and J. Moses. 2014. "Rethinking Historical Trauma." *Transcultural Psychiatry* 51: 299–319. doi:10.1177/1363461514536358

Komro, K. A., M. D. Livingston, T. K. Kominsky, B. J. Livingston, B. A. Garrett, M. M. Molina, and M. L. Boyd. 2015. "Fifteen-Minute Comprehensive Alcohol Risk Survey: Reliability and Validity across American Indian and White Adolescents." *Journal of Studies on Alcohol & Drugs* 76: 133–142.

Lowe, J. 2005. "Being Influenced: A Cherokee Way of Mentoring." *Journal of Cultural Diversity* 12: 37–49.

Lynne-Landsman, S. D., K. A. Komro, T. K. Kominsky, M. L. Boyd, and M. M. Molina. 2016. "Early Trajectories of Alcohol and Other Substance Use among Youth from Rural Communities Within the Cherokee Nation." *Journal of Studies on Alcohol and Drugs* 77: 238–248. doi:10.15288/jsad .2016.77.238

Marohn, S. 2003. "The Natural Medicine Guide to Schizophrenia." Charlottesville, VA: Hampton Roads.

Marohn, S. 2011. "The Natural Medicine Guide to Bipolar Disorder." Charlottesville, VA: Hampton Roads.

Ogunwole, S. U. 2002, February. "The American Indian and Alaska Native Population: 2000." Issued by U.S. Census Bureau. Retrieved from http://www.census.gov/prod/2002pubs/c2kbr01-15.pdf

Robbins, R., C. Stoltenberg, S. Robbins, and J. M. Ross. 2002. "Marital Satisfaction and Cherokee Language Fluency." *Measurement and Evaluation in Counseling and Development* 35: 27–34.

Sutton, M. Q. 2004. "The Cherokee: A Southeastern Case Study." In M. Q. Sutton, ed., *An Introduction to Native North America* (2nd ed.), pp. 349–359. Boston: Pearson Education.

Thomas, F. N. 1994. "Solution-Oriented Supervision: The Coaxing of Expertise." *The Family Journal* 2: 11–18.

Trujillo, A. 2000. "Psychotherapy with Native Americans: A View into the Role of Religion and Spirituality." In P. S. Richards and A. E. Bergin, eds., *Handbook of Psychotherapy and Religious Diversity*, pp. 445–466. Washington, DC: American Psychological Association.

U.S. Census Bureau. 2015. "ACS Demographic and Housing Estimates: 2011–2015 American Community Survey 5-Year Estimates." Retrieved from https://factfinder.census.gov/faces/tableservices/jsf/pages/productview.xhtml?pid=ACS_15_5YR_DP05&src=pt

Wetsit, D. 1999. "Effective Counseling with American Indian Students." In K. G. Swisher and J. Tippeconnic, eds., *Next Steps: Research and Practice to Advance Indian Education*, pp. 179–200 (ED427910). n.p.: ERIC Clearinghouse.

Chapter 13

Agnostic, Atheistic, and Nonreligious Orientations

Karen Hwang and Ryan T. Cragun

The last decade or so has seen a great deal of research on the association between religion, spirituality, and medical outcomes. This research has not been without controversy in terms of methodological and analytical issues. One under-researched area concerns the increasingly visible subpopulation of individuals who identify themselves as "nonreligious," a group that includes atheists, agnostics, and individuals who believe in god(s) to varying degrees but do not identify with one particular religion. As a result, relatively little is known about the health and quality of life within this group, particularly in comparison to religious individuals. We begin by providing definitions and demographic information on the nonreligious, then explore two topics related to nonreligion and health: (1) reasons for the neglect of nonreligious individuals and reasons for increasing attention to them; and (2) what the current research does indicate about the nonreligious, particularly about affirmatively nonreligious individuals (i.e., atheists) in contrast to passively nonreligious individuals (i.e., the religiously indifferent).

INTRODUCTION

The topic of religion and health has been the focus of much empirical research, particularly within the past two decades, but the health and well-being of atheists, agnostics, humanists, the nonreligious, and other secular individuals has received much less attention (Hwang 2008; Hwang, Hammer, and Cragun 2011). This situation is, however, beginning to change, with more attention being given to this topic (*see* Hayward, Krause, Ironson, Hill, and Emmons 2016). There are a few reasons why research on the health of nonreligious individuals has been limited to date, including the relatively low number of atheists in the general population, the relative lack of interest in atheists on the part of researchers, and the implicit stereotypes many people hold about atheists.

Definitions

Broadly speaking, *nonreligious* refers to anything that is not part of the domain of religion but is related to that domain (Cragun 2016; Lee 2012; Quack 2014). Given that the domain of religion is constantly in flux, that means the domain of nonreligion is likewise constantly in flux (Cragun 2016). Despite the flexibility of what is meant by "nonreligion" or "nonreligious," in this chapter, when we refer to nonreligious individuals we are placing individuals into that category on the basis of their self-reported nonidentification with a religion: that is, nonreligious individuals report having no religious affiliation.

Within (and without) the nonreligious population is another group of individuals of interest in this chapter: atheists. At its most basic level, the word *atheist* refers to a person who is without ("a-") belief in a god or gods ("theism"). Atheism is, then, a belief (or lack thereof) and not an affiliation. However, "atheist" is often used as a self-identifier and is sometimes reported by individuals when asked their religious affiliation, even though it is not one (Kosmin, Keysar, Cragun, and Navarro-Rivera 2009). Some scholars have noted that there are multiple ways to be an atheist (Cragun 2015). Variations among the godless range from strong or positive atheism, which is the denial of the existence of gods; to weak or negative atheism, which is nonbelief typically due to lack of awareness (*see* Cragun 2013, and Cragun and Hammer 2011 for discussions of this idea). A point of clarification may also be in order here. Atheists may not necessarily be anticlerical or antireligious. A subgroup of atheists—New Atheists—do tend to be anticlerical and antireligious, but many atheists are keen to work with liberally religious people as well (Langston, Hammer, and Cragun 2015).

Like the term "atheist," *agnostic* is often used erroneously. Like "atheist," it can be understood based on its constituent parts; "a-" means without and "gnosis" means knowledge. Thus, agnostics are individuals without knowledge on a specific topic—in this case, knowledge about a god or gods. Agnosticism is properly understood to be a position vis-à-vis belief in a god or gods which states that knowledge about such gods cannot be attained. Using this definition, someone can be both an atheist (lacking belief in a god) and an agnostic (don't believe knowledge about a god is discernible), leading to an agnostic atheist who does not hold a belief in a god or gods but also does not believe that knowledge about a god is possible. Likewise, someone could be a theist and an agnostic, holding a belief in an unknowable god. However, "agnostic" is more commonly used to describe individuals who are unsure about their belief in a god or higher power. Technically, this would be theistic or atheistic uncertainty, but that is not how it is commonly used (Kosmin and Keysar 2007). We will use *agnostic* throughout this chapter to describe both individuals who do not believe knowledge about a god is attainable and those who are uncertain in their belief regarding a god or higher power.

There are a number of other terms that are regularly used to describe nonreligious individuals, like "humanist" (individuals who adhere to humanistic principles; see later in this chapter), "freethinker" (individuals who refuse to allow organized religion to influence their beliefs and values), and "secular" (that which is not religious). We will occasionally use these terms throughout this chapter. It is worth noting that it is not uncommon to use "secular" and "nonreligious" interchangeably, even though they are not perfectly synonymous (*see* Lee 2012).

SIZE AND DEMOGRAPHICS

Although a lot of media attention has focused on nonreligious individuals who identify as "New Atheists" (e.g., Richard Dawkins, Christopher Hitchens, etc.; *see* Tomlin and Bullivant 2016), these individuals make up only a small subset of the nonreligious population (Cragun 2014). Individuals self-identifying as nonreligious can range quite widely in beliefs and identifications. According to the Pew Research Center (2015), the number of nonbelievers worldwide is estimated to be about 1.13 billion people. The greatest concentrations of atheists outside of China occur in richer, industrialized democracies such as Japan, Canada, and most of Europe, and are lowest in South America, Africa, and the Middle East (Zuckerman 2007). It is difficult to forecast the future growth of the nonreligious, but there appear to be two concurrent trends: rates of belief within developed countries are falling, while the numbers of religious believers worldwide is increasing, due largely to higher birth rates in highly religious countries (Pew Research Center 2015).

Among developed countries, the United States remains something of an anomaly, with somewhat lower rates of both nonreligion and atheism; in the United States, between 3% and 7% are atheists (Kosmin and Keysar

2007; Pew Forum on Religion 2012). However, when you include the other nontheistic perspectives on a god, the number is much larger. For instance, in the latest wave of the General Social Survey (GSS; Smith, Marsden, and Kim 2014), just 58% of Americans reported believing in a personal God without any doubts; 3.4% reported not believing (i.e., atheists), 5.6% reported not believing there is a way to find out (i.e., hard agnostic), 12.5% reported believing in a higher power but not a personal God (i.e., deism), and 20% reported believing in a God, but doubting their belief (i.e., soft agnosticism or theistic uncertainty). The variation among the nonreligious notwithstanding, they increased in number from about 14 million to 34 million adults between 1990 and 2008 and arguably include as many as 65 million American adults as of 2015 (Pew Research Center 2015). In Kosmin et al.'s study (2009), "atheists" made up 7% of the nonreligious population; agnostics accounted for 35%, deists for 24%, and theists accounted for 27% (7% either refused to answer the question or said they didn't know). In the 2014 GSS, 14% of the nonreligious were atheists, 19% were soft agnostics, 30% reported believing in a higher power, 16% reported believing sometimes or having doubts, and 21% reported believing in a God.

Demographically, prior research has found that the nonreligious are disproportionately male, young, and more likely to be single and never married (though this last characteristic is largely due to their young ages; *see* Kosmin et al. 2009; Baker and Smith 2015). Nonreligious Americans are also more likely to be non-Hispanic Whites, though nonreligion is growing among almost all racial and ethnic groups in the United States (the one exception appears to be Native Americans; *see* Sherkat 2014). In previous decades, the nonreligious were better educated than many other groups (Roof and McKinney 1987). However, as the nonreligious population has grown over the last 20 years, it has increasingly come to look like the rest of the U.S. population. For instance, as of 2014, nonreligious Americans do not differ significantly in their educational attainment or income from Protestants or Catholics (Baker and Smith 2015; Sherkat 2014). However, atheists remain better educated than the average American and have higher incomes (Baker and Smith 2015); likewise, the gender imbalance is more pronounced among American atheists than it is among the nonreligious. Additionally, nonreligious individuals are increasingly likely to have been raised by nonreligious parents (Merino 2011), are less likely to have attended religious services as children, are more likely to associate with nonreligious peer groups and marry nonreligious spouses (Baker and Smith 2009, 2015), and are increasingly likely to report little or no religious emphasis during their childhoods (Hunsberger 2006).

Politically, a majority of both the nonreligious and atheists identify as left-leaning, mostly aligning with Democrats or as political independents. Both groups are significantly less likely to identify as Republicans compared to the rest of the population. Atheists and nonreligious individuals are more likely to live in the West and Northeast than in the South (Bainbridge 2005; Beit-Hallahmi and Argyle 1997; Hayes 2000; James and Wells 2002; Jenks 1986).

WHY RESEARCH ON THE HEALTH OF THE NONRELIGIOUS IS LIMITED

The impact of religion and spirituality on physical and psychosocial well-being is an increasingly well-developed area of scholarly interest. Numerous studies have reported an association between religion/spirituality and aspects of physical and psychological well-being (Koenig, McCullough, and Larson 2001). However, nonreligious individuals in these studies have largely been ignored or been treated in methodologically dubious ways. For instance, as noted earlier, the category of nonreligious persons encompasses a variety of beliefs, from antireligious atheists to spiritual but not religious believers. Collectively, such individuals are a heterogeneous comparison group. Comparing religious groups to such a homogeneous collection of people makes it difficult to draw any meaningful conclusions.

Another way in which prior research on the religion/health linkage is problematic is that, like religion, many nonreligious systems can be regarded as an orienting worldview that is consciously chosen by its adherents (Whitley 2010). For instance, there has been relatively little research dealing with the impact of atheism—especially affirmative atheism—on physical and mental health (Hwang, Hammer, and Cragun 2011; for an exception, *see* Galen and Kloet 2010). The data that do exist are often fraught with biases and assumptions regarding nonreligious individuals (*cf.* Bradshaw, Ellison, and Flannely 2008; Ecklund 2010; Reis, Baumiller, Scrivener, Yager, and Warren 2007), such as assuming a direct and causal association between secularity and health deficits based on purely correlational findings, or interpreting an individual's atheism as an indication of anger, rebellion, or spiritual conflict (Exline and Martin 2005) rather than its own stable and cohesive worldview.

Another impediment to prior research is poor measures of secularity (i.e., how secular people are). Although there are many survey measures designed to assess religious or spiritual development (Hill and Hood 1999), there is a marked lack of assessment measures that can accurately capture the range and depth of worldviews held by nonreligious individuals (Cragun, Hammer, and Nielsen 2015; Hwang, Hammer, and Cragun 2011).

Current measures of religiosity and spirituality typically measure these concepts in terms of "high" to "low," failing to make it possible for affirmatively nonreligious individuals to answer the questions in the measures (*see* Cragun, Hammer, and Nielsen 2015, for a lengthy discussion of this problem; *see also* Hall, Meador, and Koenig 2008; Hall, Koenig, and Meador 2008). As a result, it is impossible, using most such measures, to provide an accurate enough picture of people at the low end of religiosity/spirituality scales to differentiate between the religiously or spiritually troubled and affirmatively nonreligious individuals. Research in very recent years has begun to develop measures that allow for clearer differentiation between the affirmatively nonreligious and the affirmatively religious (Cragun, Hammer, and Nielsen 2015), and there is now some research on secular identity development (Smith 2010) as well as a new measure of secular identities (Schnell 2015). However, research using these measures to evaluate the health of nonreligious individuals in comparison to religious individuals is just now beginning to come out (Cragun and Sumerau 2017).

Another problem limiting research on the nonreligious is that definitions of terms like "religious" or "spiritual" vary from individual to individual and there is no way to determine if the measurement instruments are capturing the same concepts for all individuals. Many researchers also rely on proxy variables such as attending religious services—a participation dimension that may or may not reflect actual beliefs (Hoge 1981; Sherkat 2008). Furthermore, investigators are sometimes too quick to assume causation from correlation, without considering other explanations (e.g., only relatively healthy individuals are able to go to church; *see* Sloan 2006). The bulk of the existing research on the religion/spirituality-health connection has also concentrated largely on followers of mainstream Judeo-Christian faiths, with little attention devoted to adherents of minority religions (Kier and Davenport 2004).

Another problem with prior research is that the benefits of religious involvement seem limited to those living in highly religious areas. Stavrova (2015) found that in countries in which religiosity represents a social norm (i.e., it is common and socially desirable), religious individuals report better subjective health than nonreligious individuals, and that, even within the United States, the association of religiosity with self-rated health as well as with reduced mortality largely depends on the regional level of religiosity. This suggests that the health and longevity benefits of religiosity are restricted to highly religious regions. One further shortcoming of the religion/health literature is a lack of inclusion of explicitly atheistic control subjects, or treating such individuals as statistical outliers (Hwang et al. 2011). This may be due to low participation by atheistic individuals, or inability of many assessment instruments used to measure affirmative secularity.

HEALTH AND NONRELIGION

The purported link between religion/spirituality and health has led to some speculation that reverse coding of existing measures of religiosity would reveal a "small, robust health liability" associated with exclusively secular individuals (Hall, Koenig, and Meador 2008). However, many of these instruments measure only "high" to "low" religiosity. As a result, they offer little or no information with regard to affirmatively secular individuals, or differences between atheists, agnostics, and other nonreligious subgroups, and thus lead to the erroneous conclusion that disavowing religious or spiritual beliefs must be somehow pathological. Suggestions about poor health outcomes among the nonreligious are largely unsupported by studies that deal with explicitly nonreligious individuals. The bulk of existing research does not find any significant difference between religious and secular individuals on measures of general health (D. L. Cragun, Cragun, Nathan, Sumerau, and Nowakowski 2016; Hayward et al. 2016; Koenig 1995; Speed and Fowler 2016), death anxiety (Feifel 1974), or coping with illness or disability (Makros and McCabe 2003). In their meta-analysis of 60 published studies, Hayward et al. (2016) found no significant group differences, as determined by nonoverlap of 95% confidence intervals, in subjective health, positive affect, humility, illicit drug use, or exercise between atheists, agnostics, and religious affiliates (in contrast to Gillum 2005; and Newport, Agrawal, and Witters 2010).

Speed (2017) examined the relationship between religion/spirituality, happiness, and self-rated health. Results indicated that religion/spirituality was not associated with salutary effects for all persons, and that whether a person believed in god(s), and how confident the person was in god(s)' existence, influenced his or her experience with religion/spirituality. An implication of this study is that an atheist who is confident and coherent in his or her belief system reaps the same salutary benefits from that system that religious believers experience from theirs.

Compared to religious believers, atheists are less dogmatic, less authoritarian (Galen 2009), and less likely to be obese (Cline and Ferraro 2006). In addition, religiously unaffiliated individuals have been shown to have lower average Body Mass Index (BMI), fewer mean limitations on activities of daily living (ADLs), and report suffering fewer chronic conditions than religiously affiliated individuals.

Complicating these findings are a few studies that have focused less on the affirmatively irreligious and more on individuals who switch religions. *Switching* refers to moving from either one religious group to another or leaving religion altogether. Of particular interest is switching from high-cost groups that are theologically and culturally exclusive, such as Jehovah's

Witnesses or Mormons. Data from 1972 through 2006 in the GSS reveal that people who are raised and stay in high-cost sectarian groups have better self-reported health than those raised and staying in other religious traditions, but people who leave such groups are more likely to report worse health than those who leave other groups (Scheitle and Adamczyk 2010). Some investigators (Exline et al. 2011) have proposed that, at least for some atheists, rejection of religion results from anger at God, largely shaped by problematic attachment relationships with parents (though atheists are not disproportionately likely to have poor attachments with their parents; *see* Pasquale 2010). In these studies, samples of atheists recruited from the (1) general U.S. population, (2) college undergraduates, (3) people adjusting to bereavement, and (4) cancer patients were asked about their reactions to a hypothetical god, while comparison groups of religious believers completed similar measures regarding their relationships with God. Results showed that some atheists held images of God as extremely cruel and responsible for negative events. These so-called "angry atheists" were more likely to have difficulty adjusting to bereavement and cancer, and exhibited more psychological problems than either believers or nonbelievers. However, the reported results may have resulted from a methodological artifact: whereas religious believers were asked to describe relationships with an actual god, atheists were asked to react to a hypothetical god—two entirely different tasks involving different cognitive processes.

Other Psychological and Social Influences on Health

Prejudice and Discrimination   Despite the increasing visibility of atheists and nonreligious individuals, there has been very little change in the perception of nonreligious individuals by most Americans. Population surveys by the Pew Forum on Religion & Public Life illustrate the extensive dislike and distrust Americans feel toward people who do not believe in a god. A 2014 Pew survey asked Americans to rate groups on a "feeling thermometer" from zero (as cold and negative as possible) to 100 (the warmest, most positive possible rating). U.S. adults gave atheists an average rating of 41, comparable to the rating they gave Muslims (40), but far colder than the average rating of Jews (63), Catholics (62), and evangelical Christians (61) (Pew Research Center 2014). Results from a 2016 survey (Edgell, Hartmann, Stewart, and Gerteis 2016) revealed that 27% of Americans say that atheists "don't share my morals or values." Roughly half of Americans (49%) say they would be unhappy if a family member were to marry someone who did not believe in God.

Only 54% of Americans would vote for a presidential candidate who is an atheist (Gallup 2012), far fewer than would support a candidate who is female, gay, a racial minority, or Muslim. This figure, while still high, has increased in recent years: in early 2007, 63% of U.S. adults said they would be less likely to support an atheist presidential candidate. Forty-five percent of Americans say belief in God is necessary to have good values, and about half of Americans say the growing number of "people who are not religious" is bad for American society (Pew Research Center 2013).

Anti-atheist bias can manifest at the interpersonal level as well. In 2008, the nationally representative American Religious Identification Survey found that 41% of self-identified atheists reported experiencing discrimination in the last 5 years due to their lack of religious identification (Cragun, Kosmin, Keysar, Hammer, and Nielsen 2012). Nonreligious individuals have reported experiencing various types of discrimination, including slander; coercion; social ostracism; denial of opportunities, goods, and services; and hate crimes (Hammer, Cragun, Hwang, and Smith 2012). Openly identifying oneself as an atheist or agnostic significantly increases the likelihood of reporting discrimination. A majority of U.S. atheists reported that they would face at least minor repercussions in their families, workplaces, and local communities—most severely in the Midwest and the so-called "Bible belt" region of the South (Mann 2015; Weber et al. 2012). Without the social institutions that are functionally similar to churches—secular groups (*see* García and Blankholm 2016)—that offer affirmation and solidarity with like-minded people, many individual atheists and other individuals without strong religious beliefs report feeling lonely (Lauder, Mummrey and Sharkey 2006).

There is evidence to support the idea that simply being a member of a socially marginalized minority group can itself predispose individuals to increased physical and psychological distress, a phenomenon identified as *minority stress* (Meyer 2003). Minority stress results when stigma, prejudice, and discrimination create a threatening social environment. Such stress can lead to physical and mental health problems in people who belong to stigmatized minority groups (Gee, Spencer, Chen, and Takeuchi 2007; Paradies 2006). Studies have shown that the odds of experiencing a physical health problem are significantly higher among individuals who experience prejudicial events (Frost, Lehavot, and Meyer 2015; Williams, Yu, Jackson, and Anderson 1997). Although there is little research on atheist minority stress per se, analogues can be found among the LGBT population, as LGBT individuals—like atheists—do not constitute a visually identifiable group (unlike racial minorities). As a consequence, atheists—like LGBT individuals—often feel pressure to remain "closeted" and are unable to fully express their identity in anticipation of negative social repercussions (Silverman 2001). This can lead to hypervigilance and internalized self-hatred ("I'm not one of *those* atheists . . ."), heightened stress responses, participation in unhealthy behaviors, and avoidance of healthy behaviors (Pascoe and Richman 2009). The findings discussed here may help account for the occasional differences in health found between religious and less- or nonreligious individuals in some studies.

Risk-Taking Behavior   There does seem to be evidence that nonreligious individuals are more likely to engage in risky behavior, which a recent study has shown may help explain why some people are nonreligious in the first place (Edgell, Frost, and Stewart 2017). According to Gillum (2005), people who attended religious services less than 24 times per year were much more likely to smoke than frequent attendees. Among current smokers, frequent religious attenders smoked an average of 1–5 fewer cigarettes per day than infrequent attenders. The same association was found with smokeless tobacco use (Gillum, Obisesan, and Jarrett 2009). Young adults (age 20–32) who attended religious services less than once per month or never were shown to have higher rates of smoking compared to individuals who attended religious services at least once per month (Whooley, Boyd, Gardin, and Williams 2002). In addition, nonsmokers who reported little or no religious involvement had an increased risk of smoking initiation at a 3-year follow-up (Whooley et al. 2002). In a nationally representative sample of 2004 American adolescents regarding their attendance at religious services and engagement in diverse risk behaviors, adolescents who reported being religiously "nothing in particular" were more likely to drink alcohol, smoke marijuana, or engage in sexual activity, relative to those engaging in congregationally related activities (Sinha, Cnaan, and Gelles 2007). Older atheists were shown in one study to be more likely to use substances such as alcohol to cope with the consequences of aging (Horning, Davis, Stirrat, and Cornwell 2011).

Billioux, Sherman, and Latkin (2014) examined the relationship between religiosity and HIV-related drug risk behavior among individuals from communities with high rates of drug use. Results indicate that greater religious participation appeared to be the dimension most closely associated with drug behaviors. They found that those with greater religious participation were significantly less likely to report recent opiate or cocaine use; injection drug use; crack use; and needle, cotton, or cooker sharing. A 2002 survey revealed that women who never attended religious services had more than two times greater odds of reporting HIV risk factors than those attending weekly or more, after adjusting for age and race/ethnicity (no significant association was seen in men). Individuals with no religious affiliation had higher odds of reporting risk factors than mainline Protestants (Gillum and Holt 2010).

With regard to healthy eating habits, the evidence is not so clear. Although many surveys report that highly religious people tend to eat healthier foods (Newport et al. 2010), other research has reported that atheists and agnostics have lower BMI (Hayward et al. 2016; Kim and Sobal 2004; Kim, Sobal and Wethington 2003). Furthermore, studies have found that nationwide, states with the highest concentration of church and temple goers also have the highest rates of obesity (Ferraro 1998). Cline and Ferraro (2006) found that nonreligious women had lower rates of obesity than women from Baptist or fundamentalist religions (this relationship was not found among men). Kim and Sobal (2004) found that both Conservative Protestant women and women reporting "no religion" consumed a higher percentage of dietary fats compared to Catholic women, but the association for nonreligious women became nonsignificant after controlling for social support. Although religious communities and teachings can serve as effective mechanisms for delivering healthy eating advice (Ayers et al. 2010; Resnicow et al. 2002), other church functions—such as weekly potluck suppers—can actually contribute toward greater obesity among members. Additionally, in all of these studies, effect sizes are small, suggesting marginal differences at best.

Similar associations have been found with regard to physical exercise. Gillum (2006) found that older women who attended services infrequently or never were less likely to engage in leisure-time physical activity than those who attended more regularly, even after controlling for health status. This association was not found for men or younger women. Among a sample of older Southern U.S.-dwelling adults, greater leisure-time physical activity was associated with organized religious activity but not with intrinsic religiosity (Roff et al. 2005). Another study found that individuals with highly fundamentalist religious beliefs engaged in the lowest frequency of risk behaviors (Barna 2004). It should be noted that many of these studies are subject to the criticisms we raised earlier, as they are comparing individuals who score high in religiosity to individuals who score low in religiosity and not necessarily to affirmatively irreligious individuals.

Positive Health Values Held by Both Religious and Nonreligious Individuals

As atheism (often accompanied with humanism) can be its own organizing existential system, it makes sense that certain features of most religious systems are also possessed by secular individuals. Ho and Ho (2007) have argued that atheism does not exclude spirituality. Even in largely atheistic countries, such as mainland China, people still consider spirituality to be a positive, meaningful value. Although the word *spiritual* is traditionally associated with religious experience (and for that reason objectionable to many secularists; *see* Dein 2016), the word itself is difficult to define. Interpretations range from "search for the sacred" (which may occur outside of an established religious tradition; Pargament 1999) to "subjective self-fulfillment" (Sheldrake 2007). In light of the fact that atheists and nonreligious individuals can and often do consider themselves spiritual, it is worth noting that many studies relate self-reported health not to religiosity but to spirituality (Sessanna, Finnell, Underhill, Chang, and Peng 2011). Unfortunately, measures of spirituality have often been conflated with elements of physical and mental health, making it difficult to separate spirituality from health (*see* D. L. Cragun, Cragun, Nathan, Sumerau, and Nowakowski 2016; Koenig 2008).

Related to but separate from spirituality is the fact that there is no evidence supporting the idea that important elements of the human experience are limited exclusively to the religious or "spiritual." Norman (2006) describes five such important human experiences: (1) the experience of the moral "ought"; (2) the experience of beauty; (3) the experience of meaning conferred by stories; (4) the experience of otherness and transcendence; and (5) the experience of vulnerability and fragility (p. 474). He argues that these are meaningful components of any human life, and contests claims by some theists that such experiences are by nature essentially religious. The claim that these are religious experiences is really an attempt to marginalize nonreligious individuals and the usurpation of universal human experiences by religions. The end result is either a suggestion that nonreligious and atheist individuals are either "secretly religious" but unaware of that fact, or an attempt to suggest that nonbelievers' participation in these experiences is in some way inferior. Nonreligious individuals do have "spiritual" experiences, but they frame them in completely naturalistic or materialistic ways (*see* Ecklund 2010). In fact, there is some evidence to suggest that maintaining an intimate connection with life through family, home, friends, leisure, and work is just as spiritually important to individuals as is transcendent or nontranscendent meaning-making (McGrath 2002). In short, nonreligious individuals have meaningful life experiences, just like religious individuals do, but they often do not attribute them to supernatural powers (*see* Cragun and Sumerau 2015).

George, Ellison, and Larson (2002) reviewed the social and psychological factors that have been hypothesized to explain the health-promoting effects of religious involvement. The four potential psychosocial mechanisms that have received empirical attention are health practices, social support, psychosocial resources such as self-esteem and self-efficacy, and belief structures such as sense of coherence. Yet, these qualities are not necessarily limited to just religious believers. Like believers, atheists can also have high self-esteem, high self-efficacy, and a coherent worldview (*see* Zuckerman 2008).

Much has also been written about the beneficial role of social support and community provided by religious organizations. Likewise, secular and nonreligious people also benefit from encountering other like-minded people, either in person or online. Group membership appears to serve as a buffer against the harmful effects of social rejection (Galen 2015). Galen, Sharp, and McNulty (2015) found that secular group affiliation resulted in the same social support and community benefits to health as does religious group membership, indicating that the benefits are largely derived from being part of a group and not from anything particularly special about religious organizations.

Findings such as these suggest that nonreligious individuals share many of the pro-health attributes of religious individuals, which may help explain why so many studies find only marginal differences or no differences in health between religious and nonreligious individuals (*see* D. L. Cragun et al. 2016. Additionally, there are some sociological factors that may contribute to the occasionally observed lower levels of health among nonreligious individuals and atheists, specifically the prejudice and discrimination they face and their potentially higher rates of risk-taking (which helps account for why they are nonreligious in the first place).

HOW TO APPROACH NONRELIGIOUS INDIVIDUALS REGARDING HEALTH

We approach this final section of the chapter hoping to make two contributions. First, we want to note that there are some differences in how nonreligious individuals compared to religious individuals would prefer to communicate with healthcare practitioners. Second, we raise some questions about how healthcare practitioners should interact with nonreligious individuals when it comes to offering health advice and suggestions.

Earlier in this chapter we summarized research on differences in health between religious and nonreligious individuals, but we have been unable to find any prior research that has explored healthcare communication preferences among nonreligious individuals. As a result, we looked to see if there might be some readily accessible data that could provide insights into how nonreligious individuals may differ from religious people in how they prefer to interact with healthcare practitioners. The GSS includes several questions that help shed some light on how doctors and other healthcare practitioners might want to approach nonreligious individuals. Three questions asked in 2002 provide particularly useful insights. The first question asked respondents to indicate their agreement or disagreement with the statement: "I prefer that my doctor offers me choices and asks my opinion." Responses are shown in Figure 13.1. On this question, there were not statistically significant differences between Protestants, Catholics, Jews, and the nonreligious; most individuals prefer that their doctor ask their opinion.

However, on the next two questions (see Figures 13.2 and 13.3), there were statistically significant differences in the responses. Respondents were asked to indicate their agreement with the statements, "I prefer to leave decisions about my medical care up to my doctor" and "I prefer to rely on my doctor's knowledge and not try to find out about my condition on my own." On these two items, nonreligious individuals were significantly more likely to disagree than were Protestants and Catholics (though they were not that different from Jewish individuals). Whereas pretty much all people prefer that healthcare practitioners ask their opinions, nonreligious individuals appear to be more interested in making their own decisions and in investigating medical conditions on their own than are Protestants and Catholics.

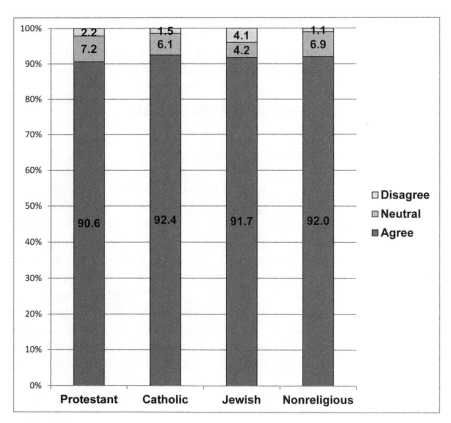

Figure 13.1 I prefer that my doctor offers me choices and asks my opinion.

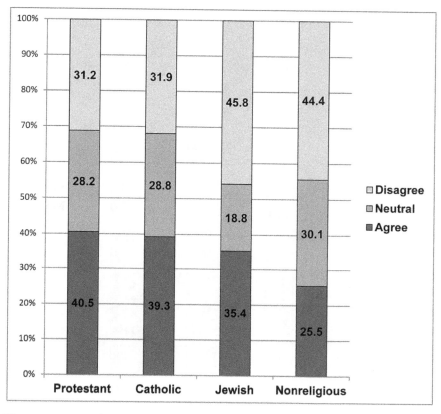

Figure 13.2 I prefer to leave decisions about my medical care up to my doctor.

Healthcare practitioners should keep these differences in mind when discussing health issues with nonreligious individuals. Specifically, healthcare practitioners should recognize that nonreligious individuals may be more likely to request additional information and may come to healthcare appointments having already investigated medical conditions. Nonreligious individuals may also be more likely to seek second opinions and to turn to scientific and peer-reviewed research to inform themselves about medical and health issues. Healthcare practitioners should be willing to share this kind of information or ways of finding such information with nonreligious individuals.

Additionally, prior research has found that nonreligious individuals, but particularly atheists, tend to be well-versed in science (Cragun 2014) and have more science knowledge than do highly religious individuals (Sherkat 2011). Building upon the earlier suggestion, healthcare practitioners should approach communication with nonreligious individuals focusing on scientific explanations. One study of patients involved in genetic

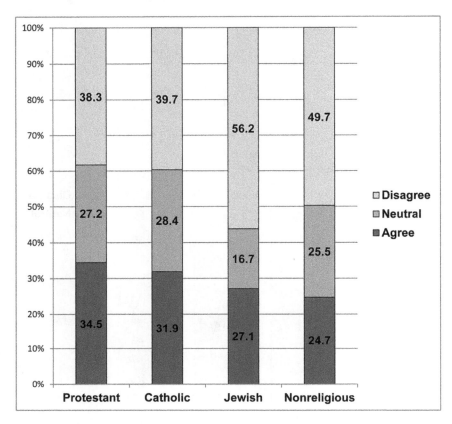

Figure 13.3 I prefer to rely on my doctor's knowledge and not try to find out about my condition on my own.

counseling sessions (Thompson et al. 2016) found that nonreligious individuals do not believe it is the job of healthcare practitioners to address religious or spiritual concerns during medical appointments and would prefer that such appointments focus on medical issues, without "wasting time" on what they perceive to be irrelevant issues, like religiosity or spirituality. Healthcare practitioners working with nonreligious issues should only touch upon religiosity or spirituality if the topic is raised by the patient and should not bring the topic up themselves.

The second issue we want to raise in relation to healthcare communication is how healthcare practitioners should think about people who are nonreligious. Based on our discussion about the sometimes detected health benefits of religiosity and spirituality, we think it is important to consider several questions. Should a physician encourage patients to embrace religious beliefs or practices that the physician believes are conducive to health or healing, even if the patient has indicated that he or she rejects those beliefs or practices? And, if a physician does encourage such beliefs, might this constitute a form of proselytizing or even coercion, given the power imbalances between physicians and patients?

Nonreligious individuals, and atheists in particular, are often quite adamant about their disbelief (Hunsberger 2006). As a result, they may be particularly likely to find the encouragement of belief to be offensive. They may also find suggestions that they should believe to be a form of coercion or proselytism (Berlinger 2004). If a nonreligious or atheist patient rejected what we are arguing are inappropriate, pro-religious or pro-spirituality suggestions, how might physicians respond? If a patient rejects advice about the possible benefits of religiosity/spirituality, does that mean such a patient is a "noncompliant" or a "bad" patient? Healthcare practitioners need to be aware that nonreligious individuals—particularly atheists—will be likely to reject suggestions that there are health benefits that derive (only or specifically) from religion, spirituality, or belief. Physicians and other healthcare practitioners should think carefully about whether the evidence for possible health benefits of religiosity, spirituality, or belief are substantial enough to warrant what would likely be perceived as discrimination by nonreligious patients.

Hospital chaplains have already begun to wrestle with this question. One of the responsibilities of professional hospital chaplains is to protect vulnerable patients against proselytizing. Some chaplains have been critical of what they perceive to be the proselytizing tendencies of some discourses in health care. We echo the concerns of hospital chaplains on this point. Given the very limited benefits that may derive from religiosity and spirituality, we believe healthcare practitioners would be misguided if they encouraged nonreligious patients to adopt religious or spiritual beliefs. Nonreligious patients are likely to perceive such efforts as discriminatory, misguided, and offensive.

CONCLUSION

In this chapter we have provided basic definitions of terms commonly used to describe nonreligious or secular individuals. We provided some information on the demographic characteristics of nonreligious individuals and atheists. We discussed at length the limitations of much of the research that finds relationships between religiosity/spirituality and health, noting that it rarely compares religious individuals to affirmatively nonreligious individuals (instead comparing individuals high in religiosity/spirituality to individuals who are low in religiosity/spirituality). Only recently have good measures of how nonreligious or secular individuals are been developed, and the differences in health observed are often marginal with small effect sizes. We summarized findings that have shown minor differences in health between religious and nonreligious individuals, but have done so carefully, noting that there are problems with many of these studies. We also explored some of the factors that may contribute to slightly worse health outcomes among the nonreligious, such as pervasive prejudice and discrimination in the United States and higher levels of risk-taking behavior among nonreligious individuals. We also noted that a growing body of research is finding that health differences between the religious and nonreligious are negligible, and that many affirmatively nonreligious individuals engage in pro-health behaviors similar to those of religious individuals.

The final contribution of our chapter was an effort to illustrate that nonreligious individuals do, in fact, have different healthcare communication preferences than do some religious individuals. Nonreligious individuals prefer greater autonomy over their healthcare decision making and are more interested in investigating the health issues they face than are Protestant and Catholic individuals. Additionally, nonreligious individuals often have greater scientific knowledge and have greater trust in science and scientific institutions than do religious people, suggesting that healthcare practitioners should focus their interactions with nonreligious individuals on scientific and medical concerns and avoid raising issues related to religiosity and spirituality unless the patients bring these topics up. It is also worth noting that there is virtually no literature examining the healthcare communication preferences of nonreligious individuals, suggesting that this line of inquiry should be pursued by future research, especially in light of the rapid growth of the nonreligious in the United States and in many other highly developed countries.

REFERENCES

Ayers, J. W., C. W. Hofstetter, V. W. Irvin, Y. Song, H.-R. Park, H.-Y. Paik, and M. F. Hovell. 2010. "Can Religion Help Prevent Obesity? Religious Messages and the Prevalence of Being Overweight or Obese Among Korean Women in California." *Journal for the Scientific Study of Religion* 49(3): 536–549.

Baker, J. O., and B. G. Smith. 2009. "The Nones: Social Characteristics of the Religiously Unaffiliated." *Social Forces* 87(3): 1251–1263.

Baker, J. O., and B. G. Smith. 2015. *American Secularism: Cultural Contours of Nonreligious Belief Systems.* New York: NYU Press.

Barna, G. 2004. *Faith Has a Limited Effect on Most People's Behavior.* Ventura, CA: Barna Research Group.

Berlinger, N. 2004. "Spirituality and Medicine: Idiot-Proofing the Discourse." *Journal of Medicine and Philosophy* 29(6): 681–695.

Billioux, V. G., S. G. Sherman, and C. Latkin. 2014. "Religiosity and HIV-Related Drug Risk Behavior: A Multidimensional Assessment of Individuals from Communities with High Rates of Drug Use." *Journal of Religion and Health* 53(1): 37–45.

Bradshaw, M., C. G. Ellison, and K. J. Flannelly. 2008. "Prayer, God Imagery, and Symptoms of Psychopathology." *Journal for the Scientific Study of Religion* 47(4): 644–659.

Cline, K., and K. F. Ferraro. 2006. "Does Religion Increase the Prevalence and Incidence of Obesity in Adulthood?" *Journal for the Scientific Study of Religion* 45(2): 269–281.

Cragun, D. L., R. T. Cragun, B. Nathan, J. E. Sumerau, and A. C. H. Nowakowski. 2016. "Do Religiosity and Spirituality Really Matter for Social, Mental, and Physical Health? A Tale of Two Samples." *Sociological Spectrum* 36(6): 359–377. http://dx.doi.org/10.1080/02732173.2016.1198949

Cragun, R. T. 2013. *What You Don't Know About Religion (But Should)*. Durham, NC: Pitchstone Publishing.

Cragun, R. T. 2015. "Who Are the 'New Atheists'?" In L. Beamon and S. Tomlins, eds., *Atheist Identities: Spaces and Social Contexts*, pp. 195–211. New York: Springer.

Cragun, R. T. 2016. "Defining That Which Is 'Other to' Religion: Secularism, Humanism, Atheism, Freethought, Etc." In P. Zuckerman, ed., *Religion: Beyond Religion*, pp. 1–16. New York: MacMillan.

Cragun, R. T., and J. H. Hammer. 2011. "'One Person's Apostate Is Another Person's Convert': Reflections on Pro-Religion Hegemony in the Sociology of Religion." *Humanity & Society* 35: 149–75.

Cragun, R. T., J. H. Hammer, and M. Nielsen. 2015. "The Nonreligious-Nonspiritual Scale (NRNSS): Measuring Everyone from Atheists to Zionists." *Science, Religion, and Culture* 2: 36–53. http://dx.doi.org/10.17582/journal.src/2015/2.3.36.53

Cragun, R. T., B. Kosmin, A. Keysar, J. H. Hammer, and M. Nielsen. 2012. "On the Receiving End: Discrimination Toward the Non-Religious in the United States." *Journal of Contemporary Religion* 27(1): 105–127.

Cragun, R. T., and J. E. Sumerau. 2015. "God May Save Your Life, But You Have to Find Your Own Keys: Religious Attributions, Secular Attributions, and Religious Priming." *Archive for the Psychology of Religion* 37(3): 321–342.

Cragun, R. T., and J. E. Sumerau. 2017. "No One Expects a Transgender Jew: Religious, Sexual and Gendered Intersections in the Evaluation of Religious and Nonreligious Others." *Secularism and Nonreligion* 6(1). http://doi.org/10.5334/snr.82.

Dein, S. 2016. "Attitudes Towards Spirituality and Other Worldly Experiences: An Online Survey of British Humanists." *Secularism and Nonreligion* 5(1). doi:10.5334/snr.48

Edgell, P., J. Frost, and E. Stewart. 2017. "From Existential to Social Understandings of Risk: Examining Gender Differences in Non-Religion." *Social Currents*, 1–19.

Edgell, P., D. Hartmann, E. Stewart, and J. Gerteis. 2016. "Atheists and Other Cultural Outsiders: Moral Boundaries and the Non-Religious in the United States." *Social Forces* 95(2): 607–638.

Exline, J. J., and A. Martin. 2005. "Anger Toward God: A New Frontier in Forgiveness Research." In E. L. Worthington, ed., *Handbook of Forgiveness* (1st ed.), pp. 73–88. New York: Routledge.

Exline, J. J., C. L. Park, J. M. Smyth, and M. P. Carey. 2011. "Anger Toward God: Social-Cognitive Predictors, Prevalence, and Links with Adjustment to Bereavement and Cancer." *Journal of Personality and Social Psychology* 100(1): 129–148.

Feifel, H. 1974. "Religious Conviction and Fear of Death among the Healthy and the Terminally Ill." *Journal for the Scientific Study of Religion* 13(3): 353–360.

Ferraro, K. F. 1998. "Firm Believers? Religion, Body Weight, and Well-Being." *Review of Religious Research* 39(3): 224–244.

Frost, D. M., K. Lehavot, and I. H. Meyer. 2015. "Minority Stress and Physical Health among Sexual Minority Individuals." *Journal of Behavioral Medicine* 38: 1–8.

Galen, L. W. 2009. "Profiles of the Godless." *Free Inquiry* 29(5): 41–45.

Galen, L. W. 2015. "Atheism, Wellbeing, and the Wager: Why Not Believing in God (With Others) Is Good for You." *Science, Religion and Culture* 2: 54–69.

Galen, L. W., and J. Kloet. 2010. "Mental Well-Being in the Religious and the Non-Religious: Evidence for a Curvilinear Relationship." *Mental Health, Religion & Culture* 14: 673–89. doi:10.1080/13674676.2010.510829

Galen, L. W., M. Sharp, and A. McNulty. 2015. "Nonreligious Group Factors Versus Religious Belief in the Prediction of Prosociality." *Social Indicators Research* 122(2): 1–22.

Gallup. 2012. "Atheists, Muslims See Most Bias as Presidential Candidates." Retrieved from http://www.gallup.com/poll/155285/atheists-muslims-bias-presidential-candidates.aspx

García, A., and J. Blankholm. 2016. "The Social Context of Organized Nonbelief: County-Level Predictors of Nonbeliever Organizations in the United States." *Journal for the Scientific Study of Religion* 55(1): 70–90.

Gee, G. C., M. S. Spencer, J. Chen, and D. Takeuchi. 2007. "A Nationwide Study of Discrimination and Chronic Health Conditions among Asian Americans." *American Journal of Public Health* 97: 1275–1282.

George, L. K., C. G. Ellison, and D. B. Larson. 2002. "Explaining the Relationship Between Religious Involvement and Health." *Psychological Inquiry* 13: 190–200.

Gillum, R. F. 2005. "Frequency of Attendance at Religious Services and Cigarette Smoking in American Women and Men: The Third National Health and Nutrition Examination Survey." *Preventive Medicine* 41: 607–613.

Gillum, R. F. 2006. "Frequency of Attendance at Religious Services and Leisure-Time Physical Activity in American Women and Men: The Third National

Health and Nutrition Examination Survey." *Annals of Behavioral Medicine* 31: 30–35.

Gillum, R. F., and C. L. Holt. 2010. "Associations between Religious Involvement and Behavioral Risk Factors for HIV/AIDS in American Women and Men in a National Health Survey." *Annals of Behavioral Medicine* 40(3): 284–293.

Gillum, R. F., T. O. Obisesan, and N. C. Jarrett. 2009. "Smokeless Tobacco Use and Religiousness." *International Journal of Environmental Research in Public Health* 6(1): 225–231.

Hall, D. E., H. G. Koenig, and K. G. Meador. 2008. "Hitting the Target: Why Existing Measures of 'Religiousness' Are Really Reverse-Scored Measures of 'Secularism.'" *Explore (New York, N.Y.)* 4: 368–373.

Hall, D. E., K. G. Meador, and H. G. Koenig. 2008. "Measuring Religiousness in Health Research: Review and Critique." *Journal of Religion and Health* 47: 134–163.

Hammer, J. H., R. T. Cragun, K. Hwang, and J. M. Smith. 2012. "Forms, Frequency, and Correlates of Perceived Anti-Atheist Discrimination." *Secularism and Nonreligion* 1: 43–67.

Hayward, D. R., N. Krause, G. Ironson, P. C. Hill, and R. Emmons. 2016. "Health and Well-Being among the Non-Religious: Atheists, Agnostics, and No Preference Compared with Religious Group Members." *Journal of Religion and Health* 55(3): 1024–1037.

Hill, P. C., and R. W. Hood. 1999. *Measures of Religiosity*. Birmingham, AL: Religious Education Press.

Ho, D., and R. Ho. 2007. "Measuring Spirituality and Spiritual Emptiness: Toward Ecumenicity and Transcultural Applicability." *Review of General Psychology* 11: 62–74.

Hoge, D. R. 1981. *Converts, Dropouts, Returnees: A Study of Religious Change Among Catholics*. New York: Pilgrim Press.

Horning, S. M., H. P. Davis, M. Stirrat, and R. E. Cornwell. 2011. "Atheistic, Agnostic, and Religious Older Adults on Well-Being and Coping Behaviors." *Journal of Aging Studies* 25(2): 177–188.

Hunsberger, B. 2006. *Atheists: A Groundbreaking Study of America's Nonbelievers*. Amherst, NY: Prometheus Books.

Hwang, K. 2008. "Atheists with Disabilities: A Neglected Minority in Religion and Rehabilitation Research." *Journal of Religion, Disability and Health* 12: 186–192.

Hwang, K., J. H. Hammer, and R. T. Cragun. 2011. "Extending Religion-Health Research to Nontheistic Minorities: Issues and Concerns." *Journal of Religion and Health* 50: 608–622.

Jenks, R. J. 1986. "Perceptions of Two Deviant and Two Nondeviant Groups." *Journal of Social Psychology* 126(6): 783–790.

Kier, F., and D. S. Davenport. 2004. "Unaddressed Problems in the Study of Spirituality and Health." *American Psychologist* 59(1): 53–54.

Kim, K. H., and J. Sobal, J. 2004. "Religion, Social Support, Fat Intake and Physical Activity." *Public Health Nutrition* 7: 773–781.

Kim, K. H., J. Sobal, and E. Wethington. 2003. "Religion and Body Weight." *International Journal of Obesity* 27: 469–477.

Koenig, H. G. 1995. "Use of Acute Hospital Services and Mortality among Religious and Non-Religious Copers with Medical Illness." *Journal of Religious Gerontology* 9(3): 1–21.

Koenig, H. G. 2008. "Concerns about Measuring 'Spirituality' in Research." *Journal of Nervous and Mental Disease* 196: 349–355.

Koenig, H. G., M. E. McCullough, and D. B. Larson. 2001. *Handbook of Religion and Health*. New York: Oxford University Press.

Kosmin, B. A., and A. Keysar. 2007. *Secularism and Secularity: Contemporary International Perspectives*. Hartford, CT: Institute for the Study of Secularism in Society and Culture.

Kosmin, B. A., A. Keysar, R. T. Cragun, and J. Navarro-Rivera. 2009. *American Nones: The Profile of the No Religion Population—A Report Based on the American Religious Identification Survey 2008*. Hartford, CT: Institute for the Study of Secularism in Society and Culture.

Langston, J. A., J. H. Hammer, and R. T. Cragun. 2015. "Atheism Looking in: On the Goals and Strategies of Organized Nonbelief." *Science, Religion, and Culture* 2: 70–85. http://dx.doi.org/10.17582/journal.src/2015/2.3.70.85

Lauder, W., K. Mummery, and S. Sharkey. 2006. "Social Capital, Age and Religiosity in People Who Are Lonely." *Journal of Clinical Nursing* 15: 334–340.

Lee, L. 2012. "Research Note. Talking about a Revolution: Terminology for the New Field of Non-Religion Studies." *Journal of Contemporary Religion* 27: 129–139. doi:10.1080/13537903.2012.642742

Makros, J., and M. P. McCabe. 2003. "The Relationship Between Religion, Spirituality, Psychological Adjustment, and Quality of Life among People with Multiple Sclerosis." *Journal of Religion and Health* 42: 143.

Mann, M. 2015. "Triangle Atheists: Stigma, Identity, and Community among Atheists in North Carolina's Triangle Region." *Secularism and Nonreligion* 4(1): 1–11. doi.org/10.5334/snr.bd

McGrath, P. 2002. "'A Spirituality Quintessentially of the Ordinary': Non-Religious Meaning-Making and Its Relevance to Primary Health Care." *Australian Journal of Primary Health* 8(3): 47–57.

Merino, S. M. 2011. "Irreligious Socialization? The Adult Religious Preferences of Individuals Raised with No Religion." *Secularism and Nonreligion* 1: 1–16.

Meyer, I. H. 2003. "Prejudice as Stress: Conceptual and Measurement Problems." *American Journal of Public Health* 93: 262–265.

Newport, F., S. Agrawal, and D. Witters. 2010. "Very Religious Americans Lead Healthier Lives." Retrieved September 18, 2011, from http://www.gallup.com/poll/145379/Religious-Americans-Lead-HealtherLives.aspx

Norman, R. 2006. "The Varieties of Non-Religious Experience." *Ratio* 19: 474–494.

Paradies, Y. 2006. "A Systematic Review of Empirical Research on Self-Reported Racism and Health." *International Journal of Epidemiology* 35(4): 888–901. doi:10.1093/ije/dyl056

Pargament, K. 1999. "The Psychology of Religion and Spirituality? Yes and No." *International Journal of Psychology and Religion* 9: 3–26.

Pascoe, E. A., and L. S. Richman. 2009. "Perceived Discrimination and Health: A Meta-Analytic Review." *Psychological Bulletin* 135(4): 531–554.

Pasquale, F. L. 2010. "An Assessment of the Role of Early Parental Loss in the Adoption of Atheism or Irreligion." *Archive for the Psychology of Religion 32*(3): 375–396.

Pew Forum on Religion. 2012. "'Nones' on the Rise." Washington, DC: The Pew Forum on Religion & Public Life. Retrieved from http://www.pewforum.org/Unaffiliated/nones-on-the-rise.aspx

Pew Research Center. 2013. "Growth of the Nonreligious." Retrieved from http://www.pewforum.org/2013/07/02/growth-of-the-nonreligious-many-say-trend-is-bad-for-american-society/

Pew Research Center. 2014. "New Pew Research Survey Explores How Americans Feel About Religious Groups." Retrieved from http://www.pewforum.org/2014/07/16/new-pew-research-survey-explores-how-americans-feel-about-religious-groups/

Pew Research Center. 2015. "The Future of World Religions: Population Growth Projections, 2010–2050." Washington, DC: Pew Research Center. Retrieved from http://www.pewforum.org/files/2015/03/PF_15.04.02_ProjectionsFullReport.pdf

Quack, J. 2014. "Outline of a Relational Approach to 'Nonreligion.'" *Method & Theory in the Study of Religion* 26(4–5): 439–469. doi:10.1163/15700682-12341327

Reis, L. M, R. Baumiller, W. Scrivener, G. Yager, and N. S. Warren. 2007. "Spiritual Assessment in Genetic Counseling." *Journal of Genetic Counseling* 16(1): 41–52. doi:10.1007/s10897-006-9041-8

Resnicow, K., A. Jackson, R. Braithwaite, C. DiIorio, D. Blisset, S. Rahotep, and S. Periasamy. 2002. "Healthy Body/Healthy Spirit: A Church-Based Nutrition and Physical Activity Intervention." *Health Education Research* 17: 562–573.

Roff, L. L., D. L. Klemmack, M. Parker, H. G. Koenig, P. Sawyer-Baker, and R. M. Allman. 2005. "Religiosity, Smoking, Exercise, and Obesity among Southern, Community-Dwelling Older Adults." *Journal of Applied Gerontology* 24: 337–354.

Roof, W. C., and W. McKinney. 1987. *American Mainline Religion: Its Changing Shape and Future.* New Brunswick, NJ: Rutgers University Press.

Scheitle, C. P., and A. Adamczyk. 2010. "High-Cost Religion, Religious Switching, and Health." *Journal of Health and Social Behavior* 51(3): 325–342.

Schnell, T. 2015. "Dimensions of Secularity (DoS): An Open Inventory to Measure Facets of Secular Identities." *International Journal for the Psychology of Religion* 25: 272–292. doi:10.1080/10508619.2014.967541

Sessanna, L., D. S. Finnell, M. Underhill, Y.-P. Chang, and H.-L. Peng. 2011. "Measures Assessing Spirituality as More than Religiosity: A Methodological Review of Nursing and Health-Related Literature." *Journal of Advanced Nursing* 67(8): 1677–1694.

Sheldrake, P. 2007. *A Brief History of Spirituality*. Marston, MA: Blackwell.

Sherkat, D. E. 2008. "Beyond Belief: Atheism, Agnosticism, and Theistic Certainty in the United States." *Sociological Spectrum* 28: 438–459.

Sherkat, D. E. 2011. "Religion and Scientific Literacy in the United States." *Social Science Quarterly* 92(5): 1134–1150.

Sherkat, D. E. 2014. *Changing Faith: The Dynamics and Consequences of Americans' Shifting Religious Identities*. New York: NYU Press.

Silverman, D. 2001. "Coming Out: The Other Closet: American Atheists." Retrieved from http://atheists.org./atheism.coming_out

Sinha, J. W., R. A. Cnaan, and R. W. Gelles. 2007. "Adolescent Risk Behaviors and Religion: Findings from a National Study." *Journal of Adolescence* 30(2): 231–249.

Sloan, R. P. 2006. *Blind Faith: The Unholy Alliance of Religion and Medicine*. New York: St. Martin's/Griffin.

Smith, J. M. 2010. "Becoming an Atheist in America: Constructing Identity and Meaning from the Rejection of Theism." *Sociology of Religion* 72(2): 215–237. doi:10.1093/socrel/srq082

Smith, T. W., P. Marsden, and J. Kim. 2014. *General Social Survey*. Chicago: National Opinion Research Center.

Speed, D. 2017. "Unbelievable?! Theistic/Epistemological Viewpoint Affects Religion–Health Relationship." *Journal of Religion and Health* 56(1): 238–257.

Speed, D., and K. Fowler. 2016. "What's God Got to Do with It? How Religiosity Predicts Atheists' Health." *Journal of Religion and Health* 55: 296–308.

Stavrova, O. 2015. "Religion, Self-Rated Health, and Mortality: Whether Religiosity Delays Death Depends on the Cultural Context." *Social Psychological and Personality Science* 6: 911–922.

Thompson, A. B., D. Cragun, J. E. Sumerau, R. T. Cragun, V. De Difis, and A. Trepanier. 2016. "'Be Prepared If I Bring It Up:' Patients' Perceptions of the Utility of Religious and Spiritual Discussion During Genetic Counseling." *Journal of Genetic Counseling* 25(5): 945–956.

Tomlin, S., and S. Bullivant. Eds. 2016. *The Atheist Bus Campaign: Global Manifestations and Responses* (Lam ed.). Leiden/Boston: Brill Academic Publishing.

Weber, S. R., K. I. Pargament, M. L. Kunik, J. W. Lomax, and M. A. Stanley. 2012. "Psychological Distress among Religious Nonbelievers: A Systematic Review." *Journal of Religion and Health* 51(1): 72–86.

Whitley, R. 2010. "Atheism and Mental Health." *Harvard Review of Psychiatry* 18(3): 190–194.

Whooley, M. A., A. L. Boyd, J. M. Gardin, and D. L. Williams. 2002. "Religious Involvement and Cigarette Smoking in Young Adults: The CARDIA Study." *Archives of Internal Medicine* 162: 1604–1610.

Williams, D. R., Y. Yu, D. S. Jackson, and N. B. Anderson. 1997. "Racial Differences in Physical and Mental Health." *Journal of Health Psychology* 2: 335–351.

Zuckerman, P. 2008. *Society Without God: What the Least Religious Nations Can Tell Us About Contentment*. New York: NYU Press.

Chapter 14

Epilogue: Religion, Science, and Health—A Question of Balance or the Space Between?

Scott F. Madey

The chapters in this book present the major religions and philosophies and how they can help our understanding of what makes us healthy and what makes us sick. The authors in several chapters explore the extant research on religion and health and others compare religion and science in the context of health.

This epilogue explores the next steps in our understanding of the relationship between religion, science, and health. The subtitle of this chapter—"A question of balance or the space between?"—puts us at a crossroads between a choice of integration or selection of a different path. The first part of this chapter addresses religion and science views toward health and illness and how religion and science are part of our health-illness orientation. I then propose a model that highlights the tension between religion and science and the possible validity and invalidity of these perspectives. Finally, I ask the reader to consider with me whether religion[1] and science vis-à-vis our health-illness orientation should be based on an integration of the two or a contemplation of and meditation on the space between them.

HEALTH-ILLNESS ORIENTATION

To understand the relationship between scientific and religious orientations and a health-illness orientation, I propose that a person's health-illness orientation is a way of identifying, monitoring, and behaving with regard to health and illness. This orientation is comprised of mental representations such as prototypes, attitudes, and beliefs regarding health and illness. It is also comprised of affect, such as energy, negative and positive mood, well-being, irritability, and frustration regarding health and illness. A third component of health-illness orientation is behavior. Behavior components in part consist of coping and compliance, self-regulation, treatment seeking, and health habits.

Perhaps the most important factor affecting health-illness orientation and its components of cognition, affect, and behavior is one's culture. *Culture* is defined as an accumulated knowledge of a people, encoded in language, embodied in physical artifacts, belief, values, and customs passed on to generations (Lewis 2002). Culture involves shared communication and social experience, norms, mores, and expected ways of thinking and behaving. Embodied in the concept of culture are self-identity, family, age, race, traditions, socioeconomic status, gender identity, religion, and spirituality (Gurung 2006). Religion and spirituality importantly promote positive health behaviors in a sociocultural context—and impact our health-illness orientation by providing it with a narrative of deep meaning. Another component of culture that has implications for our health-illness orientation is the scientific enterprise. Advancements in medicine, along with the sociohistorical-political impact of these advancements, are embodied in the representations, affect, and behaviors that comprise our health-illness orientation. This chapter focuses on two aspects of culture, religion and science, and explores the relationship between religion and science in relation to one's health-illness orientation.

The Common Sense Model of Self-Regulation

Although it is proposed that our health-illness orientation is comprised of cognitions, affect, and behaviors primarily built up from a sociocultural milieu, an organizational framework is needed. A robust model that may provide this framework and will be useful for our understanding is the Common Sense Model (CSM) of self-regulatory health behavior. Proposed by Howard Leventhal and colleagues (Cameron and Leventhal 2003; Leventhal, Phillips, and Burns 2016; Meyer, Leventhal, and Gutman 1985), the CSM was designed to help understand how people self-regulate their health behaviors. People do not necessarily need skilled medical knowledge, nor do their diagnoses and coping have to correlate with clinical or biomedical data. Thus, I propose that the CSM is the fundamental way that lay people construct their health-illness orientation.

According to the Common Sense Model, illness representations involve a complex array of identification of symptoms and beliefs about the types of symptoms associated with particular diseases, cause, timeline, and consequence. Next in this model is a selection of coping options: the options selected depend upon the content of the representation. For example, coping responses may be going to a physician, use of over-the-counter medications, or alternative medicine and therapies, to name a few. Finally, an evaluation, or appraisal of the effectiveness, of the coping response occurs. Depending upon the appraisal, the representation and/or the coping response may be altered. A second arm of the Common Sense Model involves representing emotional reactions, such as distress, fear, or anger (Leventhal, Leventhal, and Schaefer 1991). The emotional reaction also involves coping responses, such as relaxation, distraction, or substance use. Finally, an appraisal is made of the emotional coping used and its effectiveness in reducing the negative emotion associated with the identification of a particular illness or disease (Cameron and Jago 2008; Leventhal, Brissette, and Leventhal 2003).

The CSM has received much empirical support. Importantly, the CSM highlights the relationships involving emotions and potential health behaviors associated with one's representations of symptoms. An early study by Meyer, Leventhal, and Gutman (1985) found that patients who believed that high blood pressure could be identified symptomatically (e.g., flushing, palpitations, tension) were more likely to quit taking their medication when they reported feeling better compared to patients who more accurately identified that high blood pressure does not have easily identified symptoms and that continued taking of medication is part of maintenance. Perceptions by patients of their illness and the potential benefits of a timely diagnosis and their ability to interact and plan with family members for eventual health changes correlate with increased willingness to interact with a healthcare provider (Gleason et al. 2016). Conversely, patients unaware of the illness may often experience a mismatch between their symptom experiences, or perceived lack of symptoms, and the information they are subsequently given by others, resulting in increased anxiety (Chittem, Norman, and Harris 2015).

EXAMPLES OF THE CULTURAL-RELIGIOUS COMPONENT OF THE COMMON SENSE MODEL

A way to further demonstrate the Common Sense Model is to apply it to cultural-religious views of health-illness orientations. Here I explore three examples: Empacho, representativeness heuristic, and Christian fatalism.

Empacho

Hispanic medicine defines illness under two categories: Natural (i.e., *Males Naturales*) and those involving witchcraft, or supernatural origins (i.e., *Males Puesto*). Empacho is a *males naturales* (Neighbors 1969) and is characterized as a blockage of the stomach wall making it difficult for the person to digest food. Under a common sense organization, the representation of Empacho is a "cold" condition with symptoms such as vomiting, tenderness of the stomach, swollen stomach, and stomach pain. The timeline is that it can be short-lived and is usually cured with the first treatment. The consequence can be that failure to dislodge the obstruction can be fatal. The cause is believed to be an intestinal obstruction caused by eating too much, eating the wrong type of food, or eating poorly prepared food. Finally, it is controllable if caught early. The coping part of the CSM applied to Empacho would be to seek a folk healer (*curandero* or *curandera*), rolling an egg on the stomach, massage, and/or ingestion of olive oil or tea to try to dislodge the obstruction. Applying the appraisal component of the CSM, expectation of effectiveness is usually high. If the treatment works, there is a high likelihood that one will use the procedure again. If not effective, some healers may try a combination of folk and Western medicine. Under the emotional arm of the CSM, the condition may initially be distressing and require the use of prayer (*cf.* Krause & Bastida 2011), typically designed to help the patient reduce stress and anxiety.

Representativeness Heuristic

One way we understand the health-illness orientation is to look at how we judge health-related events. Our perception of the probability or diagnosis of an event (e.g., cancer) is based on the likelihood that the symptoms match a prototype or schema in memory. This representativeness heuristic is used to judge the likelihood that observed features of an object are characteristic of the category (Gilovich 1991; Kahneman and Tversky 1972; Nisbett and Ross 1980). An example of representativeness comes from the Pennsylvania Germans. An old folk prescription instructs parents not to cut a child's fingernails until the 9th week after birth. It is believed that one must "scratch" for one's existence (i.e., work hard) and that premature cutting of the fingernails may cause the child to become indolent or to engage in thievery (Brendle and Unger 1970).

Related to the concept of representativeness is the idea that like goes with like (Gilovich 1991). Again from the Pennsylvania Germans (Brendle and Unger 1970), a folk prescription to improve memory is to boil the heart of a swallow in milk and wear it as an amulet around the neck. It was presumed that barn swallows had such a good memory that they could return year after year to their old nests in the barn (it is unclear if anyone actually checked if these were the same swallows returning each year, however).

Representativeness can also lend credence to a therapy, technique, or prescription by connecting features of treatments to a model, such as the biomedical model or to alternative approaches (e.g., Traditional Chinese Medicine [TCM]). For example, magnet therapy is a popular (though unfounded) treatment approach. For many, this treatment makes sense because of the representativeness heuristic. Often these magnets are sold in oval shapes, or integrated into bandages. These features "represent" medical treatment (i.e., application of a bandage). Also, the application of magnets to certain parts of the body may trigger connection to the ideas of acupuncture or acupressure.

Christian Fatalism

Another view that affects the health-illness orientation is Christian fatalism (Brendle and Unger 1970). It is often found in many cultures and has important implications for the health-illness orientation. With regard to the Pennsylvania German culture, Brendle and Unger (1970) write that in this culture, "afflictions that come from God are believed to have a purpose. They are sent as a trial, as a punishment, or as a part of preordained order of things" (p. 13). Similarly, Lithuanian folk medicine proposes that illness is given by God so that people would not fear death (Balkute 2000). There exist many similarities among cultures' folk medicine as related to religion and treatment of disease. These similarities include attribution of cause, such as loss of soul, given by God, retribution, bewitchments, or the result of the evil eye; and treatments, such as herbals, amulets, incantations, sympathy cures, or transference.

Drawing from the work of Baumann (2003), we can extrapolate her principles of cultural assessment of health beliefs to religious beliefs. For example, the meaning and purpose of prescriptions, regimens, and treatments must be interpreted in the context of the person's religious beliefs integrated into the person's common sense models. In effect, this use of situated discourse (Kleinman, Eisenberg, and Good 1978) is important to elicit explanatory models within a cultural system. According to Baumann (2003), the importance of situated discourse is that it helps identify explanatory models within cultures; explores differences between social groups within a community; and, as a qualitative approach, accesses a rich historical, social, and political context in which individual behaviors take place (p. 245). By extrapolation, situated discourse give us an insight into a person's CSM by allowing the patient to ask questions about cause, etiology, personal impact, timeline, severity, treatment considerations, effectiveness appraisal, impact on functions of daily living, and associated emotions.

SCIENCE AND RELIGION AND THE VALIDITY-INVALIDITY OF BOTH

Religion and science have much to offer to our understanding of a health-illness orientation. For example, both have the goal of getting at the "mysteries" of our existence. It has been proposed that science and religion are becoming more connected. For example, Buddhist and Hindu thought is found to provide an insight into subatomic particles (Capra 1991), and consciousness might be discovered in the microtubules of mitochondria (Hameroff, Craddock, and Tuszynski 2014; Hameroff and Penrose 2014). Probabilistic thinking gave rise to better understanding of wave-particle theories, field theories, superstrings, and dark matter (e.g., Greene 2003).

However, both religion and science can be invalid. They can be driven by false ideology, destructive agendas, and abuse and exploitation of others. For example, an agenda-driven science created policies that led to the sterilization of thousands due to the propagation of eugenics (Stern 2007). Restrictive immigration laws were enacted because of xenophobia and the misunderstanding of intelligence by scientists (Daniels 2004). Lobotomies were performed on thousands as a way to control behavior and emotional disturbances (El-Hai 2005). The use of radiation on children with intellectual disabilities (Moreno 2001) and the infamous Tuskegee experiments (Jones 1993) speak to the destructive possibilities when science is used as part of an agenda. More recently, the Hoffman Report (Hoffman et al. 2015) exposed the CIA's agenda to recruit psychologists with the goal of normalizing the use of torture on prisoners of war. In somewhat similar ways, religious fervor can result in a search for apostates and heretics, resulting in witch hunts, inquisitions, genocide, terrorism, crusades, and to justify the continuation of cultural stratification and castes.

At least two views exist regarding the validity of religion with regard to health. One view is that alternative and complementary approaches can be validated using scientific methodology (Miller, Emanuel, Rosenstein, and Straus 2004). By extension, the same methodological requirements are to be applied when testing religious, or faith-based, treatments as would be done in any biomedical clinical trial. Methodological considerations would include the use of double-blind studies, application of appropriate control groups, and random assignment. Also, evaluations of findings should be based on sample size and characteristics of the samples used and the generalizability of the findings.

Reported results using this approach have been mixed. For example, little evidence exists that the practice of *Taijiquan* reduces risk for falls in older adults (Norwalk, Prendergast, Bayles, D'Amico, and Colvin 2001; Verhagen, Immink, van der Meulen, and Bierma-Zeinstra 2004). However, others find that the practice of *Taijiquan* can significantly reduce chances of falling in older adults (Li et al. 2012). At least one study on the use of external *Qigong* to reduce lymphoma growth in mice (Chen et al. 2002) found no difference in tumor reduction among control (no external *Qigong*), external *Qigong* performed by a master, and external *Qigong* but performed by an untrained person. Santee (in Chapter 4 of this book) also points out that the effectiveness of *Taijiquan* and *Qigong* are mixed. However, more hopeful is the evidence he presents that meditative practices and mindfulness are beneficial to health. At least, according to Santee, there is no real downside to practicing *Taijiquan* and *Qigong*. Other views are less amenable to scientific scrutiny. Santee points out that a practice such as sitting in oblivion (*zuowang*) would defy an operational definition that could be put to a scientific test.

Another view is that the "reported" effect of religious practice on health can be attributed to the placebo effect. Faith healings, for example, have been argued to be no more than a placebo effect (Gilovich 1991). Although faith healing is an element in some cultures, it can also contribute to the perpetuation of ineffective practices. The placebo effect (Macedo, Farré, and Banos 2003) draws from expectations either broadly from the culture, from interactions between patient and practitioner, or specifically from the individual. Studies show that a warm, friendly practitioner increases positive interactions with patients (Thomas 1987; Thomas 1994). Practitioners' belief that a placebo is effective results in increased effectiveness reported by the patient. Patients' faith in the treatment contributes to placebo effects (Turner, Deyo, Loeser, Von Korff, and Fordyce 1994). The scientific judgment of invalidity of the treatment would be made when a practitioner who presents as warm and caring, and believes that the treatment is effective, along with the patient's belief in the effectiveness of the treatment, results in reported effectiveness of a treatment, prescription, or therapy that in fact has no specific causal relationship to the condition being treated (Di Blasi, Harkness, Ernst, Georgiou, and Kleijnen 2001).

Thus, it should be recognized that science and medicine can also engage in practices and ideologies that are controversial, dubious, and potentially harmful. The predominance of science may normalize practices within a folk model that we call the biomedical model (Engel 1977). Placed in a social-historical context, the biomedical model has implications for how we separate normal process from pathology, regard the medical regimens and treatments applied, and define the trajectory of illness. Therefore, distinguishing the confusion between normal process and pathology becomes a predominant concern.

Medicalization of Natural Processes

Medicalization of natural processes reifies the predominant Western, biomedical model of illness, disease, and health. Per a Western biomedical model, disease is thought to be disruptive, interfering with activities of daily living. As a result, all associated physical, emotional, and psychological symptoms are interpreted within this medical model.

For example, misdiagnosis of women with heart disease occurs because symptoms of heart attack in women are inconsistent with a male model of heart attack (Martin and Lemos 2002; Shifren 2003). Similarly, menopause, if seen as a life disruption, and accompanied by anxiety and depression based on outdated sociocultural beliefs of loss of reproductive potential and value, will often result in symptoms being perceived from this perspective. For example, a medical model of menopause has created an industry (Coney 1994) that has resulted in a view of menopause as a deficiency condition (V. Meyer 2003), requiring long-term if not lifelong treatment and maintenance (Erol 2014). This view has historically resulted in use of hormone replacement therapy, but treatments such as Valium were also used based on purported psychological symptoms such as depression and anxiety (Coney 1994).

Another implication of the medicalization of natural processes is that it discourages use of alternative approaches such as mindfulness. Here too one must be careful not to ignore real pathology that would respond most effectively to traditional Western medical approaches. However, a balance would be necessary to identify conditions arising from disease or from a natural process. One consequence for the patient under a strict medical model is that he or she may always be a "patient," often for a very long period of time. This status, as it relates to timeline, would significantly change the person's health-illness orientation, thus affecting cognition, emotion, and behavior.

One could argue that the preceding examples do not invalidate religion or science, but instead simply demonstrate that practices and ideologies associated with these two are faulty, rather than directly undermining the core principles of either. However, I propose that the "hijacking" of religion and science at times tends to perpetuate agendas, false beliefs, and ideologies, and distorts and destroys the principles on which science and religion were founded. Further, as Hwang and Cragun (Chapter 13) propose, methodological problems exist when comparing religious to non-religious individuals. These include no clear operational definitions of *religious, nonreligious,* and *spirituality;* inherent prejudice and bias against the nonreligious; and the confusion of correlation with causality. Taking these problems into consideration, Hwang and Cragun, in their review of the literature comparing religious to nonreligious individuals, find little difference between the two in pro-health behaviors.

THE QUATERNIO OF OPPOSITES

To allow us to move forward in our understanding of the relationship of science and religion to our health-illness orientation, I propose a model of quaternity (Jung 1970). This four-sided model places science and religion alongside the validity and invalidity of both. Religion and science and the valid-invalid conjunctions are recognized as opposites in this proposed model arranged in a quaternio and represented as a *physis,* or cross. The proposed model is analogous to Jung's Quaternio of Opposites. Pairs of opposites, such as moist-dry, cold-warm, heaven-earth, masculine-feminine, are arranged in a quaternio with the "two opposites crossing one another" (p. 3). Jung applied the conjunction of alchemical-religious symbols to his explanation of behavior in order to understand conflicts of the conscious with the unconscious and discord within the self. As he stated in the preface to his work *Mysterium Coniunctionis* (Jung 1970), "alchemy provides psychology of the unconscious with a meaningful historical basis" (p. xiii). The process of resolving these opposites, which are often in conflict, ultimately involves transcendence beyond and "liberation from opposites" (p. 223). This liberation, according to Jung, is something akin to the *nirdvandva* of Hindu philosophy, but applied to a psychological totality of the self.

To understand the relationship between religion, science, and our health-illness orientation, I ask the reader to consider a quaternio model placing religion and science on one axis and the validity and invalidity of these perspectives on the other axis. Although an exegesis of Jung's connections of religion and alchemy to depth psychology is beyond the scope of this chapter, suffice it to say that Jung proposed that a conjunction of opposites can also represent a struggle between broader, conflicting ideologies. In the proposed model, religion and science play converse roles in the "drama of opposites . . . which is fought out in every human life" (Jung 1970, p. 166). Given this opposition between religion and science, the question then becomes whether the two can be brought together into some type of unity that ideally transcends our separate understanding of each. As often is the case, however, these two ideologies are compared and contrasted, where similarities but mostly differences are highlighted, or one is subordinated to the other. It thus remains unclear what would unite the two. The task would appear almost impossible if we follow Jung's, and the alchemists', advice to express the opposites "in the same breath" (p. 42).

A QUESTION OF BALANCE OR THE SPACE BETWEEN?

How do we begin to resolve religion and science vis-à-vis our health-illness orientation? One criticism of science's attitude toward religion, faith, and spirituality is that science often accepts a very narrow view of these concepts. Specifically, these are treated as extraneous variables and operationalized according to the rules of scientific methodology. The testing of these as variables with other variables is the product of the hypothetico-deductive, reductionistic stance of the scientific method. As a result, spirituality and religion are understood in science as moderators or mediators, and therefore not fully appreciated in a holistic way.

Drawing from similar comparisons in physics and philosophy (e.g., Jeans 1942/2009), it can be argued that the oppositions and differences that exist between religion and science cannot be resolved, as they speak different languages, have different worldviews, and include different concepts or similar concepts differently conceptualized (see Chapter 1 for additional challenges regarding science and religion). Further, it is believed that if science is to progress, it must engage a radical empiricism, discarding metaphysical explanations and holding to scientific methodology and sound statistical reasoning. It would follow that metaphysical concepts linked to religion, although acknowledged by science and found to have important implications for health and well-being, still remain separate perspectives. It is also fair to consider that science and religion are often at odds with each other regarding health. For example, strong, opposing beliefs exist on the religious and scientific side regarding abortion (Chapter 7) and the health of the mother, prohibition of medical procedures in some cultures and religious groups, and in creationism and fatalism as guiding principles in some religious views.

The easy answer is that we must begin to take a more holistic perspective regarding health-illness orientation. This idea has been around for centuries, running from Hippocrates to Engel (1977) and others. A holistic perspective offers the idea that there is a connectedness of culture, medicine, and the person that has cosmological implications. It has certainly been proposed that the laws of physics as related to subatomic particles can be attuned to Eastern thought, particularly if one concentrates on the interconnectedness of all things in the cosmos (Capra 1991). But Eastern thought also proposes that the way to health is to understand the void, or emptiness (Chapter 4).

As we move forward in our understanding of religion and science as these relate to health, the question becomes: Do we find a balance between the two, an integration of religion and science; or do we recognize that a divide indeed exists and direct our work toward contemplating the space between? In the next section, it will be proposed that a unity may not be possible— not in the way most discuss the tension between religion and science—but that we should instead to borrow from Eastern philosophical views and investigate the void, or the space between religion and science. This contemplation brings the bold assertion that from it a new, transcendent model of health-illness orientation emerges that will not be linked to our present constructs of religion and science. This notion of the void, or space between, will serve as an analogue for the gap between religion and science, and will be considered in more detail in the next section.

THE SPACE BETWEEN

The Creation of Adam

Michelangelo Buonorrati was commissioned by Pope Julius II in 1508 to paint the ceiling of the Sistine Chapel. Michelangelo created, in fresco, a stunning chronological narrative of nine stories from Genesis. One of the paintings that generated much thought was "The Creation of Adam." Depicted in this fresco is the finger of God (*spiritus*; Barolsky 2013), about to instill life and spirit into the laconically posed Adam. However, as Barolsky (2013) points out, there exists a tension in the space between the finger of God and that of Adam. Importantly, the event is "suspended forever" . . . and is the "ultimate divine *non-finito*" (p. 24). This gap is thus a place of tension requiring a resolution. Barolsky (2013) reported that scholars in the 18th century, preoccupied with science, speculated that the gap was the spark of electricity. Other thoughts turned to the idea that God as depicted in the fresco was the source of art and music, or the first artist and architect ready to instill these ideals into an awaiting Adam. Or, one could suggest the duality of body and spirit.

Barolsky (2003, 2013) speaks more closely to the goals of Michelangelo and proposes that the "Creation of Adam" embodies concepts from the Bible. One is that God is *creator spiritus*. Adam is not complete (*non-finito*) until touched by the finger of God. Within the gap resides the "awesome power of conception" (Barolsky 2003, p. 34) awaiting the finger of God to instill the spirit in Adam. An even deeper meaning is proposed by Barolsky

(2003). The creation of Adam is an allegory of the descent of Jesus—the second Adam. Barolsky proposes that when touched by God, Adam becomes alive in spirit. The first Adam thus evokes the second Adam-Jesus within the trinity: God as *creator spiritus*, Holy Spirit, and Jesus as one.

More pertinently to the ideas presented in this chapter, the gap creates a paradox, a mystery to be contemplated. Until the act is complete, or the gap is closed, one is not entirely sure of the intent. The paradox represents a popular concept in the renaissance of *discordante-concordia* (imperfection-perfection). Interestingly, Barolsky (2003) points out that the artists of this era often left parts of their work unfinished (particularly in sculptures). The idea was that the "antithesis between the unfinished area and the finished work . . . brought out by implication their very mastery of the medium" (p. 49). I would offer that the unfinished area in the "Creation of Adam" is exactly the space between the finger of God and the finger of Adam—not leading to resolution but to possibilities.

Liminal Space

Another way we can think of the void between religion and science in the proposed quaternio-of-opposites model is as a liminal space. *Limen*, or threshold in a socio-cultural context, is described as a transition, or rite of passage as one changes status in the culture from one state to another. This transition creates a liminal space of uncertainty and ambiguity. In rites of passage, the transition from liminal space to postliminal space (i.e., the initiates' integration into society with new roles and responsibilities) is usually supported by rituals where elders help the initiate across the threshold to a new status and role in society (Turner 1969; van Gennepp 1909/2004). Liminal space seems to have both positive and negative features. For example, liminal space represents a transition. This transition can imply growth, transcendence, and psychospiritual development. It can also reflect existential crisis, such as living and dying, a place where people are "betwixt and between," "neither one thing or another, or both" (Turner 1967, p. 93). Liminal space is ambiguous, uncertain, a place of dissonance, a limbo.

The concept of liminal space has been applied to understanding a person's health and illness. Liminal space from the patient's perspective has been investigated for cancer (Adorno 2015; Forss, Tishelman, Widmark, and Sachs 2004; Little, Jordens, Paul, Montgomery, and Philipson 1998; Navon and Morag 2004), organ transplantation (Crowley-Matoka 2005), cholesterol (Felde 2015), and mental health (Barrett 1998; Fischer 2012; Warner and Gabe 2004; Yuen 2011). Liminality can also describe physical spaces such as a lobby in a nursing home as the existential metaphor describing the space between old age and death (Gamliel 2000). Relatedly, discussions of transitional space from a psychoanalytic and social construct perspective focus on conflict and turbulence within an organization, between individuals, and between individuals and environment (Fischer 2012). Ambiguity, uncertainty, isolation, and conflict reside where people are "in-between" their relationship with others (Foulkes 1948/1991, p. 1191), their community (cf. Warner and Gabe 2004), and their relationship with religion and science.

Liminal Space and Health-Illness Orientation

The concept of liminal space now provides us with an understanding of the space between religion and science according to the proposed quaternio-of-opposites model, with implications for our health-illness orientation. Our health-illness orientation can be disrupted by ambiguity, uncertainty, or potential for isolation from others; or if symptoms are undiagnosed, misunderstood, or represent stigmatized diseases that potentially make the person a societal outcast. This disruption can also come from a confrontation with one's own mortality. These factors create, for the patient, a liminal space of uncertainty between choices to be made and states of existence

Implications of Liminal Space for Health-Illness Orientation

Delayed Treatment Seeking   The creation of liminal space regarding health can affect one's health-illness orientation and have implications for treatment seeking. The patient can be aware of symptoms as potentially threatening but choose not to seek immediate medical attention. Under a biomedical model, seeking treatment is considered a normative response, whereas delay, or not seeking treatment, on the part of the patient is perceived as denial or negligence, carrying with it the negative connotations of blame and irresponsibility. Granek and Fergus (2012) make this point in their investigation of the liminal space women experience in decisions to seek or not to seek a physician's advice upon detection of an abnormality of the breast (Granek and Fergus 2012). The concept of liminal space can now be connected to the CSM discussed earlier. An awareness of change of physical state could lead to worry, dismissal of symptoms, or evaluation of symptoms as something or nothing. Behaviorally, any self-regulation response is initially in limbo, carrying with it implications for timeline and type of appropriate coping responses selected juxtaposed against the socioculturally defined moral judgment of one's behavior vis-à-vis treatment seeking.

Illness Trajectories and Liminal Space   A second example of how disruptions to our health-illness orientation create a liminal space appears in an examination of illness trajectories. For example, the concept of liminal space has been utilized in organ transplantation where the patient is "caught betwixt and between the role of sick and healthy patient and normal person" (Crowley-Matoka 2005, p. 822). Similarly, one must investigate the contextual factors in illness trajectories in diseases such as cancer (Adorno 2015; Granek and Fergus 2012). These trajectories create states in which one is neither healthy nor sick, or is moving between a sick role to a dying role (Adorno 2015), or transitioning between life and death. The liminal space concept can also be understood in asymptomatic conditions such as high cholesterol (Felde 2015).

Science and Religion as Liminal Space   According to the proposed quaternio-of-opposites model, the liminal space between religion and science can be one of ambiguity, uncertainty, and communicative isolation (*cf.* Adorno 2015), thus impacting one's health-illness orientation. Here one's health-illness orientation is an in-between state vis-à-vis one's understanding and application of religion and/or science. These choices involving religion and science are part of and embodied in the person's health-illness orientation.

Many life situations are experienced in this liminal space. Perhaps the most profound liminal space is between everyday living and confrontation of our own mortality. Within this space of anxiety and uncertainty is juxtaposed our sociocultural views of religion and science.

Science as Liminal Space   It can be argued that science consists of ritualized strategies, in a sociocultural context, reflecting a *weltanschauung* (Kuhn 1996). Here, the scientist is "enculturated" into the role of being a scientist and working within the existing paradigm through which puzzles are solved (Kuhn 1996). A predominant paradigm, or model, related to health is the biomedical model, which some have argued to be a folk model of Western medicine (Engel 1977). For example, the ideal behavior under the biomedical model is that once a person detects troubling symptoms, this should result in immediate seeking of an appropriate physician (Granek and Fergus 2012).

Liminality as it relates to science can be thought of as the ambiguous space between supernatural (i.e., religious) explanations and scientific explanations of phenomena, or the transition space between unscientific to scientific explanations. Thus, a tension exists in this liminal space. This is also akin to changes in paradigms or a crisis stage, as discussed by Kuhn (1996). Even more pronounced is the liminality when science fails to explain mysterious or undiagnosed medical conditions (Nemecek 1996; Nettleton,

Watt, O'Malley, and Duffey 2005). Conditions such as lupus, fibromyalgia, and Lyme disease, where the causes were unknown, resulted in the sufferer living in liminal space of ambiguity, uncertainty, fear, and anxiety. One can argue that in some cases these can be considered temporary liminal spaces, as science eventually finds an explanation, but some remain permanently liminal. In addition, symptomless conditions can be placed in this concept of liminal space as problematic for science in relation to patient adherence to treatment and acceptance. Examples are cholesterol levels and high blood pressure. Usually, patients become aware of these conditions only through blood tests, screening, or physical exams. Not only could these symptomless conditions affect adherence to medical regimen under the CSM, but the conditions could create the liminal space between identification of illness (based on expressed symptoms) and non-illness (based on no external symptoms) as another factor affecting peoples' health choices. When confronted with an illness, the patient is traditionally faced with binary choices, an "ontological dualism" (Adorno 2015, p. 114) that constrains types of choices from a scientific standpoint.

Religion, Spirituality, and Faith as Liminal Space   Spirituality and religion can also create a liminal space of ambiguity, uncertainty, and communicative isolation (*cf.* Adorno 2015) in one's health-illness orientation. "Spiritual perspectives and practices can provide a context wherein anxieties about physical and mental functioning may be faced, felt, and understood" (Yuen 2011, p. 42). In effect, spiritual practices allow us to understand, confront, and possibly cross the threshold of that liminal space of uncertainty, ambiguity, and anxiety with regard to physical and mental health. From the standpoint of the clinician, Yuen (2011) describes the liminal space as something that "engenders an ability to listen, not just to others, but to ourselves, our innermost values, without judgment. This pairing of stillness with activity can informs [*sic*] our actions and decisions, particularly in times of uncertainty, by joining inner, heartfelt values with outer medical decisions that are rooted in time, rates, centimeters, and other metrics. This inclusion of the 'unknown' liminal moments in the clinical encounter may be a key to acknowledging the spiritual aspect of the interaction" (p. 44).

Furthermore, our understanding of religion as liminal space requires a more complete understanding of the transition from life to death. We wander along dimensions of health and life, illness and death, everyday living and mortality. The liminal space between living and dying can be one of ambiguity and uncertainty. Religion and spirituality can guide one through the threshold in ways that science cannot. However, religion as a transcendent, existential-based process may too be exemplified by uncertainty, doubt, and isolation. This crisis of faith exposes the liminal space between life and death, as exemplified by Arjuna's doubt regarding his *Dharma* (*Baghavad Gita* 1994) or by Christ's cry of being forsaken upon the cross (Matthew 27:46 [*New American Bible*], n.d.). The liminal space was resolved by an existential transcendence.

Mandorlas   Here I propose to think about religion and science within the concept of mandorla. Mandorlas are often represented by two overlapping circles (also ellipses) containing the intersection of two opposites such as male and female. In art history, it is the oval shape that enshrines a (usually) sacred figure such as the Christ or Mary, in Christian art (Brunetti 1951/1952). Mandorlas are also found in Hindu and Buddhist art (Fowler 2000/2001). The mandorla behind a Buddha figure exemplifies incandescence, a spiritual glow, and a transcendence (Suzuki 2010). The statue of the Buddha Yakushi (e.g., *Shichibutsu Yakushi*), the medicine or healing Buddha, became a popular icon during the Heian period (794–1185 CE) in Japan. During this period, a popular way to represent the Buddha was as a statue surrounded by a mandorla of 6 or 7 smaller, healing Buddhas (Suzuki 2010).

In classical Greek and Roman art and medieval art, mandorlas were often depicted as shields. A shield conveyed a victory motif where the primary figure—the emperor, victor, god—was portrayed. Over time, the victory motif of battle became an analogue to include religious victory. An example is a miniature of the ascension in the Rabula Gospels (586–587 CE). The mandorla depicts Christ's ascension surrounded by winged angels where beneath the mandorla are placed "wings, wheels, head of man, lion, ox, and eagle . . . combined to meet the requirements of the involved vision of Ezekiel" (Elderkin 1938, p. 236).

The mandorla as an intersection of opposites can also address the paradox of religion and science. Scientific thinking incorporating the concepts of force fields, probability, and quanta is linked to metaphysical understanding of Hindu and Buddhist cosmologies. In the classic, *The Tao of Physics*, Fritjof Capra (1991) describes quantum field theory as continuum "which is present everywhere in space and yet in its particular aspect has a discontinuous 'granular' structure. The two apparently contradictory concepts are thus unified and seen to be merely different aspects of the same reality" (p. 215). New Age perspectives have also connected the two and speculate that the mandorla as a symbol of an aura surrounding a figure is similar to force fields of modern science (Callicott 2000).

Yet we are still faced with the problem of resolving the two in relation to health-illness orientation. Perhaps we should consider not what each shares with the other, but rather what *emerges* from the contemplation of the two. According to Mandorla Resources International, "the Mandorla is to move beyond 'either-or' thinking—even beyond ideas of common ground or compromise—and stand in the tension of opposites long enough for something new to emerge. In the realm of the Mandorla, the whole truly yields something greater than the sum of its parts, opening doors of possibility, discovery, and creativity" (http://www.mandorla.com/resources/home .html).

CONCLUSION: INTO THE VOID

Faith, spirituality, and religion are not bound by scientific methodology. Others believe that the realms of faith, religion, and spirituality are unscientific and are not sufficient or necessary to understand health. This epilogue, however, stresses that indeed faith, spirituality, religion, and science are important in how we construct our health-illness orientation, as they all have important implications for cognition, affect, and behavior. However, religion and science are often viewed as incompatible, or at odds with each other. It has been argued that the best that science has done is to treat these variables of religion, spirituality, and faith in relation to other variables and determine the amount of variance explained regarding health. Of course, a scientist can have strong religious or philosophical views that guide his or her ethics, appropriateness of research, and application of findings; and one can cross the liminal space of uncertainty and ambiguity regarding one's health through spiritual and religious insight (*cf.* Yuen 2011). The bottom line is that to understand our health-illness orientation, one does not need a religion to do science, nor does one need a science to do religion, and both can independently address our health-illness orientation. It seems, then, that it is not an easy task to cross the threshold to a postliminal articulation of a model of religion and science.

As proposed in this chapter, religion and science, organized under a Common Sense Model of self-regulation, are important factors that make up our health-illness orientation; however, both often stand diametrically opposed to and at odds with each other. How do we resolve this paradox? The intellectual community has worked hard to look for an integration of science and religion, but this is not an unproblematic enterprise. It is proposed that another way to understand the relationship between science and religion and our health-illness orientation is to borrow from Eastern philosophy and to ponder and meditate on the emptiness or the void between religion and science. The void can also be understood as a great chasm between religion, which is based on metaphysics, and science, which is based on empiricism and scientific methodology. A model to understand this void was proposed based on the quaternio of opposites aligned along the conjunction of science-religion and valid-invalid features.

The validity and invalidity of both religion and science in conjunction with metaphysics and scientific method creates a space between the two. Contemplation of this space may be the starting point of understanding. Perhaps the space between religion and science contains nothing, but it could possibly contain everything. Religion requires a leap of faith. If indeed we are a being-toward-death (Heidegger 1927/1996), our health-illness orientation— whether or not we are consciously aware of it—contains the inevitability of our own mortality and the leap of faith needed to see beyond death. Science too is a leap of faith, requiring a belief that our practices and methods are valid while faced with the haunting specter that these practices may be based on no more than social constructs limited by time and space. Understanding our health-illness orientation involves the liminal space between religion *qua* not-science and science *qua* not-religion. One could therefore consider that any attempt at integration of religion with science is an unhealthy obsession—a product of our own irrationality—leading to emotional strain and to an unprofitable end. Perhaps the key is not to find an integration of religion and science, but rather to contemplate the space between the two, to embrace the void, so as to find hope ultimately leading to transcendence and an enlightenment of our own health-illness orientation.

ACKNOWLEDGMENT

I would like to thank Dr. Toru Sato, my colleague and friend, who called my attention to the concepts of liminal space and mandorlas.

NOTE

1. Although recognizing that the terms *faith*, *spirituality*, and *religion* have differences and similarities, I primarily use the term *religion* in my discussion, for brevity of exposition.

REFERENCES

Adorno, G. 2015. "Between Two Worlds: Liminality and Late-Stage Cancer-Directed Therapy." *OMEGA: Journal of Death and Dying* 71(2): 99–125.
Balkute, R. 2000. "Lithuanian Folk Medicine" (trans. G. Ambrozaitiene). *LABAS The Lithuanian E-Zine* 3(3). Retrieved from http://www.angelfire.com/tx/LABAS/2000/feb/medicine.html
Barolsky, P. 2003. *Michelangelo and the Finger of God*. Athens, GA: Georgia Museum of Art.
Barolsky, P. 2013. "The Genius of Michelangelo's 'Creation of Adam' and the Blindness of Art History." *Notes in the History of Art* 33(1): 21–24.

Barrett, R. J. 1998. "The 'Schizophrenic' and the Liminal Persona in Modern Society." *Culture, Medicine and Psychiatry* 22: 465–494.

Baumann, L. C. 2003. "Culture and Illness Representations." In L. D. Cameron and H. Leventhal, eds., *The Self-Regulation of Health and Illness Behavior*, pp. 242–253. New York: Routledge.

The Bhagavad Gita. 1994. W. Sargeant, trans. New York: State University of New York.

Brendle, T. R., and C. W. Unger. 1970. *Folk Medicine of the Pennsylvania Germans: The Non-Occult Cures.* New York: Augustus M. Kelley Publishers.

Brunetti, G. 1951/1952. "Jacopo della Quercia and the Porta della Mandorla." *Metropolitan Museum of Art Bulletin* 10: 265–274.

Callicott, B. 2000. "Mandorlas, Halos, and Rings of Fire." *Quest Magazine* 88(4): 124–127. Retrieved fromhttps://www.theosophical.org/publications/quest-magazine/42-publications/quest-magazine/1348-mandorlas-halos-and-rings-of-fire

Cameron, L. D., and L. Jago. 2008. "Emotion Regulation Interventions: A Common-Sense Model Approach." *British Journal of Health Psychology* 13: 215–221.

Cameron, L. D., and H. Leventhal. 2003. *The Self-Regulation of Health and Illness Behavior.* New York: Routledge.

Capra, F. 1991. *The Tao of Physics: An Exploration of the Parallels Between Modern Physics and Eastern Mysticism* (3rd ed.). Boston: Shambhala.

Chen, K. W., S. C. Shiflett, N. M. Ponzio, B. He, D. K. Elliott, and S. E. Keller. 2002. "A Preliminary Study of the Effect of External Qigong on Lymphoma Growth in Mice." *Journal of Alternative and Complementary Medicine* 8(5): 615–621.

Chittem, M., P. Norman, and P. R. Harris. 2015. "Illness Representations and Psychological Distress in Indian Patients with Cancer: Does Being Aware of One's Cancer Diagnosis Make a Difference?" *Psycho-Oncology* 24: 1694–1700.

Coney, S. 1994. *The Menopause Industry: How the Medical Establishment Exploits Women.* Alameda, CA: Hunter House.

Crowley-Matoka, M. 2005. "Desperately Seeking 'Normal': The Promise and Perils of Living with Kidney Transplantation." *Social Science & Medicine* 61: 821–831.

Daniels, R. 2004. *Guarding the Golden Door: American Immigration Policy and Immigrants Since 1882.* New York: Hill and Wang.

Di Blasi, Z., E. Harkness, E. Ernst, A. Georgiou, and J. Kleijnen. 2001. "Influence of Context Effects on Health Outcomes: A Systematic Review." *Lancet* 357: 757–762.

Elderkin, G. W. (1938). "Shield and Mandorla." *American Journal of Archeology* 42(2): 227–236.

El-Hai, J. (2005). *The Lobotomist: A Maverick Medical Genius and His Tragic Quest to Rid the World of Mental Illness.* Hoboken, NJ: John Wiley & Sons.

Engel, G. L. 1977. "The Need for a New Medical Model: A Challenge for Biomedicine." *Science* 196: 129–136.

Erol, M. 2014. "From Opportunity to Obligation: Medicalization of Post-Menopausal Sexuality in Turkey." *Sexualities* 17(1/2): 43–62.

Felde, L. K. H. 2015. "I Take a Small Amount of the Real Product: Elevated Cholesterol nd Everyday Medical Reasoning in Liminal Space." *Health* 15(6): 604–619.

Fischer, M. D. 2012. "Organizational Turbulence, Trouble, and Trauma: Theorizing the Collapse of a Mental Health Setting." *Organization Studies* 33(9): 1153–1173.

Forss, A., C. Tishelman, C. Widmark, and L. Sachs. 2004. "Women's Experiences of Cervical Cellular Changes: An Unintentional Transition from Health to Liminality?" *Sociology of Health & Illness* 26(3): 306–325. Retrieved from http://onlinelibrary.wiley.com/doi/10.1111/j.1467-9566.2004.00392.x/full

Foulkes, S. H. 1948/1991. *Introduction to Group-Analytic Psychotherapy.* London: Karnac.

Fowler, S. 2000/2001. "Shifting Identities in Buddhist Sculpture: Who's Who in the Muro-Ji Kondo." *Archives of Asian Art* 52: 83–104.

Gamliel, T. 2000. "The Lobby as an Arena in the Confrontation between Acceptance and Denial of Old Age." *Journal of Aging Studies* 14(3): 251–271.

Gilovich, T. 1991. *How We Know What Isn't So: The Fallibility of Human Reason in Everyday Life.* New York: Free Press.

Gleason, C. E., N. M. Dowling, S. F. Benton, A. Kaseroff, W. Gunn, and D. F. Edwards. 2016. "Common Sense Model Factors Affecting African Americans' Willingness to Consult a Healthcare Provider Regarding Symptoms of Mild Cognitive Impairment." *American Journal of Geriatric Psychiatry* 24: 537–546.

Granek, L., and K. Fergus. 2012. "Resistance, Agency, and Liminality in Women's Accounts of Symptom Appraisal and Help-Seeking upon Discovery of a Breast Irregularity." *Social Science and Medicine* 75: 1753–1761.

Greene, B. 2003. *The Elegant Universe: Superstrings, Hidden Dimensions, and the Quest for the Ultimate Theory.* New York: W. W. Norton.

Gurung, R. A.R. 2006. *Health Psychology: A Cultural Approach.* Belmont, CA: Thompson-Wadsworth.

Hameroff, S., T. J. A. Craddock, and J. A. Tuszynski. 2014. "Quantum Effects in the Understanding of Consciousness." *Journal of Integrative Neuroscience* 13(20): 229–252.

Hameroff, S., and R. Penrose. 2014. "Consciousness in the Universe: A Review of the ORCH OR Theory." *Physics of Life Reviews* 11: 39–78.

Heidegger, M. 1927/1996. *Being and Time.* Trans. J. Stambaugh. New York: Harper State University of New York Press.

Hoffman, D. H., D. J. Carter, C. R. V. Lopez, H. L. Benzmiller, A. X. Guo, S. Y. Latifi, and D. C. Craig. 2015a. *Report to the Special Committee of the Board of Directors of the American Psychological Association: Independent Review Relating* to *APA Ethics Guidelines, National Security Interrogations, and Torture*. Chicago, IL: Sidley Austin LLP. Retrieved from http://www.apa.org/indepen dent-review/APA-FINAL-Report-7.2.15.pdf

Jeans, J. 1942/2009. *Physics and Philosophy*. Cambridge, UK: Cambridge University Press.

Jones, J. H. 1993. *Bad Blood: The Tuskegee Syphilis Experiment* (Expanded ed.) New York: Free Press.

Jung, C. G. 1970. *Mysterium Coniunctionis: An Inquiry into the Separation and Synthesis of Psychic Opposites in Alchemy* (2nd ed., Vol. 14). Trans. R. F. C. Hull. Princeton, NJ: Princeton University Press.

Kahneman, D., and A. Tversky. 1972. "Subjective Probability: A Judgement of Representativeness." *Cognitive Psychology* 3: 430–454.

Kleinman, A., L. Eisenberg, and B. J. Good. 1978. "Culture, Illness, and Care: Clinical Lessons from Anthropologic and Cross-Cultural Research." *Annals of Internal Medicine* 88: 251–258.

Krause, N., and E. Bastida. 2011. "Prayer to the Saints or the Virgin and Health among Older Mexican Americans." *Hispanic Journal of Behavioral Science* 33(1): 71–87.

Kuhn, T. S. 1996. *The Structure of Scientific Revolutions* (3rd ed.). Chicago: University of Chicago Press.

Leventhal, H., I. Brissette, and E. A. Leventhal. 2003. "The Common-Sense Model of Self-Regulation of Health and Illness." In L. D. Cameron and H. Leventhal, eds., *The Self-Regulation of Health and Illness Behavior*, pp. 42–65. New York: Routledge.

Leventhal, H., E. A. Leventhal, and P. Schaefer. 1991. "Vigilant Coping and Health Behavior: A Life Span Problem." In M. Ory and R. Abeles, eds., *Aging and Health Behavior*, pp. 109–140. Baltimore, MD: Johns Hopkins.

Leventhal, H., L. A. Phillips, and E. Burns. 2016. "The Common-Sense Model of Self-Regulation (CSM): A Dynamic Framework for Understanding Illness Self-Management." *Journal of Behavioral Medicine* 39: 935–946.

Lewis, M. K. 2002. "Introduction." In M. K. Lewis, ed., *Multicultural Health Psychology: Special Topics Acknowledging Diversity*, pp. 1–16. Boston: Allyn & Bacon.

Li, F., P. Harmer, K. Fitzgerald, E. Eckstrom, R. Stock, J. Galver, . . . S. S. Batya. 2012. "Tai Chi and Postural Stability in Patients with Parkinson's Disease." *New England Journal of Medicine* 366: 511–519.

Little, M., C. F. C. Jordens, K. Paul, K. Montgomery, and B. Philipson. 1998. "Liminality: A Major Category of the Experience of Cancer Illness." *Social Science & Medicine* 47(10): 1485–1494.

Macedo, A., M. Farré, and J.-E. Banos. 2003. "Placebo Effect and Placebos: What Are We Talking About? Some Conceptual and Historical Considerations." *European Journal of Clinical Pharmacology* 59(4): 337–342. doi:10.1007/s00228-003-0612-4v

Mandorla Resources International. n.d. Home Page. Retrieved from http://www
.mandorla.com/resources/home.html

Martin, R., and K. Lemos. 2002. "From Heart Attacks to Melanoma: Do Common
Sense Models of Somatization Influence Symptom Interpretation for Female
Victims?" *Health Psychology* 21(1): 25–32.

Meyer, D., H. Leventhal, and M. Gutman. 1985. "Common-Sense Models of Illness: The Example of Hypertension." *Health Psychology* 4(2): 115–135.

Meyer, V. F. 2003. "Medicalized Menopause, U.S. Style." *Health Care of Women International* 24: 822–830.

Miller, F. G., E. J. Emanuel, D. L. Rosenstein, and S. E. Straus. 2004. "Ethical Issues
Concerning Research in Complementary and Alternative Medicine." *Journal of the American Medical Association (JAMA)* 291(5): 599–604.

Moreno, J. D. 2001. *Undue Risk: Secret State Experiments on Humans.* New York:
Routledge.

Navon, L., and A. Morag. 2004. "Liminality as Biographical Disruption: Unclassi-
fiability Following Hormonal Therapy for Advanced Prostate Cancer." *Social
Science and Medicine* 58: 2337–2347.

Neighbors, K. A. 1969. "Mexican-American Folk Diseases." *Western Folklore* 28(4):
249–259.

Nemecek, S. 1996. "Mysterious Maladies: Separating Real from Imagined Disorders Presents Frustrating Challenges." *Scientific American* 275(3): 24.

Nettleton, S., I. Watt, L. O'Malley, and P. Duffey. 2005. "Understanding the Narratives of People Who Live with Medically Unexplained Illness." *Patient Education and Counseling* 56: 205–210.

The New American Bible. n.d. Nashville, TN: Catholic Bible Press.

Nisbett, R., and L. Ross. 1980. *Human Inference: Strategies and Shortcomings of Social
Judgment.* Englewood Cliffs, NJ: Prentice-Hall.

Norwalk, M. P., J. M. Prendergast, C. M. Bayles, F. J. D'Amico, and G. C. Colvin.
2001. "A Randomized Trial of Exercise Programs among Older Individuals
Living in Two Long-Term Care Facilities: The fallsFREE Program." *Journal
of the American Geriatric Society* 49: 859–865.

Shifren, K. 2003. "Women with Heart Disease: Can the Common-Sense Model of
Illness Help?" *Health Care for Women International* 24: 355–368.

Stern, A. M. 2007, March. "'We Cannot Make a Silk Purse Out of a Sow's Ear':
Eugenics in the Hoosier Heartland." *Indiana Magazine of History,* 103(1):
3–38. Retrieved from https://scholarworks.iu.edu/journals/index.php/imh
/article/view/12254/18215

Suzuki, Y. 2010. "The Aura of Seven: Reconsidering the *Shichibutsu Yakushi* Ico-
nography." *Archives of Asian Art* 60: 19–42.

Thomas, K. B. 1987. "General Practice Consultations: Is There Any Point in Being
Positive?" *British Medical Journal* 294: 1200–1202.

Thomas, K. B. 1994. "The Placebo Effect in General Practice." *Lancet* 344:
1066–1067.

Turner, J. A., R. A. Deyo, J. D. Loeser, M. Von Korff, and W. E. Fordyce. 1994. "The Importance of Placebo Effects in Pain and Treatment Research." *Journal of the American Medical Association (JAMA)* 271: 1609–1614.

Turner, V. 1967. *The Forest of Symbols: Aspects of* Ndembu *Ritual.* Ithaca, NY: Cornell University Press.

Turner, V. 1969. The Ritual Process: Structure and Antistructure. Ithaca, NY: Cornell University Press.

van Gennepp, A. 1909/2004. *The Rites of Passage.* New York: Routledge.

Verhagen, A. P., M. Immink, A. van der Meulen, and S. M. A. Bierma-Zeinstra. 2004. "The Efficacy of Tai Chi Chuan in Older Adults: A Systematic Review." *Family Practice* 21(1): 107–113.

Warner, J., and J. Gabe. 2004. "Risk and Liminality in Mental Health Social Work." *Health, Risk, and Society* 6(4): 387–399.

Yuen, E. 2011. "Spirituality and the Clinical Encounter." *International Journal for Human Caring* 15(2): 42–46.

About the Editor and Contributors

DEAN D. VONDRAS, PhD (editor), is Professor of Human Development and Psychology at the University of Wisconsin, Green Bay, where he teaches courses in Adulthood and Aging and Spirituality and Development. He has contributed scholarly articles addressing associations between aspects of spiritual well-being and alcohol use in female college students; the ideological contexts of religions and their influences on health-associated behaviors; spiritual aspects of caregiving; and best practices for teaching about spirituality and developmental processes. Dr. VonDras has a special interest in the intertwining of health and psychological processes in adult development and aging, and previously served as a Post-Doctoral Fellow at the Behavioral Medicine Research Center at Duke University Medical Center, and a Research Associate in the Alzheimer's Disease Research Center at Washington University Medical Center in St. Louis. Dr. VonDras has also been recognized as a University of Wisconsin, Green Bay, Teaching Scholar, as well as a University of Wisconsin System Teaching Fellow, and has received awards for Best Practices in Teaching, and Creative Approaches to Teaching.

VIBHA AGNIHOTRI, PhD, is an associate professor and the Head of Department (HOD) of Anthropology at Nari Shiksha Niketan Post Graduate College, Lucknow University, Uttar Pradesh (India). She has several publications and has authored various books on the scholarly aspects of social sciences and astrology, her second passion after anthropology. She is also the President of the Association of Academic People Society and the Academic Association of People of Social Science. She is the Vice President of the Santosha Devi Memorial Society. Dr. Agnihotri is also a founding member of the Indian National Confederacy and the Academy of Anthropologists (INCAA) and General Secretary of Manav Kalyan Evam Vigyan Prasar Sansthan, a nongovernmental organization. She is the editor and associate editor of numerous national and international journals, including *Voice of Intellectual Man* and *The Eastern Anthropologist.* She has traveled to more than 40 countries to organize and present on various panels in World Congress across Asia, Europe, Canada, and the United Kingdom.

VINAMRATA AGNIHOTRI, MS, graduated with a bachelor's in Psychology (Hon.) and master's in Psychology from the Lady Shri Ram College and Daulat Ram College, University of Delhi, respectively. With a knack for research and acumen regarding organizational behavior, she has completed two dissertations on workplace aggression, work-family conflict, and subjective health and well-being, both at the undergraduate and graduate levels. She has twice represented India at the Youth for Human Rights Summit at Geneva in 2009–2011, and subsequently organized the International Walk for Human Rights in Lucknow and New Delhi—the first ever in India. She is the editorial assistant of the international journal *Voice of Intellectual Man* and has attended and presented papers at several national and international conferences on psychology, sociology, education, and spirituality. In addition, she is a member of various societies including the American Psychological Association, and has published in national and international journals. Currently, she is an education consultant and a career counselor working with Indian students in selection of best possible options according to their interests and aptitudes.

MONA M. AMER, PhD, is an associate professor and Chair of the Department of Psychology at the American University in Cairo, Egypt. Her research focuses on ethnic/racial disparities in behavioral health, with specializations in the Arab American and American Muslim populations. She is interested in immigration/acculturation and mental health, mental illness stigma and other cultural barriers to service utilization for diverse racial/ethnic groups, and the design of culturally valid research measures. She has developed cultural competence training programs for health and mental health practitioners working with Muslim and Arab clients. Dr. Amer has more than 35 professional publications, including 2 books: *Counseling Muslims: Handbook of Mental Health Issues and Interventions* (2012) and *Handbook of Arab American Psychology* (2015). She is the previous editor-in-chief of the *Journal of Muslim Mental Health.*

MOSES APPEL, BA, was recipient of the prestigious Psychology Award from Touro College. His work has focused on religious orientation and eating-disordered behavior, and in-group treatment for patients with psychotic disorders at the Manhattan Psychiatric Center. He is currently the Research Coordinator at the Center for Anxiety, a psychology clinic located in New York, where he is involved in various research projects on religion, spirituality, and mental health.

LEANNE ATWELL, MSW, is a licensed school social worker in a therapeutic middle school. Her MSW is from Loyola University Chicago and she has a BA in Psychology with an emphasis in counseling from Trinity International University. For more than 10 years, she has worked in the education field in different capacities, including Service Learning co-coordinator. She has been a member of a multicultural missions team working in Chicago as well as two missions teams in India. During the most recent trip to India, she co-led extensive, culturally sensitive, team-building training; helped facilitate a women's conference; and presented workshops on office management and photography. Atwell recently assisted in editing a book by Holly Nelson-Becker titled *Religion, Spirituality, and Aging: Illuminations for Therapeutic Practice* (2017).

NASIM BAHADORANI, Dr.PH, MBS, is a researcher at Loma Linda University, School of Public Health. Bahadorani is currently serving as Secretary of the Sufi Psychology Association®. She is a recipient of the Public Health Center for Health Research Dissertation Grant, and the Hulda Crooks Research and Public Health Practice Grant at Loma Linda University. Bahadorani has a master's degree in Biomedical Science, with clinical research experience in the molecular biology of a rare brain tumor called hypothalamic hamartomas, at the Barrow's Neurological Institute in Phoenix, Arizona. Her research interests include how spirituality and religious practices dynamically affect the biochemical, molecular, and biophysics pathways that induce sustainable positive changes which improve well-being, increase compassion, and ultimately result in healthy functioning.

SALOUMEH BOZORGZADEH, PsyD, is the current president of the Sufi Psychology Association®. She is a licensed clinical psychologist in private practice in Chicago, Illinois. Her training is focused on high-risk adolescents (self-injury, eating disorders, substance abuse, and suicide), and her clinical work includes a special focus on spirituality and diversity issues. In addition, she chairs a committee on Interfaith Understanding.

ARNDT BÜSSING, MD, is Professor for Quality of Life, Spirituality and Coping at the Witten/Herdecke University (Germany). His main research focus is on quality of life, spirituality, and coping (i.e., spirituality as a resource to cope; spiritual needs of persons with chronic diseases, elderly and handicapped persons; spiritual dryness in pastoral workers), and effects of nonpharmacological integrative medicine interventions to support persons with chronic diseases.

RYAN T. CRAGUN, PhD, is an associate professor of sociology at The University of Tampa. His research focuses on Mormonism and the nonreligious and has been published in numerous professional journals. He is also the author of several books.

DANA DHARMAKAYA COLGAN, MS, MA, CYI-500, is a doctoral PhD candidate in Clinical Psychology at Pacific University. Her clinical and research focus is on the science and clinical application of mindfulness: specifically, culturally appropriate adaptations and delivery models for diverse populations and the promotion of psychophysiological wellness and resilience among first responders, including physicians, primary care teams, and law enforcement officers. She received a Mind and Life Summer Research Institute Fellowship in 2014 and recently accepted a postdoctoral fellowship at The Oregon Center for Complementary and Alternative Medicine in Neurological Disorders at Oregon's Health and Science University. She has authored or co-authored eight peer-reviewed manuscripts; presented her research at state, national, and international conferences; and recently co-authored a book on evidence-based mindfulness practices within psychotherapy.

KEVIN A. HARRIS, PhD, is an assistant professor in the Department of Psychology at the University of Texas of the Permian Basin. He is also a licensed psychologist in Texas. His primary research interests include the psychology of religion and spirituality, clinical judgment, music psychology, spirituality as a character strength, and campus sexual assault prevention.

NINA J. HIDALGO, MS, is a doctoral candidate at the University of Oregon and a doctoral intern at Pacific University's Psychology and Comprehensive Health Clinic. Her clinical and research focus is on mindfulness-based interventions, health service delivery and utilization pathways, and marginalized groups. She regularly presents and facilitates workshops on diversity and multicultural issues at universities, mental health clinics, and national conferences. She is the recipient of the Promising Scholar Award and the Graduate Teaching Award from the University of Oregon Graduate School, as well as numerous other awards and scholarships in support of her work with underserved communities in the Pacific Northwest.

KAREN HWANG, EdD, received her doctorate in 2005 and completed postdoctoral training in Medical Rehabilitation Outcomes Research at the Kessler Research Foundation. She was an adjunct assistant professor at the University of Medicine and Dentistry of New Jersey before retiring and now participates in independent writing and research projects through the Atheist Research Collaborative.

JEFF KING, PhD, is a professor at Western Washington University's Department of Psychology. King is a licensed clinical psychologist and has provided clinical services to primarily American Indian populations for the past 28 years. He was director of Native American Counseling in Denver, Colorado, for 13 years. He also worked for two years among the Taos and Picuris Pueblo through the Indian Health Service. He is currently the president of the First Nations Behavioral Health Association, an organization that advocates at the national level for cultural competence and reduction in the disparity in mental health care for Native Americans and other ethnic minority populations. King is a tribally enrolled member of the Muscogee (Creek) Nation of Oklahoma.

MIRIAM KORBMAN, BA, is a doctoral candidate in the Clinical Psychology doctoral program at Long Island University-Post. She has been involved in research at Mount Sinai School of Medicine examining the role of stress-induced cravings on relapse in smoking cessation, and the Applied Research and Community Collaboration Institute (ARCC) in Suffern, New York, where she served as project manager on studies evaluating the importance of sexual and physical development education for Orthodox Jewish children as well as the efficacy of a prevention program for child sexual abuse in the Jewish community. She has also served as project manager for the Harvard Medical School Study on Judaism and Mental Health, and is co-author of several publications on topics relating to the role of religion and spirituality in mental health. Korbman's current professional interests include working with children and adolescents suffering from anxiety and related disorders, as well as disseminating evidence-based clinical treatments to children, families, and schools in the Jewish community.

SCOTT F. MADEY, PhD, is professor of Psychology at Shippensburg University of Pennsylvania. His research interests are in the areas of patient-illness perception and attainment of health goals. He is presently investigating how patient-illness perceptions form; how these perceptions change across the lifespan; and how they affect judgment, decision making, and medical compliance. Another of his research interests investigates romantic relationships and implicit theories of couples. He teaches General Psychology, Multicultural Health Psychology, History of Psychology, and the Social Psychology of Aging.

HOLLY NELSON-BECKER, PhD, LCSW, is Professor at Loyola University Chicago and a Hartford Faculty Scholar in Geriatric Social Work. Her PhD is from the University of Chicago and her MSW is from Arizona State University. Her research areas focus on spirituality and aging, with an emphasis on end-of-life concerns and diverse cultural expressions. She helped create national standards for spiritual care in palliative care and is past Chair of the Interest Group on Religion, Spirituality, and Aging for the Gerontological Society of America. She served on the National Program Committee for the Hartford Doctoral Fellows Program in Geriatric Social Work. She was awarded Fellowship in the Gerontological Society of America in 2013. The strengths perspective and positive psychological principles form the foundation for her research and teaching. She is the author of more than 50 publications as well as the book *Religion, Spirituality, and Aging: Illuminations for Therapeutic Practice* (2017).

CARL OLSON, PhD, is Professor of Religious Studies at Allegheny College. Besides more than 230 book reviews and essays in journals, books, and encyclopedias, his latest of 18 books published include: *The Different Paths of Buddhism: A Narrative-Historical Introduction* (2005); *The Many Colors of Hinduism: A Thematic-Historical Introduction* (2007); *Celibacy and Religious Traditions* (2007); *Religious Studies: The Key Concepts* (2011); *The Allure of Decadent Thinking: Religious Studies and the Challenge of Postmodernism* (2013); *Indian Asceticism Power, Violence, and Play* (2015); and *Religious Ways of Experiencing Life: A Global and Narrative Approach* (2016). While at Allegheny College, Professor Olson has been appointed to the following positions: Holder of the National Endowment for the Humanities Chair, 1991–1994; Holder of the Teacher-Scholar Chair in the Humanities, 2000–2003; Visiting Fellowship at Clare Hall, University of Cambridge, 2002; and elected Life Member of Clare Hall, University of Cambridge 2002.

DÉSIRÉE POIER, MSc in Public Health, is a research associate at the Professorship of Quality of Life, Spirituality and Coping at the University of Witten/Herdecke (Germany). Her research focuses on the evaluation of movement-orientated interventions of integrative mind-body medicine.

PAUL E. PRIESTER, PhD, is a professor in Counseling Psychology in The School of Professional Studies at North Park University. Dr. Priester completed a master's degree in Rehabilitation Counseling from the University of Iowa and a PhD in Counseling Psychology from Loyola University, Chicago. His research interests include: the role of spirituality in recovery from addictive disorders; research-based methods to prevent drug use in young adults; integrating spirituality into the counseling process; multicultural counseling; the measurement of Islamic religiosity; and the use of popular films as an adjunctive tool in counseling. Besides his academic interests, he operates an organic farm (Happy Destiny Farm) in Two Creeks, Wisconsin, with his wife (Katherine); three children (FP, the Real Paul, and Margo) and his Treeing Walker Coonhound (Comet).

DAVID H. ROSMARIN, PhD, ABPP, is an assistant professor in the Department of Psychiatry at Harvard Medical School, part time, and Founder/ Director of the Center for Anxiety. He is a board-certified psychologist, clinical innovator, and prolific researcher who has authored more than 50 peer-reviewed publications and 100 abstracts focused on spirituality and mental health. Clinically, Rosmarin provides behavior therapy for patients presenting with anxiety, affective, psychotic, personality, and somatoform disorders, while attending to relevant spiritual factors in treatment. His work has received media attention from ABC, NPR, *Scientific American*, the *Boston Globe,* and the *New York Times.*

SHANNAN RUSSO, BS, is a MSW candidate in Loyola University Chicago School of Social Work, specializing in Health Social Work. She is also a candidate in the Loyola Law School Child Law and Policy program. She obtained a BS in Psychology and Criminal Justice from Baldwin Wallace University. Russo interned with Heartland Alliance in the Chicagoland area. Russo also interned with the Veteran's Health Administration at Jesse Brown VA Medical Center in both the Palliative Care and Suicide Prevention departments.

MOHAMMAD SADOGHI, PhD, is an assistant professor in the Computer Science Department at Purdue University. Previously, Sadoghi was a Research Staff Member at IBM T.J. Watson Research Center for three years. He received his PhD from the Computer Science Department at the University of Toronto in 2013. He was the recipient of the Ontario Graduate Scholarship and the NSERC Canada Graduate Scholarship. Broadly speaking, his research focuses on high-performance and extensible Big Data Management Systems. He has more than 40 publications in leading database conferences/journals and holds more than 30 filed U.S. patents. He is the recipient of EPTS Innovative Principles Award (2012) and ESWC Best In-Use Paper Award (2016). He has served as the PC Chair (Industry Track) for ACM DEBS'17, the Co-chair of Doctoral Symposium at ACM/IFIP/USENIX Middleware'17, and the Co-chair of Active Workshop at IEEE ICDE'17. Since 2017, he has been serving as Vice President and Technical Director of the Sufi Psychology Association®.

ROBERT SANTEE, PhD, is Professor of Psychology at Chaminade University of Honolulu, where he teaches undergraduate classes in psychology, undergraduate classes in Chinese thought/religion, and graduate classes in counseling. He has a PhD in Educational Psychology and a PhD in Philosophy with a general focus in Asian thought and a specific emphasis in Daoism. He has presented a number of papers on Daoism in China. He is certified as a Martial Arts (Wushu) instructor (Jiaolian) in Fujian, China. He is a nationally certified counselor. He is the author of *An Integrative Approach to Counseling: Bridging Chinese Thought, Evolutionary Theory, and Stress Management* (Sage 2007) and *The Tao of Stress* (New Harbinger Press 2013).

Index

Page numbers followed by *t* indicate tables and *f* indicate figures.

Medicine (*cont.*)
  biomedicine, 105, 116; Buddha,
  350; Elder, 304; folk, 338–339;
  Greco-Roman, 164; herbal, 105;
  Hindu system, 32; Hippocratic,
  229; Hispanic, 338; ideologies re,
  341–344; internal, 33, 74;
  Lithuanian, 339; mind–body, 55;
  modern, 7, 117, 187–188, 273;
  preventive, 75; psychosomatic
  form, 117; sacred, 281;
  shamanistic, 289, 300–301, 304;
  Sufi influence in, 219, 221; toll
  of practicing, 31; Traditional
  Chinese, 80, 90, 339; Western,
  56, 80, 90, 279, 338, 348
Medicine men/women, 267, 277, 279
Medicine Wheel, 269*t*, 297, 303
Meditation: addiction to, 57; adverse
  health outcomes, 57–58; Ayurvedic,
  33–34; Buddhist, 44–45, 55, 57, 62,
  64; Catholic characterization,
  158–164, 173; chakra-focused, 34;
  concentration-based, 49; Daoist,
  79, 85, 91; on God, 37; on God's
  work, 250; healing through, 250;
  heart, 214; holy, 156; Jain, 36–39;
  mindfulness and, 49, 52, 56–58,
  91, 174; movement, 215; moving,
  90; nonspecific, 57–58; reflecting,
  162; Rastafarian practice, 244;
  relaxation-based, 57; silent, 162;
  sitting in oblivion, 91; on space
  between health and illness, 35;
  Sufi characterization of, 211–215,
  219; Transcendental (TM),
  57–58; true meaning of, 214;
  walking, 52–53. *See also* Qigong;
  Zikr
Menopause, 53, 170, 342
Mental health: effects of social/
  community processes, 126,
  133–134, 278; effects of spiritual
  activities/orientation, 31, 35, 53,
  120–121,126, 138–139, 140, 143,

197, 199, 237, 255, 265, 282, 288,
  304, 313, 346, 349; historical
  trauma and, 295; in Jewish
  population, 137–138; prayer for,
  250; professional concerns,
  129–131, 137–138, 190, 193, 247,
  255, 263, 280, 289, 301; stigma, 127,
  141, 317
Michelangelo, 345
Middle East, 254, 256, 311
Middle Path, 43–44, 48, 59–61, 65
Mind/heart as source of distress,
  82–85
Mindful Awareness, 50–51, 53
Mindfulness, 2, 39, 44–58, 61–62, 64,
  91, 174, 250, 341–342, 362
Mindfulness-Based Eating Awareness
  (MB–EAT), 51
Mindfulness-Based Interventions
  (MBIs), 55–58, 64
Mindfulness-Based Relapse
  Prevention (MBRP), 51–52
Mindfulness-Based Stress Reduction
  (MBSR), 55, 64
Mindfulness Training, 16, 55
Mohawk, 268, 274
Monks, 109, 111, 155–156, 220;
  Azumahito, 99; Benedictine, 156;
  Bodhidharma, 62; Buddhist, 112;
  child, 112; Christian, 165; Greek
  Orthodox, 158–159, 167, 173;
  Kōbō Daishi, 109; Kūkai, 109,
  Yōgō, 100
Monogamy, 59
Monotheism, 39, 120, 151, 245–246,
  257, 298
Mood, 57, 336; state, 57
Morals, 193, 208, 316: behavior, 89,
  167; beliefs, 218; choice, 87–88;
  codes of, 116, 249; contextual,
  87–88; ethics, 157; etiquette, 199;
  failures, 99; imperative, 7–8, 131;
  interpersonal behavior, 86, 88;
  issues, 254; judgment, 296, 347;
  law, 156; laxity, 166; life, 86;